About The Author

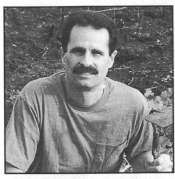

When John Thomas began his pursuit of agelessness, his *calendar age* was 27 while his *real* age—his **bio-electric age**—was 39. Today, John is 51 years on the calendar, yet his bio-electric age is only 19! Thomas is living proof that you can reverse aging.

John was heavily influenced by the exemplary lives of Dr. Paul C. Bragg and Jack LaLanne. He spent twenty-four years researching every aspect of the aging process while he applied what he had learned in his own life.

While preparing to enter the medical field, Thomas realized that science asks the *wrong* questions and generates sterile answers. It knows aging only by its *symptoms!*

John was encouraged to write *Young Again!* because he does not age. You might say he got the job by default. Time stands still for John.

For a book like *Young Again!* to be *meaningful,* the author would need to have *personally* "lived" the subject matter AND be *living* proof that aging reversal and rejuvenation are possible and within the reach of anyone sincerely desiring to experience them.

The author would need a broad background in the sciences, philosophy, politics, history, and nutrition. He would need to think "low tech" and write in a style that would insure *communication* with the reader.

John wrote this book to help the lay person—and the practitioner—who needs practical information and answers to their health problems. It was NOT written for "experts" who claim to have answers, but who can't demonstrate proof in their lives or that of their patients.

Young Again! is a *testimony* to anyone who wants to experience the MIRACLE of agelessness. It is mosaic of nature's secrets pieced together for the very first time.

Young Again! encourages everyone to talk the talk AND walk the walk! This book was written for you.

Thoughts From Patricia Bragg

What a masterpiece! *Young Again!* is the best of the best! It will help millions of people.

We are a nation of half dead people! Cancer, heart trouble, high blood pressure, osteoporosis, etc. The health of our people is slipping fast. The question is why?

Good health is something that cannot be purchased from a doctor or in a bottle of pills. Good health is the product of a healthy lifestyle. America needs to know more about how to achieve health and vitality. Staying youthful, no matter what your age, is central to the health message and to the message of this book.

My father, Dr. Paul C. Bragg N.D., Ph.D. was a teenager dying of tuberculosis when he *chose* a life of health. Dad was ninety-seven years "young" when he died of a surfboard accident. During his life, he helped thousands of people find the path to agelessness. One of those people was Jack LaLanne.

Jack was a sickly boy. His health was so poor he was forced to drop out of school. Dad's message changed his life. Today, Jack LaLanne is a legend. He is living proof that the health message really works.

Dad said the world was lacking strong, courageous men and women who were not afraid to buck the trend of commercialism in the food industry and in the healing arts—people who could stand tall.

Here we have a strong crusader who *believes* in the health message and who *lives* what he preaches. John Thomas' wonderful book is his gift of love to the world.

Now, dear reader, it is your turn to experience a life of boundless energy and health. The keys are in your hand. Read and follow this book and it will change your life. *Young Again!* is the most thorough and concise message ever written on the subject of healthy living.

No excuses. You know right from wrong. Remember, what you eat and drink you become. It's either sickness or it's health. It's time to choose. Now! Today!

Young Again! is truly a personal guide to ageless living. I am honored to be a part of it.

young AGAIN!

How To **REVERSE** *The Aging Process*

John Thomas

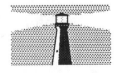

Plexus Press
Kelso, Washington
USA

young AGAIN!
How To Reverse The Aging Process
By John Thomas

Published by:

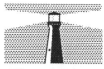

• Plexus Press •

Plexus Press
P.O. Box 827
Kelso WA 98626-0072
Phone (360) 423-3168
Fax: Requires voice contact
SAN# 298-1440

Cataloging-In-Publication Data

Thomas, John
Young Again! How to Reverse The Aging Process / by John Thomas
p. cm.
References: p.
Includes index.
Includes glossary.

ISBN 1-884757-76-6
1. Aging. 2. Rejuvenation. 3. Longevity. 4. Health. I. Title
RA776.75.T56   1995
613.04—dc20   94-65131

Printed in the United States of America

20 19 18 17 16 15 14 13 12 11 10 9 8 7 6 5 4

DEDICATED TO...

Robert McLeod—You will meet Bob in Chapter one. He became my mentor, a living example, and a good friend.

Dr. Paul C. Bragg N.D., Ph.D.—Paul Bragg was the point man of the health movement in the United States. Millions of people owe their lives to him. He served his fellow man well, and his Creator to the fullest. Paul Bragg saved my life!

Charles Walters—Charlie is the editor of Acres USA. He taught me to winnow the wheat from the chaff. He helped me establish the link between "live" food and "live soil." His editorial pen is the harbinger of TRUTH in matters of agriculture and national economics. He is another Thomas Paine!

Diane DeFelice M.S., R.D.—Diane was my upper level college nutrition instructor. She is unselfish in her effort to help students make the connection between diet, lifestyle and good health. She helped me realize that *Young Again!* simply had to be written.

Patricia Bragg N.D., Ph.D.—Patricia *challenged* me to write this book. She also challenged me to pick up the baton her father handed to her and to Jack LaLanne. Patricia is the daughter of the great Wizard—"Paul Bragg." Patricia is a mighty force in the health movement worldwide. She is a voice crying in the wilderness!

Jack LaLanne—Beginning in the 1950's, Jack LaLanne became "Mr. Fitness." He is a living example of the benefits that accrue from a healthy lifestyle and regular exercise. Jack has been the point man in the fitness industry for over forty years! He deserves our applause and thanks. Many people have been blessed by his work.

Leonard Ridzon—Of all the people I have met in 51 years, this farmer makes me think more than any other. Leonard is a simple man, but he isn't simple. He sees the Creator's handiwork and asks questions to whoever will listen. His questions can hold a pack of doctors at bay; they seldom risk an answer. And when Leonard talks, you had best be listening. He says as much *between* the lines as he does in words. Thank you, Leonard!

Publisher's Note....

TABLE OF CONTENTS

Acknowledgements

The author would like to take this opportunity to acknowledge and thank the following people who were involved, directly and indirectly, in bringing this book to fruition and/or to the attention of the public.

Robert Stephan D.D.S., Dr. John Briggs, Dennis Higgins M.D., Robert C. Atkins M.D., Julian Whitaker M.D., Linus Pauling M.D., William Campbell Douglass M.D., Edward Arana D.D.S., Hal Huggins D.D.S., Dr. Helen A. Guthrie, Dr. Roger Lent, Joseph Kramer M.D., Ignaz Semmelweis M.D., Thomas Gerber M.D., Arnold Lorand M.D., Max Gerson M.D., Dr. Carey Reams, Drs. Paul C. and Patricia Bragg, Dr. Bernard Jensen, Dr. Guenther Enderlein.

Bob Mcleod, Jack LaLanne, Charles Walters, Mitchell May, Tom Valentine, Christopher Bird, Charlette Gerson Straus, Gar Hildenbrand, Matt Kilts, Burt Stoker, Kyle McLain, Bob Greenebaum, Bud Curtis, Walter Grotz, Dean Stonier , Bob Allen, Merlyn Anderberg, Diane DeFelice, J. Carmen Robinson, Leann Sutton, Ray and Carolyn Teagarden, Lynette Goodwin-Lynch, Carol Arana, Dan Poynter, Nancy Poehlann, Frank and Kay Morrow, Michelle Cooley, Hanna Campbell, Barbara Rosengrant, Dan James, Doreen Hettinger, Marva Matheny, Brian Ulrich, Sheila Fickenscher, Sandy Herman, Merilyn McConaghy, Nancy Ohuche, Linda Berthof, Linda Torretta, Al Primm, Ellen Rosbach, John Murphy, Werner and Janice Gerhardt, Tom Mahoney, Rita Ryan, Bob Pike, Bill McMahan, Cathy Cameron, Keith Ries, and to my personal family as well as the family into which I was blessed to have been born.

Special thanks to Elizabeth Beryl and Patricia Borgstrom for their assistance in editing and clarification, and to Terri Lonier for her help and kindness.

Cover by Juan

Introduction by Robert B. Stephan D.D.S.

Man's ways are the antithesis of Nature's ways. They have little resemblance to the natural healing process. Nature provides the basis of life and the potential to help man correct his disease causing tendencies, but drug based medicine has chosen to increase health care productivity rather than identify the constraints which inhibit good health.

Allopathic medicine seems to be infatuated with technology, powerful drugs, and the suppression of symptoms. It prefers to *cut, poison,* and *burn,* when less would do. Medicine's world is physical and chemical.

We are moving away from this physical and chemical based system of disease care and into the realm of energy and spirit. This is not a new movement, but a rediscovery of ancient wisdom. It is a mix of "proven" wisdom combined with technology.

As we move away from a *disease* care system and into a *health* care system, we will need a compass and a road map to navigate by if we hope to find our way through the maze of exploding knowledge and rediscovered tradition that is fast approaching us.

Young Again! serves the dual purpose of a navigation tool and a survival manual. It is easy to read and it is a very complete gathering of information. It will guide you to a healthy, vibrant life *and* it will take you where Western Allopathic doctors fear to tread.

It is a divine privilege to be involved in the march to a preferred future, and it is a great pleasure to have John Thomas' wonderful book to use as a fount of information in my position as a Holistic Biological Dentist. Discover in this book the joy and path of good health!

Dr. Robert B. Stephan, D.D.S., B.S., F.A.P.D.
Spokane, Washington
Holistic Dental Association, Board of Directors
International Academy of Oral Medicine and Toxicology
American Academy of Biological Dentistry
Occidental Institute, Research Faculty
Environmental Dental Association

Introduction by Dr. John A. Briggs

Our body is an incredible work of art. Unfortunately, it does not come with an owner's manual—as does a car—that tells us *how* to care for our body.

Consider the master mechanic. He has knowledge of the workings of his car. He knows how to protect his investment. His world is a world of regular maintenance and mechanical details. He avoids the pitfalls of ownership through individual responsibility. He knows *how* to maintain his car's youthfulness and vigor.

The medical world is not like the world of the master mechanic. In my practice, I have seen people with the full range of health related problems—problems directly related to modern living—problems that could be avoided if people only had an owner's manual.

These people come to me willing to spend their fortunes. They have tasted the bitterness of disease and old age—they cry out for good health. They also DREAM of regaining the health of their youth.

I help them as best I can. I point the way, but my time is limited as is their money. What these people really need is an owners manual for the care and maintenance of their body. I have wished for such a manual.

My wish was fulfilled when John Thomas wrote *Young Again!* It contains all the information my patients need to maintain their youth and vigor.

Young Again! arms the reader with practical, valuable information. This book is correctly aligned with the concepts of Naturopathic medicine. It will help the reader to stay young no matter what their age.

Thomas' research is exhaustive. He has a thorough working knowledge of the healing arts. Most importantly, he drives home his points with simple examples designed to help the reader understand.

Read this book and follow the information it contains. If you do, you too can achieve the radiant health I observed when John Thomas first introduced himself.

Dr. John A. Briggs
Naturopathic Physician
Clatskanie, Oregon

Foreword by Charles Walters

"People can be fed to live peacefully or fight, to think or dream, to work or sleep, to be virile or pathologic, physically, mentally, and spiritually developed or retarded, and for any possible degree of advance or variation within the mechanical limits of the organism."

This was the late Albert Carter Savage speaking during the early years of WW II, and Winston Churchill took him seriously. After all, the health of England's fighting men was all that stood between the freedom of Englishmen and Hitler's thirst for world domination.

It was realized that food had to carry a fair complement of minerals in order to confer health, and the idea that vitamins could function without minerals was at least as strange as the concept that coal-tar drugs—capable of making a healthy person ill—could make a sick person well.

These few thoughts came to mind when John Thomas' manual *Young Again!* arrived on my editorial desk.

Individual health is too important to be left in the hands of physicians, but how can a person make informed decisions to not only preserve health, but to conquer sickness as well? Most books deal with individual problems—single factor analysis, we call it—but leave unanswered the silent killer in our lives, namely *shelf life.* For it is shelf life in the grocery store that annihilates the quality of life for the consumer.

When most of today's senior citizens were still youngsters, strange words in type too small to read became an indispensable part of almost every label. First came the emulsifiers and stabilizers—carrageenan in cheese spreads, chocolate products, evaporated milk, ice cream and dairy products. All evidence of mutagenicity, carcinogenicity, and teratogenicity remained neatly tucked away in the scientific literature.

Dioctyl sodium sulfosuccinate became the wetting agent of choice, even though infants suffered gastrointestinal irritation and reduced growth rates as a consequence of its use. There were also dozens of flavorings and colors other than Red Nos. 2 & 4, all inimical to sustained human health. Aspartame (Nutrasweet) is a sweetener with approximately one hundred sixty times the sweetness of sugar. The problem is that people with phenylketonuria can't handle it. It accumulates in the system and causes mental retardation and even death. Cereals, chewing gum, and gelatins are loaded with it.

As shelf life for foods improved, strange anomalies in the population multiplied. The public prints became filled with reports of bizarre crimes (youths dumping gasoline on old ladies and setting them on fire, for instance) and asylums for the insane became a growth industry, finally to emerge with credentialed practitioners and a new nomenclature—mental health!

Did shellac—a food grade version of furniture finish—used as a confectioner's glaze have anything to do with this? Or xylitol, a sugar substitute that is a diuretic and causes tumors and organ damage in test animals? Or propylene glycol alginate, or oxystearin (a modified glyceride), or glycerol ester of wood rosin, or guar gum? All annihilate lesser life and whittle away at human health a bit at a time!

John Thomas' message in his manual on health is clear and to the point. Witless science has worked its mischief, but we are not helpless. We have only to take command of our own health and make sensible judgements without reference to higher approved authority.

Young Again! has little to do with mirror image vanity and everything to do with the "mechanical limits of the organism," as Albert Carter Savage put it, meaning the human body.

Young Again! has to be read with a box of marker pens handy. It is a matchless narrative and an encyclopedia of health. It covers the secrets of the ancients and projects forward to encompass the range of the electromagnetic spectrum. The advice—page by page, chapter by chapter—may not entirely reverse aging, but it is certain to put the process on hold.

Charles Walters
Editor, Acres USA
Kansas City, Missouri

Aim High!

All of us wish to improve our health. Hopefully, that is the reason you are reading this book.

My approach to health and longevity is more than a simplistic approach. I have chosen to provide the reader with as much information as possible.

It is not my intent to be absolute or overzealous. Few people will be able to comply 100% with all of my recommendations. Yet even the smallest steps will bring improved health. The reader is encouraged to advance in personal knowledge at his/her own pace. Do not feel doomed because you can't do everything that is recommended. Please realize that the material presented represents the BEST we can shoot for—the goal—the ideal!

The ideal world of health is a lifestyle that includes wholesome food, pure water, proper exercise, adequate rest, low stress, a clean body, and a strong mind. These things are worth striving for, yet, the *perfect* lifestyle is very difficult to live in a world where disease and human suffering are the norm.

Hopefully, this book will help each person find a middle ground where they can enjoy the best health life has to offer consistent with their own circumstances.

Life is not perfect. We live in an imperfect world. We fall short of the ideal. We are constantly subject to events and circumstances beyond our control or choice.

Yet, each day, we Do have the opportunity to make "choices" that affect our lives and health—and that of those those around us—for good and for bad. We must strive to make the best choices we can.

The reader is reminded that good health is a cumulative state of being that is worth striving for.

NEVER forget that the *alternative* to good health is a sorry existence. Poor health cheats you of your happiness and your life.

Aim high and do the very best you can. Good health is worth the effort!

1

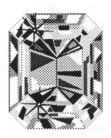

Something Of Value

"If you want to look and feel as I do when
you are my age, you must begin now!"
Robert McLeod

It was a strange place for me to meet the person who would become my mentor. Stranger still were the circumstances—a restaurant meeting room in San Bernardino, California in 1971. The event: A district sales meeting for ARCO (Atlantic Richfield Company), formerly Richfield Oil Company.

Having graduated from college the previous September, I stood in awe of the grandeur of it all. The Company, the oil industry, and all that.

We had instinctively corralled ourselves into groups based on our position on the corporate ladder. Barnyard pecking order they call it.

And as a few of us were talking, I overheard my immediate superior and his cronies laughing and poking fun in a rather contemptuous way at one of their peers—a man named, Bob McLeod.

McLeod was not socializing with people of his own level ("status inconsistent" the sociologists call it). Instead, his peers had shunned him. As I listened to their gossip, something caught my attention.

"You know," one of them said, "McLeod is a vegetarian. He doesn't eat meat. He's...real strange!" "Yah! He's into health, whatever that is," said another.

It was difficult to compare McLeod to this arrogant, egocentric bunch of executives. I could NOT account for the differences between the *group* and the stranger, McLeod.

McLeod looked young. His smile, his eyes, his laugh—nothing squared with someone of forty-nine years. His hair was vibrant! His stomach trim and slim. I liked what I saw!

The executives, well, they all looked twenty years older than McLeod. Paunchy stomachs, grayed hair, bald heads, fat, cigarettes blazing, and booze. Many were ready for their gold watches. But by this time in history, gold watches had been replaced by the old glass hand, a slap on the back and the epitaph on the grave stone, "He was a good old boy!"

McLeod Knew

McLeod knew something they did not, for he was forty-nine years "young" and the others, who were in their late thirties and early forties, were, well,....older!

I took my first step into the world of ageless living as I navigated in McLeod's direction. Life would never again be the same for me. I was destined to be there on that day, at that moment, and Bob McLeod was destined to become my mentor. God works in strange ways!

I introduced myself to this forty-nine years *young* enigma and as we talked it became crystal clear that he was a very special human being.

Immediately, my mind was made up! "When I reach forty-nine, I am going to *LOOK* and *FEEL* like Bob McLeod!"

"It's a long story and you are going to have to search it out for yourself, but I would consider it a privilege if I can assist you," he said.

Instant friends we were! Fellow travelers for sure! Our paths only crossed a few times in the months that followed. When they did, he would take me under his wing and point the way.

"If you want to understand how I have managed to look and feel twenty years younger than I am, you will have to study. I recommend you begin by reading a book by Dr. Paul C. Bragg, entitled, *The Miracle of Fasting.*

"You will not find all the answers there, but this book is a good place to start," he said.

Six months after meeting Bob, I left the company and lost ALL contact with him until August of 1993. He still looks *young and vibrant!* If you saw him on the street today you would guess him to be in his late forties. Not too bad for someone age 69 years YOUNG!

Twenty-four years have passed and now it is my turn. As I approach fifty-one years *young*, I am here to tell you that you CAN stop that clock! You CAN reverse the aging process—if you truly desire to do so.

Fear

People are reluctant to venture out, to break new ground, to sail uncharted waters—particularly when it involves being *different.* Perhaps it is social pressure. Perhaps they think they are giving up *something of value.* Regardless, fear and ignorance are the primary stumbling blocks that keep people from following the path of good health. Instead, they hang onto old bad habits that become the glue with which they seal their grave(s).

All of my peers at that fortuitous meeting are well on their way into old age. All of them were past their anabolic PEAK at that time. Today, most of them suffer from degenerative conditions and some of them are dead. Regardless, all of them are old beyond their years. This is a sad and unnecessary epitaph.

People do not think "they" are going to get old. They know they have to die, but it is the other guy who gets old, never them. One day they wake up and look in the mirror, and their mind says, "Heh! Better enjoy it while you can! Time is short!" As friends grow old and die, the image in the mirror is confirmed—disease and old age have arrived.

It's important that the reader understands diseases and conditions. A disease is simply a condition that medicine has "officially" given a name. When we have a disease we have a condition. A condition is something that alters our lifestyle and prevents us from enjoying life as we normally would.

We do not CATCH diseases. We DEVELOP conditions. Disease should be hyphenated. It should be spelled "dis-ease," and we will do so for the remainder of this book to drive home the point. We die of conditions, not dis-eases!

How we define our condition(s)—dis-ease—will greatly influence our attitude about aging and our ability or inability to take control of our lives and remedy the forces that cause the bio-electric body to grow OLD.

It's Your Decision

Would YOU like to become *Young Again?* All that is required is that you complete this book and apply its lessons in your life. If you want to experience the **miracle** of reversing the aging process, you MUST *visualize* the end result in your mind's eye.

The miracle is available to *anyone* who wants it, but it is NOT free. You will become acquainted with the price as each chapter unfolds.

Once you understand HOW you become old, you will understand HOW to become *Young Again!*

PREVIEW: *In the next chapter, you will discover that you have four different ages. You will also determine your anabolic PEAK and learn about its significance in your life.*

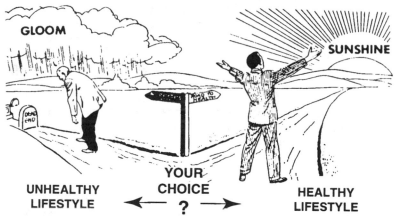

GLOOM

SUNSHINE

UNHEALTHY LIFESTYLE ← **YOUR CHOICE ?** → **HEALTHY LIFESTYLE**

The choice of which road to take is up to the individual. He alone can decide whether he wants to reach a dead end or live a healthy lifestyle for a long, happy, active life.   – Paul C. Bragg

"In this book, the author goes a long way to provide hope that, in a world beset by health threatening pollution of all kinds, we are afforded some tools with which to build healthier, longer, and perhaps happier lives."
Christopher Bird, *The Secret Life of Plants*

2

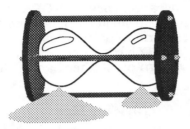

young Again!

*"Youth is a wonderful thing. What
a crime to waste it on children."*
George Bernard Shaw

Old age flows out of days filled with new hopes and new dreams of good times to come. Good times that go unfulfilled because our body fails to keep up with our mind.

An old body with a young mind is a phenomenon where conflict and misunderstanding abound. It is a condition where the body we once knew becomes *lost* in Time and unable to communicate with the mind. Flip sides of the same coin: a young mind, an old body. Each expresses itself in a different language with no interpreter to translate.

Aging does not occur by accident. It occurs through ignorance. People become old because they do not know HOW to stay young. They are becoming old much faster than they once did. This is particularly true among the young. The young are experiencing the ONSET of old age by age twenty-four. Diseases that were once the domain of the old now belong to those young in years.

Despite the statistical claims of the *experts*, life expectancy is *not* greater today than it was yesterday. The statistics used to support this claim of greater life expectancy have been skewed by the number of children reaching adulthood. At one time, half the population of the United States died prior to reaching age twenty. Those deaths held life expectancy down. The *statistical* rise in life expectancy over the last fifty years has caused a gullible public to accept medicine's false claim of greater life expectancy. This is a serious mistake.

We are NOT better off today than we were yesterday. Degenerative conditions have replaced infectious conditions. Moreover, contagious conditions are on the rise and are returning with a vengeance. They are MORE than an old enemy returned. Their return spells ill for those who are unprepared and unwilling to conform to nature's plan.

A long, HEALTHY life is what we were meant to experience during our sojourn on Mother Earth. That is what this book is all about.

Dividing Line

At my initiation into the study of aging in 1971, it was considered difficult to turn the body's biological clock backward if someone had *survived* thirty-five years of NORMAL living. If we made the same statement today, we would have to reduce age thirty-five down to age twenty-four. The dividing line between youth and the ONSET of old age is falling—fast!

When we are young, our health is at its peak and the body is able to repair itself quickly and easily. The word *anabolism* best describes this state. Anabolism means the absence of breakdown in body tissues. It also implies normal body repair of muscle, skin and bones. It is a *building up* process.

As we age, body functions slow and we become fragile. Injuries do not heal as quickly. *Catabolism* best describes this state. It means the breaking-down of body tissue. It is the opposite of anabolism.

Catabolism releases energy. It is a kind of *self-digestion* where the body lives off the energy released from the digestion of its own tissues. This is bare-bones energy used to meet the body's *minimum* energy needs. Energy produced through catabolic activity is starvation energy. Catabolic activity can keep us alive, but it should NOT be equated with health and longevity. Catabolism has its roots in death.

When we are young we are anabolic. When we are old, we are catabolic. Of course, there are degrees within these two categories. In this book, when we use the words *anabolism* and *catabolism* we are referring to the OVERALL condition or direction of the bio-electric body and its implications to the aging process.

The age twenty-four dividing line we spoke of earlier is our **anabolic PEAK.** It is that point in Time when the young begin their slide into old age. Some people experience their anabolic peak earlier than age twenty-four. For others it comes a little later. The *point* is that its onset is arriving much to soon.

Once Upon A Time

There was a time when it was uncommon to see the first signs of old age until the fortieth or forty-fifth year—unless one was subject to hardships beyond the norm. Obesity, gray hair, balding, loss of sexual drive, wrinkled skin, and diminished vitality are all classic *SIGNS* of old age.

Before we can erase these signs of old age, we need to understand *why* they occur. We also need to understand *how* they express themselves. When we become AWARE of the passing of *TIME*, we also become aware of the invisible forces of aging—forces that cause the young to wake up old.

When we reach our **anabolic peak,** we are at the crossroads of Time. We are caught between the wonder of youth and the approach of old age.

Aging initiates quietly and without notice. It is a self-ordained process that speeds the passing of Time and hastens our date with death.

Change The Script

Life does NOT have to be this way! We can change the script if we *choose*—no matter what our age! We can *reverse* our course if we are willing to learn and then act upon our new-found knowledge.

It is not the idea of growing old that people fear. Rather, it is the idea that old age will *cheat* them of the enjoyment of the things they once took for granted. For most, the thought of old age gives rise to visions of a dead-end street, loneliness, pain, suffering, and finally death.

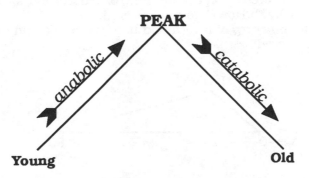

Anabolic Peak—That point in time when our youth is spent and the onset of old age has begun.

When I chose the title for this book, I wrestled between *Forever Young* and the present title, *Young Again!* The former title did not fit those people who are on the *anabolic* side of the pyramid. They will not read this book because they cannot grasp the meaning of the word *old.* Their world is *young.* They are never going to get old—or so they think.

Only those who realize that they have *passed* their anabolic peak understand the implications of the word *OLD.* To them, the idea of becoming *Young Again!* is only a dream.

Hosea proclaims, "My people are destroyed for lack of knowledge." However, it is not knowledge that mankind lacks, but the wisdom to discern the difference between false knowledge and truth. *Old age* and *old* are not necessarily synonymous. They do not have to mean the same thing.

The Doctor

When we are dying, we hear the pronouncements of medicine "Nothing can be done!" "Accept that which cannot be changed!" and other expressions designed to worm their way into our consciousness. These expressions numb our wits and excise our will to live.

Oral pacifiers, these pronouncements! Empty words, designed to help us accept and rationalize the phenomena of life and death.

In the beginning—when poor health manifests itself— the medical folks talk of recovery. In time, recovery gives way to high-tech jargon and HOPE.

For the terminal patient, who has cast himself or herself before the altar of science, medicine quickly exhausts its mumbo-jumbo, turning instead to steely words that chisel our name on the tombstone.

The doctor announces death's call. The patient answers that call with forced preparation and/or frustration and the questions "Why?" "How?" go unanswered.

The *mystery* of health and happiness, life and death goes unanswered.

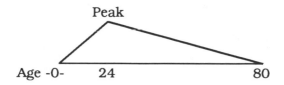

Peak

Age -0-   24   80

Aging Pyramid—note how far left of center the anabolic peak is located. In this case, it is shown at age 24.

The Clergy

Religious training convinces us that we have an "appointed time" and to "accept what God has foreordained"—soothing words that placate our emotions and numb the reality of the moment. Few people dare to question religion's pronouncements. There is little quarter for rationality here.

Instead, we elevate to dogma that which we do not understand. We blindly follow our beliefs, never pausing to question "Why?" and "How?" life slips between our fingers.

We give up. We grow old. We accept what we have been taught, and we die decades ahead of Time because medicine said, "Sorry!" and our religious leaders offered us little consolation—except a "hereafter."

The balance of society attempts to buffer the "Why?" and "How?" with cynicism set to music in songs like Peggy Lee's, *Is That All There Is!* Because we do NOT know where to find the answers, we keep dancing, pausing only to break out the booze.

Our inability to winnow truth from lies is *not* totally our fault. We have been schooled to accept the flood of distortions that emanate from our societal organs—government, newspapers and universities. They are bullhorns—all of them—wired to the halls of Science, the present god of our civilization. Science has become a cult, a national religion, but science fails to answer *"Why?" and "How?"*

Pilgrimage

Daily, we *voluntarily* make the pilgrimage to Science's cultic altar, paying homage to the idea that cause and effect can be explained using single factor analysis. We accept the *theory* that there is "a" bug responsible for every dis-ease, "a" pill for every ailment.

We are told we have a built-in alarm clock that signals our time to die, when longer days—good days—filled with health and happiness are within our reach if we will only act and accept our greatest gift of all—good health!

Science and medicine blame the bacteria and viruses for our health problems. Religion blames Eve for bringing the curse of sickness and death upon Adam and mankind.

Instead of taking responsibility, we prostrate ourselves before the *Altar of Science* and pay homage with the fruits of our labor. We buy medicines and pills that treat our symptoms and leave the causes untouched, and more importantly, *unidentified!*

Palliation is a term that comes to mind. It says much

about medical science in a few syllables. It means relief of signs and symptoms without curing the underlying dis-ease.

Drugs produce change in body function. They are prescribed to prevent, diagnose, or cure dis-ease. *Palliation* is the fourth reason pharmacology texts give to justify drug administration. Palliation *tricks* the patient and leads the physician astray.

How different life would be if people had a correct knowledge about dis-ease and the aging process, and then acted upon that knowledge. Sadly, mankind lives in a medically induced stupor, where the "Why?" and "How?" of life and death, health and disease goes unanswered.

Make no mistake, 99% of the aging process is under our direct, personal control. We can possess and maintain a young body AND a young mind—if we wish. This book was written to answer the "Why?" and "How?" and to point the way to the path of ageless living.

What Is Your Age?

How we define age can make a big difference in our *attitude* toward life. Our attitude dictates our daily actions. Our actions in turn draft our physiological future and our *bio-electric age.*

Age can be defined on the basis of chronological age, mental age, functional age, and most importantly, *bio-electric* age. *Carefully* review each.

Calendar age is how old we are in years upon this earth. We celebrate our calendar age each year with a birthday party. Unfortunately, we celebrate in *past tense* and in the *negative* by defining age in years *old,* instead of years *young!*

Mental age is defined by the way we think. Mental age is our perspective on life. It is a kind of mental cohort effect. A mental cohort is a "mental" time capsule where the person's mind is *stuck* in a time period in the past say in the time of the Great Depression when a person grew up. Many older people are living proof of a *mental* cohort effect. These are people who are mentally young, but *physically* old.

Most of us know someone like this. Perhaps a loved one. Regardless of how young this person thinks, it is obvious that their body long ago passed its anabolic peak—losing cadence with their mind. *Old* body, *young* mind. Not a very exciting prospect is it?

Functional age is based on our ability to function. *Nursing* and bogus *holistic* medicine define functional health as our ability to experience normal, everyday desired activities. These bogus medical definitions say *health* can include one or more degenerative dis-eases, while *wellness* is based on the way we perceive ourselves, regardless if our present limitations have suspended younger, healthier lifestyles.

These are plastic definitions. Plastic definitions bother me because they lead us astray! Medicine's and nursing's present definitions of health and wellness *dodge* the issues and causes of aging and dis-ease! They are dead end statements.

We can only experience *peak* health in the ABSENCE of dis-ease. This book teaches you HOW to achieve that goal every day of your life for as long as you desire to live.

Reversing your *bio-electric age*, which is your body's *actual age*, is what this book is about. Your bio-electric age can be measured. You will learn HOW to manipulate it. You will measure your own personal *bio-electric* age in a future chapter. This should motivate you to finish reading this book so you can learn what you need to know to become *Young Again!* When you learn how to control the factors that influence your bio-electric age, the destructive effect of Time is neutralized. When you *LOOK, THINK,* and *FEEL* young, you are *Young Again!*

PREVIEW: *In the next chapter, you are going to determine your REAL age and identify those things that are causing you to become old before your time. The information you provide will become YOUR foundation for the balance of this book. Are you ready?*

Brown Eyes Green
We are taught that eye color, balding, and diabetes are genetic. But, these things are NOT true.

Children are **born** with blueish eyes **before** they change to brown or black. Men **with** hair become bald after they **lose** it. People **become** diabetics!

All of my life, I have had dark brown eyes. Now, the're greenish. Men who have been bald for years, now have hair. People with diabetes no longer suffer with it.

These people took control of their lives and did what needed to be done. They cleansed their bodies and flushed the stones from their livers. In the process, their 'genetic' problems vanished! So can yours (see Source Index).

Who's In Control?
Question medical authority. Get up off your knees. It's YOUR body and YOUR life. You should be in control.

NORMAL COLON AND SICK COLONS

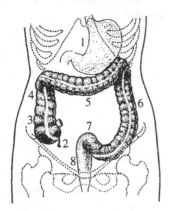

A. The Normal Colon

The normal colon in the proper position in relation to other structures: 1) stomach 2) appendix 3) cecum 4) ascending colon 5) transverse colon 6) descending colon 7) sigmoid flexure 8) rectum

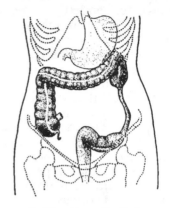

B. The Spastic Colon

The colon in spastic constipation.

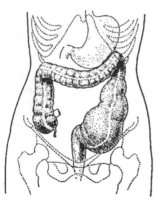

C. The Engorged Colon

The colon in engorged constipation.

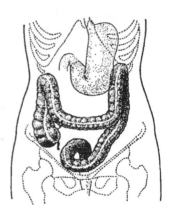

D. The Sagging Colon

Ptosis, or sagging, of the transverse colon, accompanied by displacement of the stomach.

Programmed To Die

We *program* ourselves to die, by our actions, words, and thoughts. And as we *resonate* a message of death, the reaper takes our friends and siblings, signaling the time is near. We do our best not to disappoint.

3

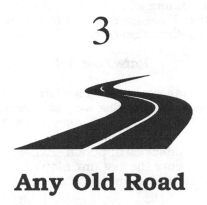

Any Old Road

*"If you don't know where you're going,
how will you know when you get there?
If you don't know how you got there,
any old road will NOT take you back."*
John Thomas

Aging is considered to be part of the normal life process. In actuality, it is the *abnormal* part of the process. Normal growth takes us from infancy to our anabolic peak. Abnormal aging takes us from our PEAK to our grave.

Aging follows a procession of Time-related events. Events we identify with descriptions like: gray hair, menopause, balding, diabetes, wrinkles, loss of physical strength, and obesity. These events are only EFFECTS that document the passing of Time. They are also SIGNS of aging!

The aging process can be slowed. It can be stopped. It can be reversed. These things are possible if we have the necessary understanding and are willing to act. Informed action is *the* controlling factor.

Most people speed the aging process and the passing of Time by choosing to ignore the SIGNS along the way. This shortens their days on the Earth and they age by default.

Instead, let us choose to *re-experience* Time, NOT by reliving our experiences, but by *reliving* Time itself—Time that we have already spent.

Aging and Time are related, but they are not the same. Aging is the result of Time poorly lived, whereas Time is the *vehicle* of aging. For example, dis-eases like cancer are the product of Time *poorly* lived. Cancer causes the passing of Time to accelerate. When this occurs, our body experiences a slump in its *bio-electric* balance and we become OLD! Think of dis-ease as Time in motion. Dis-ease *warps* our concept of Time! Aging is Time's trail (confirmation of metabolic deterioration).

Rate Yourself

The following age and Time-related "tasks" will *personalize* each of the age categories we discussed in chapter two. Each will lend the concepts of *aging* and *Time* a tangible meaning.

Use an erasable pen or pencil. *Estimate* and place *your* age on each line. Leave the last line blank until *after* you have scored your *bio-electric* age at the END of this chapter.

Mental Age	0_____	80 yrs
Calendar Age	0_____	80 yrs
Functional Age	0_____	80 yrs
Age You Feel	0_____	80 yrs
Bio-electric Age	0_____	**100 yrs**

Signs & Symptoms

Time poorly lived produces SIGNS and SYMPTOMS of *bio-electric* aging and dis-ease. Signs and symptoms represent *change* and diminished function in the vital organs and glands.

Symptoms of dis-ease are *subjective* changes in body function that are NOT apparent to an outside observer—like nausea, anxiety, pain, dryness of mouth, anorexia (loss of appetite). Symptoms sometimes go unnoticed by the host. Symptoms, however, indicate *subtle* alterations in body tissues, hormones, and fluids. Slow-down gives way to shut-down.

Aging initially occurs in the *"invisible"* realm—of the "electric" body. Eventually, it is seen in the mirror, or confirmed by the doctor's diagnosis.

Time Made Visible

Signs are apparent to an observer. They are *external* events. SIGNS of aging and/or dis-ease can be observed and measured. Signs will support a doctor's diagnosis of a morbid condition. Signs of dis-ease cause the host to become acutely aware of change in normal body function—like fever or inflammation. Hence, a sign is the *confirmation* of aging and the passing of time. *Signs are Time made visible!* Signs are *bio-electric* Time capsules.

Signs are NOT *normal* events in the life process. They represent dis-ease and pathology. When we think of them as *normal*, we diminish their impact on our consciousness and we compound their effect on the aging process.

Dis-ease—and its signs—is like the unwelcome guest who drops in. Its presence *appears* to cause temporary upset. However, when it departs, dis-ease leaves its *shadow* upon us. Sometimes the effects are self evident—as when we can no longer do the things we once did. More often than not, the effects of dis-ease are delayed until old age removes its cloak and we realize that Time has slipped away.

Damage to the vital organs is dis-ease's epitaph. Dis-ease should be our cue to change our lifestyle and begin the aging reversal process.

Charting Your Bio-electric Age

The following list is your key to *your* bio-electric age. Additionally, it is the brush and canvas you will use to determine *how* and *why* your *bio-electric* age is what it is. This list is your *personal* road map to ageless living. It points the way back in *bio-electric Time* —if you absorb the simple lessons contained in the balance of this book. Each item on this list will be fully developed.

Each item reflects an assigned point value that is based on its long term **cumulative effect**. Most items are unisex and apply to both sexes while the male/female list applies to the respective sex only. *Contributing factors* that accelerate the aging process are also listed.

NOTE: This list is not a diagnosis of a particular dis-ease condition. Rather it is a list of markers. It gives you a close approximation of your *"bio-electric age"* providing you are honest with yourself.

Check the boxes that apply. Serious *past* health conditions should be counted if they have left their mark or are of recent vintage. If you are under care, or take medications for a condition, it should be counted. Complete this exercise NOW and again after you have completed the book when you better understand the significance of each item on this list. Each item will add direction and meaning to your quest for agelessness.

Please **do not** diminish or pass judgement on the items listed. The list is comprised of signs, symptoms, effects and contributing factors.

Let me assure you that every item deserves your

attention. Their cumulative effect can easily BLOCK your path to becoming *Young Again!*

Signs, Symptoms & Contributing Factors
Of Bio-electric Aging

Unisex

Gout	40	☐
Eyes: •Crows feet around eyes (mild)	8	☐
•Crows feet (heavy)	15	☐
Skeletal Muscles: Deterioration of, loss of	20	☐
•Soft or flabby	12	☐
•Cramps/charleyhorse	18	☐
Stomach (gut): Paunchy	8	☐
•Pot/beer belly	40	☐
Eyebrows: thick, bushy	15	☐
Nose & Ear hair (external)	18	☐
Clothes: Trousers/pants & Shirts/blouses		
•Progressively larger after age 24	20	☐
Daily Energy: Erratic, not level	25	☐
Body Odor: Requires deodorant	20	☐
•Overpowers deodorant	40	☐
Bad Breath: Chronic	30	☐
Teeth: •Decayed	40	☐
•Require cleaning more than once a year	15	☐
•Cleaning required once a year	25	☐
•Cleaning every 3-6 months	40	☐
•Mercury amalgam fillings	80	☐
•Root canal(s) present in mouth	40	☐
•Gingivitis (inflamed gums)	30	☐
Nails: finger/toe		
•Weak; break easily; spots; heavy ridges	20	☐
•Slow growth	30	☐
•Thickening of toe nails	40	☐
Hearing: Poor; early onset; progressively worse	30	☐
Skin:		
•Dry, scaly (includes dandruff)	10	☐
•Psoriasis/seborrhea (scalp or body)	50	☐
•Wrinkled (hands, face)	10	☐
•Fat bumps on back of upper arms	10	☐
•Pimples & acne	30	☐
•Sweat-do not sweat much	10	☐
•Brown *liver* spots over body	40	☐
•Bruise easily	20	☐
•Heavy oil secretion	15	☐
Hair, Mustache, & Beard:		

•Predominantly gray/white 30 ❑
•Bald head 30 ❑
•Loss of body (leg) hair 60 ❑
•Slow hair growth 30 ❑
•Head hair (once wavy, now straight) 40 ❑
•Gray or white pubic, axillary, or leg hair 40 ❑

Physical Activity:
•Inability to perform hard physical work 20 ❑
•Pain/inflammation during/after work 20 ❑
•Abnormal sleep/rest required to recover 30 ❑
•Gain w/o increase in clothes size 30 ❑

Weight:
•Gain w/o increase in food 20 ❑
•Unexplained large weight loss 40 ❑

Mental:
•Short or long term memory loss 20 ❑
•Fatigued; can't face day 30 ❑
•Foggy, can't gather thoughts 30 ❑
•Need coffee to get/keep going 20 ❑

Stools:
•Lack of medium dark brown color 30 ❑
•Hard, dry 20 ❑
•Defecation requires strain/effort 20 ❑
•Food transit time between mouth and
 toilet over 24 hours 40 ❑
•Preceded by foul gas 20 ❑
•Black or red blood (hemorrhoids) 15 ❑
•Less than a "complete" stool 20 ❑

Sickness/dis-ease:
•Often feel sick w/o fever 20 ❑
•Colds more than once a year 15 ❑
•Succumb to flu most years 10 ❑
•Diagnosed degenerative dis-ease 80 ❑

Eyes:
•Require reading glasses 8 ❑
•Sensitive to sunlight 20 ❑
•Inability to adjust to dark 20 ❑
•Brown spots in iris 30 ❑
•Shadows under eyes 8 ❑
•Drooping eye lids 8 ❑
•Eye lids don't open/close evenly 20 ❑
•Macro degeneration 30 ❑
•Retinitis/tunnel vision 30 ❑

Cheeks:
•Sunken, hollow 8 ❑
•Jowls distended and inflated 25 ❑
•Flushed with spider capillaries 40 ❑

Joints:
- •Joint pain (general) — 20 ❑
- •Diagnosed arthritis, bursitis, rheumatism, or variations thereof — 60 ❑

Stature:
- •Physical height less than your lifetime peak — 60 ❑
- •Hunched-back (mild) — 40 ❑
- •Hunched-back (severe) — 80 ❑

Minor Wounds:
- •Scab drop-time for minor wounds requires over 1 week — 20 ❑
- •Subject to secondary infections — 30 ❑
- •Scars form easily — 40 ❑

Capillary Blood:
- •Fails to form a "pearl" when finger is pricked i.e. blood flows instead of forming a crown or pearl — 30 ❑
- •Color is dark red; not bright red — 30 ❑
- •*Less* than instantaneous color return to finger/toe nails when squeezed and released—both sides — 40 ❑
- •Dizziness due to poor blood flow — 30 ❑
- •Suffer w/sticky blood (Rouleau effect) — 50 ❑
- •Use of blood thinners/aspirin — 50 ❑

Respiratory (lungs):
- •Heavy breather — 30 ❑
- •Difficulty catching breath — 40 ❑
- •Suffer with water on lung — 80 ❑
- •Angina-tightness — 40 ❑

Colon/Bowels:
- •Constipation (chronic) — 50 ❑
- •On/off-irregular habits — 30 ❑
- •Alternating diarrhea/constipation — 30 ❑
- •Ongoing appendix problems — 50 ❑
- •Appendix removed — 20 ❑
- •Colitis — 40 ❑
- •Diverticulitis — 40 ❑
- •Colostomy — 60 ❑
- •Parasites — 50 ❑

Sexual:
- •Impotent/frigidity — 50 ❑
- •Painful climax/ejaculation — 30 ❑
- •Lack of interest — 40 ❑

Blood circulatory System:
- •Heart Attack — 40 ❑

•Stroke 40 ❑
•Low red blood cell count (chronic) 40 ❑
•Low hemoglobin level 30 ❑
•Diagnosed arteriosclerosis 50 ❑
•Diagnosed atherosclerosis 50 ❑
•Poor circulation 30 ❑

Lymphatic System:
•Nodes chronically swollen/painful in
  groin/armpits/throat 50 ❑
•Lymph nodes surgically removed 50 ❑
•Cancer of lymph system (lymphoma) 90 ❑
•Spleen surgically removed 60 ❑

Fat:
•Increase in subcutaneous surface fat 30 ❑
•Body weight at top of "normal" scale 30 ❑
•Body weight 10% over normal
  (unless solid body muscle/athletes) 50 ❑
•Total fat intake over 20% of diet 10 ❑
•Use of ANY margarine spreads 30 ❑
•Use of soy/canola oils or products 60 ❑
•Elimination of all fat from diet 30 ❑

Urinary:
•Chronic albumin in urine 50 ❑
•High urea level in urine 40 ❑
•Low specific gravity urine 30 ❑
•Prone to kidney stones 40 ❑
•Generally dark urine color 25 ❑
•Foul urine odor 30 ❑
•Sweet urine odor 50 ❑
•Inability to hold bladder 10 ❑
•Dribble, poor flow, can't release 40 ❑
•Volume is small (less than 4 oz) 35 ❑

General Metabolic:
•Drink less than 1/2 gal water/day 40 ❑
•Drink with your meals 20 ❑
•Drink chlorinated/fluoridated H_2O 60 ❑
•Substitute soft drinks for water 60 ❑
•Failure to drink at least 8 oz of
  H_2O every two hours 30 ❑
•Failure to drink at least 12 oz of
  H_2O every 15/30 minutes during
  hard physical activity 20 ❑
•Use fluoridated toothpaste 30 ❑
•Use common deodorants 30 ❑
•Drinking water comes from tap 50 ❑
•Drinking water source is bottled,

distilled or common filtered 30 ❏
•Regularly use aspirin or aspirin
substitute medications 40 ❏
•Regularly take Rx drugs 40 ❏
Liver & Gallbladder:
•Diagnosed for or prone to
gallstone formation 60 ❏
•Diagnosed for or prone to
hepatitis, mononucleosis,
Epstein-Barr, malaria, or
Chronic Fatigue Syndrome 60 ❏
Saliva:
•Dry mouth 20 ❏
•Must drink liquids to swallow 30 ❏
Body Temperature:
•Chronic low grade fever &/or below
normal temperature 35 ❏
•Cold hands and feet 60 ❏
•Sensitive to frigid temperatures 30 ❏
•Inability to handle hot weather 30 ❏
Connective Tissue:
•Diagnosed w/systemic lupus 90 ❏
•Diagnosed myasthenia gravis 90 ❏
•Have a diagnosed disorder 20 ❏
•Stiff joints/loss of flexibility 20 ❏
•Lack of energy 40 ❏
•Must eat often to have energy 30 ❏
•Subject to mood swings/energy drops 30 ❏
•Meals slow energy & brain function 20 ❏
•Sleepy/listless after lunch meal 20 ❏
Stress and Headaches:
•Inability to function under stress 30 ❏
•Regularly stressed-out 40 ❏
•Chronic headaches 40 ❏
Gastrointestinal Tract:
•Cramping after meals 30 ❏
•Chronic gas 50 ❏
•*Foul* gas 40 ❏
•Bloated abdomen after meals 50 ❏
•Diagnosed for colitis, diverticulitis
Crohns' dis-ease 60 ❏
Cancer:
•Diagnosis of any cancer 90 ❏
•Taken chemo/radiation therapy 75 ❏
•Bone cysts/tumors etc. (benign) 30 ❏
•Cysts or tumors of any kind 50 ❏
Tobacco:

•Smoke or chew 50 ❏

Tongue:
- •Coated, pasty white-daytime 40 ❏
- •Coated upon rising in morning 20 ❏
- •Heavily grooved 40 ❏

Sleep:
- •Sleep less than 7 hours per night 7 ❏
- •Sleep less than 6 hours per night 30 ❏
- •Sleep broken; usually interrupted 20 ❏
- •Sleep with windows closed 30 ❏
- •Sleep under electric blanket 50 ❏
- •Abnormal sleep patterns (Walking Legs etc)60 ❏

Dietary:
- •Don't use multi-vitamins/minerals 20 ❏
- •Use common vitamins/minerals 20 ❏
- •Take calcium supplements 20 ❏
- •Lump in throat (difficulty swallowing) 50 ❏
- •Pulse picks up after meal 10 ❏
- •Vomit often 40 ❏
- •Eat when nervous 30 ❏
- •Excessive appetite 30 ❏
- •Increased appetite w/o weight gain 30 ❏
- •Acid foods upset stomach 30 ❏
- •Nervous stomach 20 ❏
- •Always hungry 30 ❏
- •Poor appetite 25 ❏
- •Milk causes indigestion/bloating 20 ❏
- •Spicy foods a problem 20 ❏
- •Greasy foods cause indigestion 50 ❏
- •Eat lots of snacks 30 ❏
- •Time between meals under 4 hrs including snacks 25 ❏
- •Devour food...fast eater 30 ❏
- •Salt food 30 ❏
- •Eat lots of alfalfa sprouts 20 ❏
- •Food not home grown 40 ❏
- •Eat restaurant food regularly 50 ❏
- •Eat lots of junk packaged foods 40 ❏
- •Own/use a microwave oven 50 ❏

Computer:
- •In front of more than 1 hour daily 8 ❏
- •Closer than 30 inches from face to monitor 30 ❏

Florescent-Mercury—Sodium vapor Light:
- •Use for work light 20 ❏

Electric price scanner: 20 ❏

Cellular Telephone (use regularly) 30 ❏

Radar:
      •Work with radar (police/military)   40 ❑
Electronic Equipment:
      •Work with on daily basis   30 ❑
Smoke Detector: Sleep/work under   20 ❑
Exercise:
      •Lack of aerobic activity 3x week   30 ❑
Basal Metabolic Rate: Low   30 ❑
Wake-up: Slow; requires several hours   40 ❑
Resting Pulse Rate: above 75   20 ❑
Blood Pressure:
      •Resting pressure above 90/130   30 ❑
      •Resting pressure above 80/120   10 ❑
Sleep Patterns:
      •Insomnia (can't sleep)   20 ❑
      •Hypersomnia (sleep all time)   40 ❑
      •Narcolepsy (involuntary daytime
         sleep lasting about 15 minutes)   40 ❑
Emotions:
      •Keyed-up, can't relax   30 ❑
      •Moods of depression/melancholy   40 ❑
      •Highly emotional   30 ❑

Females Only

Menstruation & Menopause:
      •Easily fatigued   20 ❑
      •Premenstrual tension (PMS)   30 ❑
      •Painful/dificult menses   30 ❑
      •Depression before menstruation   20 ❑
      •Oaries removed   80 ❑
      •Frigid/loss of sexual desire   40 ❑
      •Menses irregular-missed often   40 ❑
      •Acne worse during menses   30 ❑
      •Painful breasts   30 ❑
      •Body painful to touch   30 ❑
      •Ovarian cysts   40 ❑
      •Hot flashes   40 ❑

Male Only

Impotentence: (inability to get/hold an erection)   60 ❑
Prostate: (inflammation of)   40 ❑
      •Removed   80 ❑
      •High PSA count   60 ❑

Urination:
- •Difficulty releasing/dribbling   40 ❑
- •Night urination frequent   40 ❑

Legs:
- •Pain inside leg or heels   30 ❑
- •Leg spasms, cramps at night   20 ❑

Total Score.. _____

Divided by .... 248 |‾‾‾‾‾‾‾‾‾

Your *bio-electric* "reference score" is........... _____

Add your points together and divide your score by 248 to obtain your *bio-electric* reference score. Example: If your score is 1965, divide by 248 to obtain a **reference score** of 7.92. Next, use the conversion scale to convert your reference score to your *bio-electric* age of 70 years. This is your **"real"** age!

Bio-electric Score Conversion Scale

The number on the left is your reference score. The number on the right is your *bio-electric age.*

.18 = 18	.22 = 20	.30 = 22	.33 = 24
.66 = 28	1.1 0= 30	2.42 = 35	2.86 = 40
3.30 = 45	3.96 = 50	4.40 = 55	5.28 = 60
6.60 = 65	7.92 = 70	8.81 = 75	11.0 = 80+

Your bio-electric age *should* motivate you to evaluate your lifestyle and the peculiarities of your particular body.

DO NOT panic or feel hopeless if your bio-electric age is older than you think it should be.

Remember, it took your entire life to reach your present *bio-electric* age. Allow yourself a little time to undo the damage. *Circle* your age and *transfer* your score to the chart earlier in this chapter. You should re-calculate your *bio-electric age* every year to determine if you are aging or growing younger. Your *bio-electric age* is a VERY important reference number.

Think About It!

If your *calendar age* is twenty-seven years and your bio-electric age is thirty-nine years—as mine was when I began the reversal process—you are losing the battle.

Consider the impact each additional *bio-electric* year exerts upon you. The younger you are, the less effect a few extra years will have. BUT, if you are already thirty-five, forty, fifty, sixty or MORE *bio-electric* years OLD, a few extra years can mean a lot and they must not be ignored or written off.

The older you are, the faster Time flies and the faster you become old! You "know" you are in trouble when the SIGNS appear. Most signs appear between *bio-electric* age thirty and fifty five. Heart attacks, arthritis, gray hair, obesity, cancer, hysterectomy, stroke, multiple sclerosis, nerve deterioration, impotence, etc.

Time is NOT on your side if your bio-electric age is equal to or greater than your calendar age.

There is NO time to waste! Don't look back! Make yourself finish this book and apply what you learn! The answers you SEEK are contained in these pages.

My calendar age is almost fifty-one, but my bio-electric age is holding at nineteen years YOUNG! Time is standing still for me—and it will do the same for you too—if you desire it.

No one's situation is hopeless!The *bio-electric* body has AMAZING resiliency! Follow the steps outlined in this book and your body will heal itself. Let your body prove to you that you can become *Young Again!*

ACTION STEPS TO AGELESS LIVING
1. **Evaluate your score.**
2. **Review the items checked.**
3. **Complete your study of this book.**
4. **ACT upon your new knowledge.**
5. **Recalculate your score once a year.**
6. **Learn to GUARD your words and thoughts.**
   Read *Your Body Believes Every Word You Say*
   (see Source Index).

Each thing you do to improve your health—no matter how small—will produce big benefits. Several small steps produce benefits far beyond the total of the individual steps. The combined effect is called *synergistic*.

PREVIEW: *In our next chapter, you will meet a few great people of science; get a glimpse of the behind the scenes maneuvering within medicine; be offered an explanation of mankind's present environmental dilemma.*

All Played Out
Life is like a record player that spins in three speeds: 33, 45, and 78. At 33 life is great. At 45 you're not so sure. At 78, you're all played out. To avoid becoming a 78 at **45,** all you have to do is change your lifestyle to 33!

Homeopathic Medicine Works!

Homeopathic medicine works at the **subtle energy** level of our existence. It does this by manipulating the body's bio-electric energy fields with substances called *remedies*.

Remedies treat dis-ease by altering vibratory frequency. They are NOT drugs in the traditional sense. Some remedies are very specific, others very general. Some treat substance problems. Others treat conditions.

Mercury toxicity (from mercury dental fillings) is a treatable with the correct choice of bioresonant remedy. A yeast infection is a systemic *condition* that responds similarly. Foreign viruses, bacteria, and serum proteins, like those used in vaccines for immunizations, can be buffered so that a child's response will not get out of hand and destroy the nervous system, immune system, hearing, or damage mental faculties.

Homeopathy uses substances whose energy *footprint* is the same or similar as the offending substance. If the *whole* body is sick, systemic frequency must be reestablished. It is very important that remedies provide complementary *biogenic* and *nutritional* support and *vitalized* to 9x, 20x, 30x, 100x, and 200x potentcies. Universal *sarcodes* that work at the "cellular" level have greater effect than specific tissue remedies.

***Potentiation* energizes a substance and makes it more powerful than it originally was.** *Succussion* (shaking or pounding of a substance so it will vibrate at a specific frequency) and *dilution* are employed to bring about *resonance* and *transference*—processes that involve the manipulation of Hertz rate.

Hertz (Hz) rate and frequency are related. When you hear the word Hertz, think "beat." The wavy horizontal line on an oscilloscope represents *beats*. Electricity in the USA is 60 cycles or beats per second. Thus, sixty seconds to a minute, sixty minutes to an hour, etc.

Earth has a wobble in her axis—like a wheel out of balance—heavy on one side. The wobble creates a beat, a thump, a vibration as it spins. The wobble is Earth's Hertz rate or frequency. Until recently, Earth's Hertz rate was 7.8. Today it is about 8.1. By year 2012, Earth changes are expected to bring about a Hertz rate of 13.

Balance **your** Hertz rate with homeopathic remedies that clear your body of stray frequencies. Good health is reflects vibrational harmony (see Source Index).

The Priesthood

Whenever a system becomes *complex*, a priesthood of *experts* soon appear. They have an agenda, a code, and their own special vocabulary. And in the people, this spawns resentment, followed by skepticism as to the system's fairness.

Learn the rules of the game. Structure your life so you can stay out of harms way. Seek simplicity. Avoid complexity. *Stay away from the priesthood of experts!*

Juice Capsules & Tablets

Next to fresh, live, home grown food, juice capsules and tablets are a wonderful way to put a garden in your kitchen and life.

Add them to your daily diet, take them when you travel. Combine them with *harmonic* pollen, *biogenic* liver, or Klamath algae, and an apple and you've got a nourishing and inexpensive meal.

Amazing Youth

It's amazing to see the changes that take place in young adults as fat turns to lean muscle mass between ages fifteen and nineteen.

Adult hormones kick in. Muscle is built without effort. Boys become strong as mules. Girls become shapely. And if teens are reasonably healthy, they enjoy good health in spite of the abuse they deal themselves.

But as adults, we fail to maintain our vital organs. Our tissues become toxic. We fail to supplement our diet with hormone precursors to keep a young appearance. We resist doing load bearing work and aerobic exercise. We refuse to train our minds to focus, focus, focus.

Adults appreciate the wonder of youth after it has slipped away. Those who discipline their mind and lifestyle can get it back. It's called *reversing the aging process!* Please answer these questions. **How long do you want to enjoy perpetual youth? Are you willing to make the changes in your lifestyle that are necessary to keep what good health you have left, and get back that which you have lost?** You deserve an answer.

4

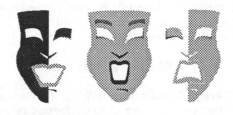

See What You Look At

Said Dorothy to the Wizard:

"You're a very bad man!"
"Oh no!" responded the Wizard.
"I'm just a very bad Wizard!"

It is difficult to comprehend aging without some understanding of the forces at work within science and medicine that blur our vision and confuse our thought processes. When understood, the reader will grasp why he or she is discovering the path to ageless living in this book instead of from the media or the medical system.

The truly Great Wizards of science and medicine are a breed of their own. They are often light years ahead of their time. They are also a problem for those who want to control and manipulate society. There have been many of these great people in science and medicine. Many of them lived out their lives on the fringe—away from mainstream medicine and science. We hear little about them, but the impact of their vision is all around us—often with another's name on their discoveries. A few hardy souls chose to function *within* the system. Their insight usually created craters that could neither be denied nor erased by the powers that be.

I refer to these people as WIZARDS. Wizards understand medical science's loss of direction and the dilemma of TRUTH vs. theory.

Medicine's tragic loss of direction did NOT occur by accident. It was foreordained. It is a tale of manipulation and *behind the scene* control.

By painting the historical landscape of a few great men and women of real medical science, we will better understand our present medical dilemma. At the same time, we will gain valuable insight into the process we call aging. Let's take a look at a few of history's Wizards.

The Great Wizards

Dr. Carey Reams was a Wizard. Reams had a sixth sense about nature and the energy forces of life at the sub-atomic level. He exhibited the instincts necessary for genius to express itself.

Like others before him, Reams knew that science and medicine had lost their way. They *refused* to see the obvious, choosing instead to face down TRUTH with calls for endless studies, procedure, and proof!

Reams *dared* to expose the connection between diet, lifestyle and dis-ease. He used simple, inexpensive testing procedures that only called for the pH of the urine and saliva plus the mapping of the blood capillaries in whites of the eyes. Reams chose NOT to follow allopathic medicine's path of profits. He knew that health and vitality are a *gift* from God. He tried to give that gift to the world. He suffered professional ridicule and legal abuse for his efforts.

Dr. Linus Pauling was a Wizard! He gave us his monumental discoveries about vitamin C. He also suffered professional ridicule for the TRUTH he heralded. Dr. Pauling was the harbinger of the fantastic DNA molecule discovery in 1954, and was gentlemanly enough to congratulate Watson and Crick's presence at the finish line *minutes* before himself.

Millions of people are indebted to Dr. Pauling. He was a wonderful scientist and a monument to TRUTH. Truth separates a good scientist from a poor one. Truth comes before personal fame and fortune. Dr. Pauling was a servant to mankind. Medicine and science would do well to emulate him.

Dr. Guenther Enderlein was a Wizard. He is responsible for the scientific and clinical documentation that proved that the blood is NOT a sterile medium. He discovered that protein based microorganisms build-up in the blood, the most toxic and deadly stage being when fungus appear in the blood. Enderlein was the first person to use body fluid pH to determine the presence of cancer in the body. The famous professor Dr.

Wilhelm Pfeffer of the University of Leipzig tested Enderlein's understanding of life with the question, "What is the difference between plant and animal?" Enderlein responded, "There is NO difference!" His discoveries proved he was correct.

Rene M. Caisse, R.N. was a Wizard. Rene was Canada's "cancer nurse." She reconstructed and resurrected an old North American Indian herbal recipe that "cured" thousands of people of all types of cancer.

Rene was a good student and a keen observer of nature's ways. She understood the *energetics* of vibrational medicine at the subtle energy level and she tempered her understanding with compassion for other human beings. Rene was hounded by health officials, but her TRUTH lives on.

Thanks to Rene's foresight (she died in 1978), her formula—and her *exact source* of "high resonance" herbs are still with us. Rene's tea is the ONLY *vibrational* product to ever be imported into mainland China specifically for the treatment of diabetes, cancer, and other degenerative conditions.

Dr. Max Gerson was a Wizard. His discoveries are of tremendous importance to the aging process. He immigrated to the United States from Germany in the 1920's. He was an excellent example of "low-tech" medical brilliance. Gerson leveled cancer's playing field by using uncommon good sense, instinct, and inexpensive therapies.

What made Gerson unique was that his therapies worked. He cared about people. He was an astute observer. He *cured* cancer with simple, inexpensive modalities and therein was the *rub*. Gerson was hounded mercilessly by the American Medical Association and various state medical boards because his work threatened medicine's dogmatic position on the nature of cancer. He died in 1959 tired and overworked.

Rachel Carson was a Wizard. She was the lady scientist who took on the military industrial complex by herself. In 1959, she wrote the book, *Silent Spring*. Rachel was the beginning of the *legitimate* environmental movement. Her findings shattered Science's litany of lies and brought the evils of pesticides into focus. She was proclaimed a witch and was burned at the stake before and after she died in 1964. Her epitaph reads: TRUTH!

Dr. Ignaz Semmelweis was a Wizard. He has particular significance to medical science and our story. He was a physician in Budapest during the middle 1800's.

Semmelweis made the mistake of confronting a thoroughly entrenched male dominated profession that had only recently wrestled away control of the healing arts from female healers—midwifery in this case. His contribution to medical science was a simple one, but it involved the use of uncommon good sense—a dangerous commodity in the face of arrogance. He said, **"Doctors, wash your hands between each patient!"** There had been unrelenting outbreaks of childbirth fever (Puerperal Fever) among women and hundreds of deaths in area hospitals.

The year was 1840, not so long ago. His detractors laughed good Dr. Semmelweis from the scene. They destroyed his reputation by character assassination—a ploy that leaves neither trail nor record of those in bloody robes. They asserted professional ostracism—a time-tested tool of the trade. Today, they resort to *reprimand* and *loss* of a physician's license to practice—putting a doctor out of business. Ostracism, licenses, and belittling are *subtle* maneuvers that are used to this day to CONTROL physicians who dare to step out of line.

This codicil is offered to stimulate the reader's perspective. *A doctor's status derives from the State. When the State grants its permission, the professional is created by way of a license. The doctor is a political being that exists at the whim of the State.*

Licenses are supposed to protect the public. *More often than not, they are a mockery that does little more than soothe. Behind the scenes, the professional boards and medical organizations badger and control the doctor who "sees truth" and dares to challenge scientific and medical dogma.*

History provides us with a long list of good Wizards—Galileo and Copernicus for example—who were driven out and destroyed. Control is the name of the game. Control is ALWAYS carefully maintained despite brush-fire political events that are provided for their therapeutic effect. Keep these thoughts in mind as future chapters unfold. In history, nothing happens by accident!

The history books tell us Dr. Semmelweis *suggested* that doctors should wash their hands between patients. They tell us *nothing* of the political maneuvering by his peers, nor of the women who died, nor of the money that was siphoned from those who prostrated themselves at medicine's altar.

How It Happened

It is helpful to understand how science and medicine lost their way. Hopefully, the author's explanation will also explain why mankind is at war with Mother Earth.

Let us go to the roots of Christianity, for it is there that we will find our clue. And God said to Adam, *"Take dominion over the Earth and every living thing thereon."*

This one command, credited to Deity, has done more to

pillage the Earth and its inhabitants—plant, animal and man— than any words ever put to task. The problem isn't the command, but the *interpretation* and *implementation.*

Misunderstood and certainly *misapplied,* the biblical edict to *"take control of Nature and hold dominion over Her"* set the course and destiny of history from the time of Christ, to Isaac Newton and the present day order.

By *blaming* the sin and fall in the garden on Eve— instead of acknowledging that BOTH male and female made their own choice—*man* dogmatized jurisdiction over woman and proclaimed WAR against Nature and the Earth. It was done in the *name* of GOD. Mankind's present dilemma is the result of blame instead of mutual respect for life.

Adam & Eve

"Power and dominion OVER nature," shaped science and its tributary, medicine, into the cult it is today. Man over God. Man over the Earth. Man over Woman—for it says, "Eve caused Adam to sin."

Interwoven in this tragic story was the shift from mankind's original primeval state as a *matriarchal* society to that of a *patriarchal* one. No longer would the blood line flow through the woman. Instead it would flow through the man. No more would Woman be exalted and recognized as the *giver* of life. Instead, she would be looked upon as the *ONE* who caused *man* to sin in the garden.

"And from this day forward, you will experience pain in childbirth as a REMINDER of your transgression." And so, Woman became the villain. A commodity to be controlled, bought, sold, and most importantly, *"blamed"* for Adam's transgression—which was Adam's own choice.

It was into this arena that Dr. Semmelweis wandered. Little did he realize that the powers behind the scene did not care about Puerperal Fever. It was profitable business. "So what if some women die as long as *we* control access to *choice* in medical care, *access* to God, and, of course, control over the *creation* of money."

Control is the name of the game. If we want to take control of our lives, we must recognize that in matters of health and longevity, things are NOT what they "seem." Recognition of this fact allows us to take control of our own destinies.

TRUTH in medicine causes problems and the greater medicine's *backlash* to a Wizard's discovery, the greater the probability that TRUTH is on the loose.

In the business of medicine and science, TRUTH prospers OUTSIDE the mainstream—out on the fringe. The fringe is where we will be taking our lessons in reversing the aging process. On the fringe you can become *Young Again!*

PREVIEW: *In our next chapter, you will become acquainted with the "energy forces" that CONTROL the aging process and you will learn HOW to identify them.*

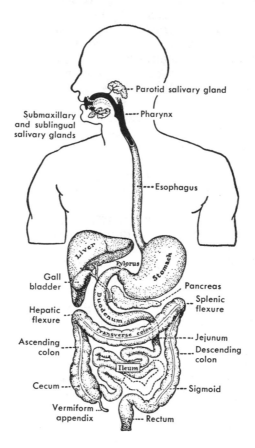

Visceral Organs Of The Abdominal Cavity

Dark Circles Under The Eyes
Circles under the eyes are a SIGN of liver overload, kidney malfunction, under hydration, lymphatic congestion, and systemic tocxicity. A change in lifestyle can eliminate these problems and add life to your years!

5

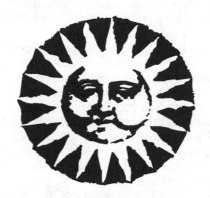

Energy And Matter

*"Reason, of course, is weak when measured
against its never-ending task. Weak, indeed, compared with the follies and passions of mankind,
which, we must admit, almost entirely control our
human destinies, in great things and small."*

Albert Einstein

Little in life is seen in polarized terms of black and
white. This is particularly true in the healing arts. For example,
consider the differences in the following modalities (therapies)
of healing presently in use.

Allopathic medicine (allopathy) attempts to heal using chemotherapy, which is *"chemically induced"* restoration of
health. It also includes surgical intervention, emergency medicine, and *palliation.* This is the predominant medical modality
practiced in the western world today. It relies on chemical
drugs to "badger" rather than to assist the *bio-electric* body to
heal itself. Allopathy believes that "opposite cures opposite."

Homeopathic medicine (homeopathy) is the exact
opposite of allopathic medicine. It was called the medicine of
"similars." Homeopathy focuses on *unfriendly energy fields* in
the body that vibrate at anti-life frequencies—frequencies that

create stress in the vital organs and imbalances with the system. Homeopathy uses vibrational "remedies" instead of chemical drugs. Remedies are potent energy substances that are *tuned* to the SAME vibrational frequency as the offending substance. Remedies **erase the signature** of the offending field which returns the patient to health or homeostasis (*homo*- the same. *stasis*-cause to stand; fix).

Chiropractic considers dis-ease to be the result of the incorrect alignment of the spinal column and the nerve plexus issuing therefrom. Poor alignment negatively influences the vital organs served by the central and peripheral nervous systems. Chiropractic has much in common with other vibrational modalities. This is the reason we often find chiropractors wearing several hats at once. Chiropractors are held in contempt by medicine. The reason: a good chiropractor is trained to be results and patient oriented, AND they are very open to alternative healing modalities.

Network Spinal Analysis (NSA) is a new form of chiropractic that integrates various "levels" of care in such a way as to *unfold* and *awaken* spinal energy flow. Healing occurs as a by-product of the freedom of the *body-mind* to utilize its natural, self-regulatory and self-expressive capabilities. In other words, healing is not the direct product of chiropractic, but of the "forces" of life itself *at the subtle energy level.*

The purpose of NSA is to determine the appropriate *timing* and *application* of mechanical forces to the tissues *before* chiropractic adjustment. NSA enables patients to release *non*-productive neurological patterns that block healing. NSA allows the *whole* person to express and experience their body's own self-intelligence and vital energy force.

[Insert] It is the author's belief that NSA brings about healing by helping the patient to become *aware* of negative energy *memory* patterns *at* and *below* the cellular level, and to "erase" them from the tissues. To learn more, read *The Twelve Stages Of Healing* (see Source Index).

Network Spinal Analysis produces significant improvement in patient self-awareness and ability to make life changes. This promising new healing modality was developed by Donald Epstein D.C. and is offered to the public by highly trained healers under the trade name *Network Chiropractic.* Call (303) 678-8101 to locate a Network practitioner in your area, or if you are a practitioner, to obtain training in this new modality.

Psych-K is wonderful new vibrational therapy. It helps people to deal with subconscious "beliefs" that direct their behavior. It is based on the idea that beliefs are the basis of our attitudes, and from these attitudes we develop behavior patterns—good and bad—that dictate our actions.

Psych-K helps people "reprogram" their subconscious mind similar to erasing a cassette tape and recording a new message. It increases self-confidence, releases old doubts and fears, and rids people of unwanted stress—and it works!

Psych-K is helping thousands of people who have heretofore been beyond the reach of traditional therapy. It is effective because it works at the *subtle energy* level of our existence. It was developed by Robert Williams, M.A. and is taught in business and public workshops nationwide. To learn more about this exciting modality, call (303) 756-9725.

Acupuncture seeks to manipulate energy flow within the autonomic and somatic nervous systems. It manages pain by opening nerve meridians (nerve pathways) or by blunting the flow of negative energy (pain). Acupuncture uses tiny needles—or their electronic equivalent—to block or manipulate energy flow and encourage healing.

Bio-magnetics heals through the use of magnetic energy. This promising modality has broad application for people who desire *personal* control over their health. It is an inexpensive therapy with great promise.

Therapeutic bio-magnets vary in size and shape and are used in everything from bracelets and seat cushions to shoe inserts and mattress pads. They are particularly useful in nullifying the effects of stress and 110 volt electrical current.

Therapeutic magnets are *stored* energy fields that favorably influence the body and promote healing. Therapeutic magnets use DC (direct current) vibratory energy to "restructure" energy fields in the body, manipulate pain, and promote healing. They modify blood and lymph flow by altering the magnetic "footprint" of the energy fields (see page 60).

Therapeutic magnets help balance positive and negative energy fields in and around injured or inflamed tissue. Millions of people have found relief and return of health by through magnetics—especially in Japan where it is used widely. In the USA, the medical establishment says magnetic therapy is quackery. The fly in the ointment is the patient who enjoys relief (see Source Index).

Vibrational medicine is a composite description that takes in dozens of healing modalities that rely on the manipulation of *energy* fields to obtain healing. It recognizes that health and sickness are manifestations of energy forces at the subtle energy level of our existence, and that healing requires that balance be established in the "whole" person.

Vibrational medicine is a *blend* of Western and Eastern thought and it is rendering wonderful results. There is no question that this form of medicine IS replacing the Frankenstein called "allopathic" medicine.

A few examples of vibrational medicine are the cold laser, photo-luminescence, MORA therapy, Network Chiropractic, therapeutic magnets, qi gong, tai chi, DEEP breathing, traditional chiropractic, homeopathy, and the use of BEV and SUPER ionized Mikrowater BEV water. These heal naturally by avoiding the trauma of surgical intervention and by promoting energy flow within the *bio-electric* body.

Compare The Difference

Allopathic medicine is based on the *Newtonian* view of reality. Sir Isaac Newton saw the world as an elaborate mechanism. Newton so influenced allopathic medicine that for the past three hundred years, the body has been viewed as a grand machine that takes its orders from the brain, central, and peripheral nervous systems. This view has now shifted to a new model that sees the body as a flesh and blood biological computer. Nuts and bolts have given way to circuit boards and switches. These approaches fall short of the reality of life at the **subtle energy level** of our existence.

The Newtonian approach fails to account for the energy forces like spirit, intuition, conscious and subconscious mental thought, biofeedback. These forms of pure energy compose our *sixth* sense. They belong to the Fourth Dimension because they are NOT physical. They CANNOT be measured by length, width, and height—the First, Second and Third Dimensions. They belong to the world of metaphysics (meta: beyond).

Paradigm Shift

Vibrational medicine (VB)views the physical body as the *signature* or *footprint* of the invisible "electric" body. Vb is based on Einstein's view of matter, which says, "matter will release energy when taken apart." For example, the splitting of an atom in an atom bomb. This is a MAJOR *paradigm shift* from Western medicine's approach to healing. The word *paradigm* means *para*-beside, *digm*-an example that serves as a model.

The Einstein model sees the human being as a network of energy fields that co-exist and commingle together, and the body as condensed energy resonating at healthy or sick frequencies. (Mother Earth frequency is between 7.8-8.1 Hertz.)

Vibrational healing comes from the *manipulation* of these pure energy forces—one neutralizing the other, rather than one **overpowering** the other. Conventional drug therapy uses negative energy drugs—to **force** the body into submission, thereby bypassing its innate intelligence.

Vibrational medicine does not endorse the Germ Theory

of Disease. Instead, it recognizes that the TERRAIN of the bio-electric body controls the bacteria and viruses, and not the other way around. The bio-electric body is a composite terrain.

Secondly, present day drug therapy is a mixture of *hoped for* therapeutic effects and KNOWN adverse effects—the good *hopefully* outweighing the bad! Vibrational medicine avoids the use of drugs, opting to use energy forms that are more therapeutic and less traumatic to the bio-electric body.

Drugs are drugs! They alter body function in negative ways. For example, arthritis medications are extremely potent negative-chemical energy. They do violence to the body and the liver and kidneys in particular. They ease the patient's suffering through *palliation* (the relief of signs and symptoms without cure of the underlying causes).

Health Through Manipulation

An example of energy manipulation could involve running a magnet over a computer disc or cassette tape. The magnet would neutralize the *energy* stored on the disc by cancelling the other frequency and *erasing* its signature.

If the energy message on the disc were a dis-ease condition in the body, a positive change in one's health would occur when the offending energy field is *neutralized*. Whenever positive energy forces gain the upper hand, the body returns to a state of health. Since life is energy, and energy is matter, we must conclude that life and energy are manifestations of the same phenomenon. Vibrational medicine's focus is energy.

Magneto Hydro Dynamics (MHD) is a relatively new field of vibrational medicine. Its focus is in the field of dentistry at the "consumer" level through prevention of dental problems.

Plaque formation on the teeth is the primary cause of cavities. Prevent the formation of plaque and you prevent cavities. MHD works extremely well on bleeding gums and periodontal (gum) dis-eases.

MHD uses a simple sink appliance to pumps water through an **electromagnetic** field where hydrogen ions are freed from the H_2O molecules. These ions carry a positive (+) charge. When the processed water is flushed against the plaque on the teeth, or under the gum lines—the negatively (—) charged plaque is dissolved and washed down the sink. MHD is an inexpensive "in home" dental modality for your family's teeth—and your dog's teeth, too! Use it to reduce your dental bills and avoid periodontal dis-ease. We will discuss it in more detail later (see page 204 and Source Index).

Radionics is used by some alternative farmers. It involves broadcasting *energy* frequencies into the surrounding area where it will be picked up by soil, plants, animals and microbes. Compare this practice to a radio station that transmits a melody that is picked up by our radio so we can hear and enjoy it. Properly used, radionics produces highly nutritious food while controlling weeds and insects.

Biodynamics is homeopathic agriculture. It is the *medicine of "similars"* applied to the soil. It involves the use of minute amounts of biodynamic *horn* manure and other *remedies* diluted in pure *energized* BEV type water in such a way that an *energy fusion* takes place. Applied to the soil, a single PINCH of manure dramatically influences soil, microbes, crops, and weeds. Fresh cow manure packed into a cow's horn and left buried between the Equinoxes (September—March) absorbs cosmic *energy* and undergoes a fundamental ENERGY transformation. This *tuned* energy matter is no longer manure, but a totally new, different, and potent energy force field.

Medicine & Science Conflict

Medicine and science are threatened by these paradigm shifts because they conflict with textbook mentality. They challenge theory that has been elevated to the status of *LAW* by way of the mumbo-jumbo called the *scientific method.* Misuse of the scientific method has gotten us into a lot of trouble. It should be abandoned because it shackles individual creativity. Vision MUST precede inquiry rather than the other way around.

Because vibrational medicine is replacing old dead theories with models that are bringing RESULTS, it behooves each of us to learn as much as possible about these new fields of thought and *apply* them in our daily lives wherever possible. Reversing the aging process relies heavily on the manipulation of *energy* fields within the bio-electric body.

Becoming *Young Again!* involves the application of vibrational medicine at the layman's level. Given the TOOLS and knowledge, we can produce amazing results in our lives and in the lives of our loved ones at minimal expense—and minimal risk!

This book provides a basic overview of the knowledge needed to bring about vibrational healing. Application of the techniques discussed and the response each person experiences is *unique* to each individual.

New View

The universe is composed of but two things: *ENERGY* and *MATTER.* Our body is matter. It is also energy. If this is true, then medicines and drugs, which are matter, must also be energy—and they are! However, they are NEGATIVE energy—energy that manipulates illness in the short term at the expense of health and longevity in the long term. No one can deny the advances allopathic medicine has made—especially in the replacement of body parts and in emergency medicine. But there is a negative side also. We must realize that all medications and surgical intervention carry *substantial* risk.

The *combined* effect of personal neglect, dis-ease and drugs accelerates aging in the youngest of people. Aging is a cumulative process.

Energy Shift

When we choose to ignore a healthy lifestyle, an energy *shift* occurs. This results in dis-ease and illness. Reversing the aging process involves learning how to manipulate these forces so these shifts either do not occur, or are quickly returned to normal. When we talk about having an ageless body, we are talking about a body where the positive energy forces are in control—a body that does NOT require perpetual jump-starts with drugs and surgery—to keep it going.

Everything we do; everything we eat; everything we drink involves some form of ENERGY that influences the *bio-electric* body. We must learn HOW to decipher what is good for us and what is not. By learning HOW to identify these forces, we can also learn HOW to manipulate them *without* the use of drugs or invasive surgery.

Dis-ease is a manifestation of negative energy forces in the body. Vibrational medicine elevates aging and dis-ease above crap shoot status, and offers the ordinary person CONTROL over their health and life.

We *must* recognize that we are more than hunks of flesh and blood, more than biological machines, and more than spiritual beings *trapped* in our bodies during our time on Earth. We are *energy*, and as such, we are part of the cosmos, and yes, we are created in the likeness of God who is also *ENERGY*—positive, beautiful energy!

Anions & Cations

Anions and **cat**ions are usable forms of energy that are released when a chemical reaction takes place—as in our gut and liver when we eat food. The release of energy opposites— one (+) the other (-) produces the electrical activity that grants permission for life.

All matter is a combination of (+) and (–) energy forms. For example, it is the energy *pattern* of anions and cations that gives us steel. When steel is fashioned into a spoon, we identify it as a *steel* spoon. When matter are altered through fusion, we may get lead or gold instead of steel. Break the bonds that hold a substance together and energy is released. That energy will be positive or negative.

Good & Bad Energy

The terms *positive* and *negative* energy mean the same as *good* and *bad* energy. *Good* energy is "right-spin" energy and *bad* energy is "left-spin" energy. We know good energy from bad energy by its EFFECT on our health and the bio-electric body.

Positive energy has a particular *spin* of its own—it *spins to the right*, meaning clockwise. NEGATIVE energy *spins to the left*, meaning counter clockwise.

Solar energy is **an**ionic energy. It is life-giving energy. The Earth's spin is the product of **an**ionic, clockwise, right-spin energy entering the Van Allen Belt (ozone layer). As these energy particles penetrate the ozone layer they are deflected and bombard the Earth causing it to spin. When Van Allen theorized this belt in 1948, he was laughed down by the *experts*. Later he was vindicated when NASA lost contact with astronaut John Glenn as he passed through this belt(ozone layer) on his return to Mother Earth.

Anionic energy can *pass through* matter. It is also very comforting and soothing. Have you noticed the difference in the heat produced by a wood fire compared to the heat produced by gas or electricity? If you have lived in a cold climate, you know that wood heat is wonderful heat and warms you clear to your bones.

Wood heat is **an**ionic energy; it comes from the Sun. Its effect is *right-spin* and it warms us because the **an**ions released by oxidation (burning) of the wood pass through our body and warms the cells. This is similar to how a microwave oven works—with one very important exception. Microwave energy is left-spin energy and VERY destructive to life forms.

Right-spin positive energy keeps you young. Left-spin negative energy causes you to become old. The former keeps you on the *anabolic* side of the pyramid as illustrated in chapter one. The latter puts you on the *catabolic* side. One spins RIGHT, the other spins LEFT. We are interested in the way these energy forces affect living things and HOW they influence the aging process. Please check your understanding by reviewing the following drawings.

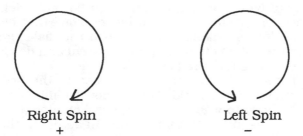

Right Spin
+

Left Spin
−

How To Determine The Spin

There are several ways to determine the spin and/or predict the effect a substance will have on the bio-electric body.

For instance, look at a bottle of vitamin E and you will see that the word tocopherol (chemistry for vitamin E) is preceded by the letter(s) d or dl.

"d" means that when infra red light is beamed through the tocopherol, the light is bent to the *right* or clockwise. This vitamin E has life giving energy. "dl" tocopherol is the opposite. "D" energy builds health and vitality. However, when "d" vitamin E is mixed in SOY or CANOLA oil as the carrier, it becomes detrimental to the body.

Those things that exert a negative influence on the body must be *neutralized,* disposed of quickly, or isolated. This applies to BOTH food and non-food substances like drugs, food additives, colorings, salts, and other noxious substances which we will discuss in more depth later.

Neutralize

The word **neutral** doesn't mean much to most people. It's kind of a *neutral* word. We must be more specific in its use. When we say that the body must *neutralize* toxic or left-spinning substances we mean that those substances which exert a negative influence on our body must be **de-energized** by the body.

To de-energize something requires energy. Please recall our magnet and cassette tape example. These are *stored* forms of energy. The magnet's energy buffered that of the cassette tapes energy because it had an opposite spin.

The body handles negative energy in similar fashion. Consider a potato—which is a natural form of stored energy. It is stored carbohydrate energy, put there by the plant for future needs. Depending on how the potato was grown, it may produce positive or negative effects in the body. All potatoes or carrots or peaches or apples are not equal!

A negative energy potato causes the body to forfeit some of its reserve energy to process and *de-energize* that negative energy field. If it is unable to accomplish the task, the toxic energies in the potato circulate in our system and do violence to our vital organs and the bio-electric body.

A left-spin substance turned loose in the body has **momentum.** It is like a boulder rolling down a hill. Stopping it requires the body to waste *vital* force and creates an energy deficit and a loss in health and vitality. In addition, the body may be FORCED to store some or all of the toxic energy or suffer further damage to the system. When the body is forced fed left-spinning energy fields, vital force is squandered. The effect is *catabolic* and it makes us OLD!

Back to the *spin.* When we say *right-spin,* I want you to think "good for my body." When we say *left-spin,* I want you to think "bad for my body." It might seem like oversimplification, but that's the way it is.

Kinesiology

Kinesiology is another way to determine a substance's spin and effect. It is the study of fluid dynamics (the movements of fluids). In the case of vibrational medicine, Kinesiology is concerned with the dynamics of blood and lymph flow in the bio-electric body.

Kinesthetics is muscle sense, the sense of perception of movement, weight, resistance and position. This is a textbook definition. It is sterile and meaningless.

Kinesthetics is also known as **Dynamic Reflex Analysis** or simply, muscle testing. Many alternative health practitioners use it to diagnose and heal their patients. Dynamic Reflex Analysis is *results* oriented. It is **not** sterile.

Kinesthetics is a useful diagnostic technique. It can be used to determine the EFFECT that a substance will have on the body. Kinesthetics involves gain or loss of strength in the fingers or limbs. It's a good testing procedure, but it requires training to become skilled in its use.

Muscle testing is influenced by heavy metal contamination in the tissues, as from mercury amalgam fillings in the teeth. Muscle testing accesses the body through the *autonomic nervous system* which is short circuited in the presence of heavy metals. (We will explain in more shortly.)

To summarize, substances exert one of two subtle energy EFFECTS on the bio-electric body and health. They are: Good • Positive • Right-spin, or Bad • Negative • Left-spin.

How To Test

All that is required is another person and the food, drug or vitamin that is being tested.

First, form a ring with the thumb and middle finger of your dominant hand. Next, have your friend attempt to gently but firmly pull those fingers apart. It is important that he or she NOTE the amount of effort it tales to *separate* the fingers. Then place the item in question in the opposite hand and repeat the exercise. In general, if it is good for the body, the fingers will become STRONGER. If it is bad, they will become WEAKER. You can place the item in question in the mouth if by yourself.

Sometimes, however, the body will give false signals because it *instinctively* KNOWS that the substance will produce a healing crisis and force the bio-electric body to cope, cleanse, and heal. Rejuvenation—like growth—can be painful and the body seeks to minimize pain—especially when it **knows** that its owner doesn't really desire healing or is unwilling to cope.

The above procedure can also be done by extending the dominant arm so it is level with the shoulder. Again, place the questionable item in the other hand. Have the other person gently but firmly pulling DOWN on the extended arm while you RESIST! Compare the results before and after and you have your answer! It is wise to cross check using other means.

Other Examples

People who drink too much alcohol have a sick liver. So will those suffering from hepatitis or mononucleosis. You can test them easily. Have them extend their arm. Next, pull down on the arm to get a feel of their strength. Then, pull down with one of your hands while at the same time you touch their liver area (just below rib cage on right front). If they have a weak liver, they will LOSE all of their strength and their arm will go down easily. They cannot resist!

My friend recently bought some tomatoes at the super market—the kind that grow mold before you get them home. I tested him using the above procedures. The results: *Total loss of strength!* They were returned to the store. If he had eaten them, he would have put a negative substance into his body and weakened his bio-electric status—and his aura—which is a reflection of the vitality of the body's vital organs and glands.

Foucault's Pendulum

A pendulum is one of my favorite ways to measure right and left spin energy. A pendulum is an antenna. It works just like the antenna of a radio station or the one on the roof of your house, except that it is a moving antenna. Antennas can send OR receive electrical signals.

All substances emit energy signals! The body has an energy signal and it has a "spin." If it comes from a body that has HIGH vitality, the spin will be to the right. The opposite is also true. This energy is also known as the body's "aura." Rocks, drugs, food, and human bodies all have auras. Kirlian photography can capture a picture of the body's energy aura.

When a pendulum is suspended by a string, horse hair, or chain, the pendulum will "spin" left or right when held over a substance like food, drugs, water, etc. Some pendulums are far more sensitive than others.

The pendulum's spin reflects the "status" of the energy field of the substance being checked. For example, white sugar emits a left-spin signal and the pendulum picks it up and spins accordingly. Here, the sugar is the radio station that transmits the signal. The pendulum is the receiving antenna. The body is the receiver and interpreter. That is all there is to it! No hocus pocus or spiritual voodoo are involved.

Learning to use a pendulum **and** vibration chain requires practice. *The Pendulum Kit* and *Vibrations* are very good instructional works on the subject.

Other Vibrational Therapies

Therapeutic Touch involves the transfer of positive energy transfer. It is used in the fields of nursing and massage therapy. Here, energy from a healthy person is used to buffer a sick or weak person's energy fields.

Laying on of hands as used in many religious circumstances is a variation of therapeutic touch. We will develop this subject in a future chapter.

Scars

While having my mercury amalgam fillings removed, my dentist noticed a one inch scar under my chin and asked when and how it got there. After I told him, he asked me to do the finger exercise we just described, only instead of placing a substance into my left hand, he had me touch the scar with my left hand. BINGO! No strength!

The EFFECT the scar was exerting was strong because it was directly in the path of a major *energy* meridian that flowed from my abdominal chakra (energy source) to the top of my head. It was *blocking* the flow of that energy.

Scar tissue is a negative energy field. Scars are recorded

in the skin's holographic memory. (*holo*-light reflected around a central object; *graph*-a record; *ic*-pertaining to.) A scar is a magnetic *energy* message like the information on a cassette tape or computer disc—no difference!

To *erase* the effects of the scar's negative energy field the dentist injected a homeopathic *remedy* along its length and instantly *full strength* returned to my joined fingers.

Trauma to the skin produces scars. Scars occur when the bio-electric body is under stress. In my case, the scar was a result of a fall when I was in a low (negative) energy state. Every organ of the body, including the skin, has *functional* cells called parenchyma cells. If these cells are traumatized when we are in a period of poor health or under stress, scars result.

Scar tissue formation in the vital organs and glands alters function and accelerates aging. A body with limited vitality is like a car driving on a flat tire. The further you go, the more damage you do to the tire and the vehicle.

Aging is the CUMULATIVE effect of negative energy forces on the bio-electric body.

Energy fields are *real!* They underwrite all of our life processes. They are the key to life's mysteries. They control aging. We must come to understand them and learn how to interpret and deal with them in our daily life.

It is very important that the reader understands that we live in a world of energy phenomena. Every person should develop the dowsing skills needed to take control of their life.

From a mental standpoint, we dowse when we use our intuition to guide us in dealings with people, things, and events—so why not in medicine, healing, and dietary choices? You will learn more about the effects of energy fields on the physiology of the bio-electric body as we progress.

PREVIEW: *Our next chapter is an overview of "high-tech" modern medicine and its magic bullet" promises. It will help you see the futility of relying on medicine's quick-fix techniques and appreciate the value of good health.*

Erase **Those Scar Memories!**

Holistc healers use *Procaine* to erase scar memory and open energy meridians blocked by scar tissue.

Procaine is the trade name for *novocaine* that dentists use to numb the nerves in your mouth. It is harmless and breaks down into two B vitamins. Procaine should be applied several times a day over a period of a week to completely erase negative energy memory.

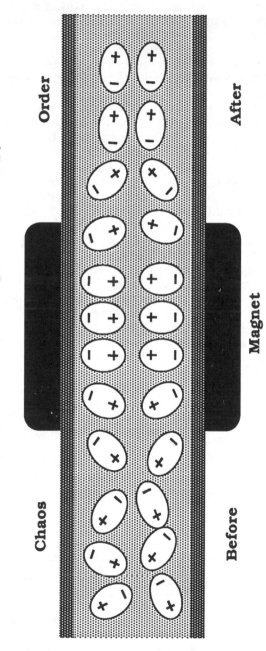

Healing Effects Of Magnetic Therapy

Chaos

Order

Before

Magnet

After

Molecular Massage Of Ionic Sea Minerals
In Blood & Lymph Fluids

6

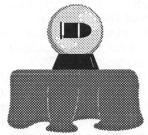

Magic Bullets

"We know life only by its symptoms"
Albert Szent-Györgyi
Discoverer of vitamin C

Allopathic medicine is no closer to understanding the *essence* of life today than it was a hundred years ago.

It understands little about basic functions like sleep, growth, pain, aging, and healing. Medicine attempts to manipulate these functions, but it does NOT understand them.

At the same time, we labor under an endless procession of new drugs and high-tech equipment concocted for the treatment of degenerative conditions like cardiovascular disease, cancer, and arthritis, just to name a few. These conditions are *technology* driven. They require ever more expensive diagnostic equipment and a long line of *experts* to operate it.

We have substituted "high-tech" medicine for the "take the pill, solve the problem" approach of yesterday. We have substituted the dis-eases of *civilization* for the contagious maladies of the past. The problems of dis-ease and aging are still with us despite our drive for technology.

High-tech medicine has become an extension of our national consciousness. It is the same "magic bullet" approach used in the movies. We incorrectly equate medicine's heroic efforts with true healing. Magic bullet technology masks our health problems and allows them to grow worse. Magic bullets blur our vision and numb our reason. They cause us to accept life on *marginal* terms instead of enjoying PEAK health.

Yesterday & Today

Yesterday, medicine knew us as people. Today, we are numbers in a cattle line—stripped of our human dignity. The difference is the *system*. The system has quashed the human being on both ends of the continuum. The doctor is denied training in nutrition and vibrational medicine. The patient gets neither. Modern medicine has substituted technology for dignity. It believes in "magic bullets."

Medicine does NOT understand dis-ease at the subtle energy level. Medicine attempts to diagnose it with tests, X-rays, CAT scans, and Magnetic Resonance Imaging. It has "trained" people to take refuge in *magic bullets* and *hope* instead of dealing with the root causes of degenerative dis-ease.

Daily, newspapers gush with glowing reports of a promising new Flash Gordon therapy. Just as fast, people fill the stalls—like cattle in the slaughter yards—waiting for the *magic bullet* that will cure their misery. Desperate people doing desperate things, ignorant as to the cause of their agony.

Poor Health • Life Of Simplicity

Poor health isn't a sin, but it's awful inconvenient and terribly expensive. There's a better way.

A life of simplicity allows you to take control of your life and health. It's the drive for money and things that stands between us and a life of simplicity. We must evaluate what is *really* important and learn to *walk away* from the rest.

If we lose our health chasing a dollar, we lose. Even if we catch lots of dollars, we still lose. When we fail to take care of our greatest treasure—our health—we end up giving our dollars to the doctors and hospitals. When we become desperate, we give our money to whoever we think will ease our pain.

We partake of *magic bullet* mentality because it offers us a quick fix to our problems. People like smoke and mirror technology, but it's a **past tense** approach. Magic bullets treat dis-ease instead of preventing it.

We are confounded by *high-tech wizards* in white coats. We seem unable to see that there is NO difference between empty promises and an bucket full of empty hope. *Magic bullets* have become an excuse—a salve for an old body.

Just because you enjoy good health today, it does NOT mean you will enjoy it tomorrow. This is the assumption that people in every generation make over and over again. It is an erroneous assumption that causes us to wake-up OLD! **It is *foolish* to squander good health today with no thought of tomorrow.**

Do whatever you need to do to get your *bio-electric* reference score under ".33" and you will enjoy a long and healthy life. Time stands still when you are truly healthy.

Good health does not *forestall* degenerative dis-ease. Instead, it means that you will NOT have to experience the hell that comes with old age. By learning how to take care of the *bio-electric* body, you avert dis-ease and enjoy **perpetual** good health. When you are *Young Again! YOU* are in control and you do NOT need medicine's "magic bullets"!

PREVIEW: *In our next chapter you will learn WHY food fails to supply the ENERGY you need to stay young and WHAT you can do about it.*

The 65% Watery Human Being

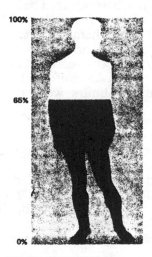

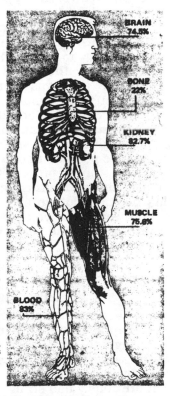

THE 65% WATERY HUMAN
The amount of water in the human body, averaging 65 per cent, varies considerably from person to person and even from one part of the body to another (right). A lean man may have as much as 70 per cent of his weight in the form of body water, while a woman, because of her larger proportion of water-poor fatty tissues, may be only 52 per cent water. The lowering of the water content in the blood is what triggers the hypothalamus, the brain's thirst center to send out its familiar demand for a drink.

"Pure Water Is The Best Drink For A Wise Man" – Henry Thoreau

Spider Bites

Spider bites are serious business. Some people experience severe reactions to thm. Others suffer loss of limbs and body parts. We are concerned with the energy forces that determine these differences.

In front of me is a story about a lady in Southern California who was bitten by a Brown Recluse spider, went into a coma, and awoke six months later missing her arms, legs, nose, and ear. Medicine has no *magic bullets* with which to treat most spider bites. I know.

Here is "my" story. I awoke at 2 a.m. with my hand throbbing and swollen. I was in *severe* pain. My hand looked like a balloon! Quickly, I shredded an organic potato, combined it with some Epsom salts and made a poultice with plastic sandwich wrap. The poultice "drew" the poison into two boils. My physician could not help me!

I visited my "holistic" dentist. He duplicated the energy frequency and "footprint" of a *homeopathic* remedy in his MORA frequency generator and applied the "invisible" energy to my hand and body—cancelling the spider's venom at the *subtle energy level* of my being. Instantly, the pain was gone. No limbs were lost. I regained full use of my hand.

Had I depended on allopathic medicine, I could have lost the use of my hand or worse. Fortunately, I was in superb health and the spider's venomous energy field did not cause permanent damage to my hand.

This story is proof of the effectiveness of vibrational medicine and authentication of the "energy" focus of this book. In future chapters, we will develop the "energy" thesis upon which peak health depends.

Peak health is the best buffer against dis-ease.

Toxicity & Wavy Hair

What does chemotherapy, wavy hair, water on the lung, and appendicitis have in common? Toxicity!!

Chemotherapy causes hair loss because it overloads the skin's waste processing capability. When hair regrows, it usually comes back wavy—even where the person previously had straight hair.

Systemic toxicity is behind wavy hair. It disguises blue and green eyes as brown and black. It dulls the hair and dims the brilliance of beautiful eyes.

7

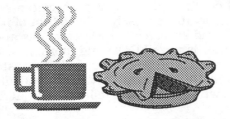

Death By Chocolate Pie

*"Chew your liquids and chew your
solids until they are liquid."*
Dr. Paul C. Bragg N.D., Ph.D.

"Death by Chocolate Pie" read the sign. It reminded me
that all food is NOT equal.

Some food is *alive* and promotes health, while other
food is *dead* and promotes death. We are concerned with the
differences in food and their influence on the aging process. We
are specifically concerned with food's *energy footprint.*

Water has a similar story to tell, but there is a fundamental difference between food and water. Foods are listed in
nutrient tables and are rated, one against another, based on
their nutrients. But water is NOT classified as a food because
it contains NO nutrients—that is, it contains no proteins, fats
or carbohydrates.

We are told that water is water, but there is MUCH more
to the story. Water is more than just "wet." Water has a
signature that powerfully influences life and health. Its *signature* is reflected in the direction and intensity of its spin.

Water is considered a *necessity* of life because we
cannot live without it. Oddly, the *experts* tell us to limit *food*
intake. Then in the same breath they tell us to drink as much
water as we desire without regard to the type of water or its
vibrational MEMORY as reflected in the hertz rate at which it
vibrates. Water is food, and like food, and all water is not equal!

We pick and choose our food on the basis of personal

taste, appearance, color, and aroma. Yet, we fail to make an issue about the water we drink. We do not consider water food. Water IS food. Water is THE most important food we put into our body. Water is not important for the nutrients it contains—it contains none. Water is important for the *ENERGY* that it *should* contain. Extremely pure water—water whose vibrational memory more closely reflects that of Mother Earth is what water—and specifically BEV water—is about.

BEV water is pure FOOD and more. It also has right-spin characteristics that people can feel and taste. It is **body friendly** because it energizes, hydrates, and detoxifies the system. People who drink it will tell you it is "different!"

Live Food

Traditional food that is *biologically active* has a right-spin *signature* and it produces right spin effects in the body. It contains enzymes, charged ionic minerals, vitamins, and positive energy that are absolutely necessary for good health. These components of "live" food are the foundation of life itself. Let's discuss enzymes.

Enzymes are biochemical proteins. Some enzymes are *catalysts.* A catalyst accelerates a reaction, or causes a reaction to take place that either would not occur or would occur at a much slower rate if it were not present.

Enzymes can be compared to oxygen's effect on a fire. No oxygen, no fire. Without oxygen, fire can neither start nor continue. "True" catalysts are used over and over. They are neither altered or destroyed in the reaction. An example is the platinum and rhodium used in catalytic converters on cars. These *noble* metals convert toxic gases like carbon monoxide to carbon dioxide and water. They do it through a series of oxidation and reduction (redox) reactions. *(In future chapters, you will learn how use redox reactions to your benefit.)*

In the body, most biochemical catalysts are consumed, altered or destroyed in the reactions they fuel and must be continually *manufactured* by the body. The liver is our PRIMARY enzyme and catalyst manufacturing organ, and therefore will always be a player in any health disorder.

The constant formation of new enzymes requires tremendous amounts of *right-spin* energy that must come from substances that are "live" and friendly to the bio-electric body. Dead food and dead water are negative energies. They are left-spin energy forces that fail to contribute to health, and instead block or neutralize the positive effects of food and water that has a right-spin energy *footprint* and *signature.*

Biocatalysts

Biological catalysts cause reactions to occur millions of times faster than what would occur if they were not present. Without biocatalysts, life as we know it could not exist.

Vitamins do not work unless all of the needed major *and* minor (trace) minerals are present in the body in balanced form. In biochemistry, vitamins are called *cofactors* because they work WITH minerals and enzymes. Because most vitamin supplements are synthesized (man-made) despite claims to the contrary on the label, they are useless at best and damaging to the vital organs at worst. Moreover, most mineral supplements are **useless** because they are in "elemental" form. (We will develop these points as we go along).

Your best source of biologically active vitamins and minerals is garden fresh food. Most vitamin supplements do not come from **real** food. And because synthesized substances are negative energy substances, the body must either *neutralize* them or *store* them in body fat to protect the vital organs.

When we have **EXCESS** toxins and wastes in the system, biochemical reactions slow and blood and lymph circulation becomes difficult. **Excess** wastes and toxins interfere with vital organ function and hormonal balance, and their accumulation leads to "systemic" (whole body) degeneration and rapid aging. Waste removal is expedited with Yucca extract, fresh lemon, lymphatic self massage, enhanced proanthocyanidins (PAC's), colon therapy, and BEV water.

Cooked Food

Cooking denatures enzymes. Denatured enzymes can't do their job because they have LOST the characteristics that caused them to work. Cooking food seldom improves quality. Improper cooking totally destroys food value and enzymes.

I am not suggesting you to stop cooking your food, but I am suggesting you that you eat plenty of fresh, raw, (and preferably) home grown vegetables and fruit—perhaps 50% of dietary intake.

Avoid high heat and cook no longer than necessary. Use steam kettles instead of submersing food in water. Use stir fry methods. Avoid microwave ovens—they alter food enzymes, destroy vitality, and cause the food to take on a vibratory signature that is anti life. Avoid table salt, additives, flavor enhancers, and dyes. These substances *zap* the bio-electric body's energy fields and block crucial biochemical reactions. When you eat them you **cheat yourself** of good health.

Metabolism

Metabolism is a term that comes to mind. It means *biotransformation* and refers to the way food molecules are transformed into energy molecules in the body's energy pathways. Metabolism involves *fusion* reactions that join individual atoms into right spin *energy* molecules. This is the opposite of the kind of energy produced by nuclear fission (atom bombs/ nuclear power plant wastes, microwave ovens). Fusion reactions are right-spin and anabolic—they build up! Fission reactions are left-spin and catabolic—they tear down!

Metabolites are the waste products of biochemical reactions. Dissected the word looks like this: *meta*-beyond. *bol*-tranformation. *ite*-product of. Hence, a product that is **beyond** transformation. Metabolites are waste. When we speak of metabolic wastes, we are talking about toxins and/or metabolites. Included in this definition are man-made chemicals of organic synthesis (poisons like pesticides and herbicides).

Animal Protein

Industrialized man eats high on the hog. He eats too much animal protein and not enough fruits and vegetables.

Animal proteins come from the top of the food chain. If animals are healthy, their proteins will reflect a right-spin *signature* and their proteins will sustain us. But if they are not healthy, their proteins will have a left-spin signature and they will cause us to become sick and age prematurely.

Most animal proteins now represent *left-spin* energy in the form of concentrated metabolic and environmental wastes. Sick animals concentrate negative energy. Animals suffering from environmental stresses and excesses (bad food, air, water, and habitat) become sickly just like humans.

Food energy derived from sick animals brings on dis-ease in man a thousand times faster than does food energy from sick fruits or vegetables.

Animal proteins can be an excellent source of *energy and nutrients.* At the same time they are a two-edged sword and must be used sparingly and wisely. The problem has to do with *quantity* of meat eaten (includes fish and fowl), how *often* it is eaten, the *level* of metabolites and poisons in the animal's tissues, the ability of the liver, skin, lungs, and kidneys to process the wastes, and lastly, transit time from the mouth to the toilet. (We will develop these points as the book unfolds.)

In his wonderful book, *Fatu Hiva,* Thor Heyerdahl tells how he and his wife, in 1937, lived with the last surviving cannibal of the Marquesas, an island chain twelve-hundred miles northwest of Tahiti. The cannibal told them that human flesh is different than other animal flesh. It is "sweet." and I would add, so is the flesh from a toxic cow that was in a *catabolic* state and sick when it was slaughtered. Toxic meat and fish have more flavor. Toxins are more concentrated in the animal's fats than in the lean tissues for reasons we will discuss in great detail later.

The Food Chain

Here is an example of what is meant by the statement, "animals are at the top of the food chain."

A rabbit eats food that is contaminated with pesticides. The poisonous residues are stored and concentrated in its flesh and fatty tissues. One day the farmer decides the rabbits are out of control and uses a toxic chemical to poison them. Next, an eagle comes along and eats from the carcass of the dead rabbit. Thus the poisons in the rabbit are now in the eagle's body—hence the poisons moved UP the food chain.

When we eat sick meat, fish, and fowl, we become the eagle and the poisons and metabolites concentrate in us. If you are going to eat animal proteins, eat them from healthy animals and in limited amounts.

Negative energy food from any source—animal or plant—is sick food. Sick food must be dismantled and *neutralized* by the body. Left-spin food causes the body to squander vital energy that is needed to keep us healthy and young. When we eat sick food, we lose more than we gain!

Animal Proteins & The Bowel

Animal proteins MUST be eliminated from the intestines within twenty-four hours. If they remain in the gut longer than this, they putrefy and release extremely toxic, organic poisons. Substances like indoles, skatoles, and phenols. These set the stage for dis-ease, premature aging, and cancer.

Indoles, skatoles, and phenols are WHOLE molecules that are absorbed directly through the intestinal wall. Most molecules are broken down into pieces before they are absorbed, thus offering us some protection. Not so with hundreds and toxic organic compounds—be they natural or synthetic.

Potatoes absorb toxic compounds from raw, non composted manure. These toxic molecules pass **directly** into the potatoes tissues—**whole and intact.** When the potatoes are boiled, a sharp nose can identify the kind of manure that was used to grow them—pig, cow, or chicken.

Toxic molecules that are absorbed in this fashion

bypass our safety net and are a threat to our health. Toxic wastes—in the gut of a constipated person—provide the perfect environment for degenerative conditions like cancer, arthritis, diabetes, and cardiovascular to develop and progress.

Mastication

This is why chewing our food (mastication) to the point of creating liquid food from solid food is so very important—especially, if you are going to eat meat, fish, fowl, or cheese.

Eating more than one or two ounces of animal protein a day will cause you to become OLD. Limit your intake of animal protein. Eat plenty of fresh fruit and vegetables. These good habits will help you to become *Young Again!*

PREVIEW: *Our next chapter deals with digestion, junk food, and WHY it causes us to become old.*

Collard Greens

Collard greens are easy to grow and thrive anywhere in the USA. You can grow them in pots, in a flower bed, or in the garden. They are a "non" hybrid.

Eaten raw in a salad or served in plain leaf fashion, they are sweet and crunchy. They promote a healthy colon, and will stretch your food budget.

Collards winter over if planted in the summer and mulched with straw during the winter. In the spring, they come to life and produce fresh salad greens long before other vegetables can even be planted.

Insects don't attack collards. Pick the lower leaves and plants will keep producing for you. Enjoy!

Comfrey Greens

Comfrey greens are heavenly! Comfrey roots produce copious amounts of leaves that make fantastic spinach when lightly steamed or stir fried and drenched with olive oil and apple cider vinegar.

Each March, comfrey grows freely. It is rich in nutrients. The pulverized roots heal ulcers. The FDA does not like comfrey, but people—and animals—do!

Chickens and milk goats relish comfrey. Comfrey is good for the colon. Everyone should grow comfrey. Plant comfrey once, and you'll have comfrey forever!

Water! The *Essence* Of Life!

Water has memory! It "absorbs" the *frequencies* of the contaminants it carries and it **continues** to *vibrate* at those frequencies until contaminants are removed and their memory erased.

Contaminants are *energy* fields that leave their *footprint* on water by causing the molecules to *vibrate* at frequencies that are *unfriendly* to the body.

Conventional approaches to water purification are *incomplete*. Methods like distillation, reverse osmosis, carbon block, ceramic cartridges work at the mechanical level only. They are good as far as they go, they just don't go far enough.

The BEV process, on the other hand, is a Fourth Dimension approach that delivers water that tastes good and *feels different* in the body. People like it because it *awakens* natural harmonic frequencies *at* the cellular level and below.

BEV water *reprograms* the electrical *rhythm* of the body. It causes body cells to *dance*. Its energy *frequency* is body friendly. Its electromagnetic *signature* is complete. **BEV water is *music!***

The BEV process "voids" waste energy fields in water and alters hydrogen and molecular bond angles so molecules can "**dance**" and become *liquid music* and *electronic food* to the body.

BEV theory and application *transcends* traditional water testing and comparison techniques. It defies Newtonian physics. BEV water must be experienced to appreciate its profound significance to human health and longevity. **BEV has captured the *essence* of life on planet Earth in liquid form.**

The BEV process is a "proprietary" process. A full discussion of the theory and application of BEV, its relationship to aging and dis-ease is available in manuscript form.

BEV water is made in the home using BEV processing equipment. The process we call BEV focuses on biologically *friendly* DRINKING water. Next to the air we breathe, we consume more water than any other commodity. *Make sure the water you put into your body is spelled BEV!*

"Water Is MORE Than Wet.
Water Is FOOD!"

Are You Feeling Overwhelmed?

Making the transition from the "normal" good old' American diet to a healthy one can be challenging.

New ways to healthfully prepare food as well as learn about new and strange food types represent a challenge for conventional cooks. The person eating "strange" new food doesn't appreciate tampering. Unless the cook has the full cooperation and support of the participants, it is best to go slow.

Mix brown rice with white rice. Use liquid ionic sea minerals, powdered kelp, and other healthy substitutes in place of table salt. If meat comprises a big part of your diet, cook less of it and make it less often.

Invest in a good vegetarian cook book! There are several good ones available. Lindsay Wagner's *High Road To Health* is good. *Foods That Heal* is superb! (see Source Index).

Visit a health food store or food co-op and buy a supply of basic staples like brewers yeast, lentils, wheat germ, wheat bran, flax seeds, whole wheat flour, sesame seed, and Bragg Liquid Aminos. Ask for help.

Experiment with a few basic dishes. Mix them among your other dishes on the dinner table. Home made bread is a good addition to the diet and most families will appreciate it.

Make home made waffles, pancakes, and bran muffins. Use real maple syrup mixed with barley malt syrup to cut costs, yet retain a nice flavor.

Fresh garden vegetables and casserole dishes go together well. Home grown food will convert anyone.

Definitely AVOID soy oil, canola oil, and Tofu. Avoid all prepared foods. They are a guaranteed ticket to the grave. Convert your family one step at a time!

Popcorn • Oil • Salt • Brewers Yeast

Popcorn is a good food—as long as it isn't cooked in soy or canola oil and covered with salt. And for a real treat, try some brewers yeast sprinkled on your popcorn. It adds zest, and you won't need any salt. You'll love it!

"If we eat wrongly, no doctor can cure us. If we eat rightly, no doctor is needed."

Victor Rocine

8

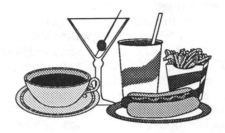

Junk Diets & Stress

"There is no such thing as 'junk food', only 'junk diets'!"
Dr. Helen A. Guthrie

All food contains energy. It is the nature of that energy its electrical *footprint* that determines what effect—good or bad—it will have on the *bio-electric* body. To understand the aging process, we must concern ourselves with the "spin" of food energy. The direction of spin as well as the intensity of the spin determines foods ability to satisfy hunger, build, and maintain healthy tissues and bones.

Nutritive tables measure nutrients. It is assumed that if we eat food is listed on a nutrient table that we will be nourished. It is also assumed that ALL nutritive food energy produces positive results in the body. These assumptions are INCORRECT.

We hear a lot about junk food because we are inundated with it. People identify junk food with quick snacks and fast food. Their association is correct. But instead of calling it junk food, let's call it bio-junk (food) because it better describes it.

Bio-junk food is composed of left-spin energy, and it greatly accelerates the aging process. If the body cannot break down or eliminate bio-junk energy from the body, it isolates it from the rest of the system. The body does this by entombing the toxic energy in body FAT that it makes specifically for this purpose. (We will develop this point in the obesity chapter.)

Dead Is Not Dead

Bio-junk food alters biochemical reactions because it has a energy **signature** of its own. In the process, it damages critical body pathways and cripples cellular activity. Bio-junk food has the ability to multiply its original sphere of influence by transferring its vibratory *footprint* to the body. It does this at the subtle energy level of our existence. Bio-junk food is the equivalent of "poison. It contains *radiomimetic* qualities that mimic the effect of nuclear *radiation* on the tissues. People who eat eventually see the effects in the mirror.

Bio-junk food has the ability to CHANGE its *footprint* after it enters the body. Its presence in the GI tract triggers *bastard* reactions that form **free radicals** in the system. Free radicals do damage to the vital organs, and especially to the liver and kidneys. The energy *footprint* of these substances is so volatile that they react with the body's energy fields the moment of contact. They continue to interfere with normal metabolism UNTIL their presence is eliminated. In other words, they have a life of their own while in the system. It is impossible to keep toxic substances from entering the system because they are ubiquitous. We can, however, neutralize their effects with enhanced PAC's and remove them with Yucca extract.

A "bio-junk food diet insures the accumulation of toxic energy fields in the tissues, lymph, and blood.

The Kidneys

The kidneys are crucial to good health, and it behooves us to pay attention to anything that negatively affects them. Bio-junk food causes tremendous long-term damage to the kidney's nephrons (blood filters). The kidneys are second only to the liver in their ability to rid the body of waste, and a decline in function is a prerequisite for the establishment of cancer or the manifestation of other degenerative dis-ease.

Taoist tradition teaches that the urinary system (kidneys and bladder)is related to the Water Element. They believed that *Jing*—the very **essence** of life—is contained within water. They believed that careful management of the Water Element was the key to youthfulness.

BEV water helps keep the kidneys young and speeds the disposal of metabolic wastes. A weak liver will shift the load onto the kidneys. However, the kidneys were NEVER meant to do the liver's job!

Digestion & Liquids

If Pavlov's dog is any indication, digestion is initiated through visual and mental stimulation BEFORE food enters our mouth. In other words, the flow of digestive juices in the mouth, stomach, and intestine are linked to vision and thought.

Digestion begins in the mouth when we chew and mix food with saliva. The flow of saliva and digestive juices are dependent on fluid hydration levels in the body. When we drink our share of water, we secrete enough saliva to begin the breakdown process we call *digestion*. Saliva also lubricates food so it can be comfortably swallowed.

It is important to TRAIN ourselves to drink a glass of water every hour or our awake day. This habit maintains perfect fluid volume levels and moves waste out of the system. It is also the key to *avoiding* the need to drink liquids with meals. **Drink plenty of water throughout the day so you can avoid liquids 1/2 hour before and one hour after meals.**

If we fail to drink enough water throughout the day, a shortfall of digestive juices is experienced, limiting digestion. Drinking water or other liquids with meals does NOT help digestion or make up for low body hydration levels. We do NOT want liquids in the stomach at mealtime. What we DO need is **undiluted** digestive juices full of enzymes and acids.

Cold liquids are hard on the body in general, and the stomach and digestive organs in particular. When cold fluids are taken with a meal, they retard and even STOP digestion. Correct temperature is one of the necessary prerequisites for chemical reactions—like those in the stomach—to occur. Low digestive temperatures create a perfect environment for the development of degenerative conditions like colitis, diverticulitis, constipation, irritable bowel syndrome, and appendicitis.

Digestive juices are MORE than water. They are powerful "right-spin" energy fields. Liquid foods taken with meals dilute them and stress the system. When correct hydration levels are maintained throughout the **entire** awake day, meal time stress on the digestive organs and glands is greatly reduced. High body fluid levels speed the flow of digestive juices from the stomach and intestinal walls, liver, and pancreas. The liver and pancreas secrete their juices through ducts directly into the intestinal duodenum that drains the stomach. Secretory cells line the stomach and intestine and depend on sufficient body fluid levels to do their job.

Dr. Franz Morell, of Germany, spoke of the primary purpose of saliva in digestion. *"[saliva's] purpose is to coat and protect food enzymes so they will neither be damaged by nor do damage to the stomach and GI tract. Exposure to digestive juices at the wrong time during digestion derails biochemical catalysts. Nature designed things such that it takes 5-10 minutes to eat an apple, but only 5 seconds to drink the juice."*

Hormones & Hydration

The ability of the **"ductless"** glands to secrete hormones, and the blood to transport them is dependent upon proper hydration. These glands secrete their products directly into the blood. They have NO ducts.

The *ductless* glands—and their hormones—control aging and vitality. As we age, we experience a SLOW-DOWN in hormonal activity. In Time, these glands go into **shut-down**. When this occurs, the doctor provides a diagnosis.

At the heart of the *slow-down, shut-down* scenario is the buildup of metabolic waste in the tissues and fluids, which is linked to water intake. Waste slows vital organ function and leads to an early grave. **SIGNS of aging seen on the outside of the bio-electric body indicate trouble on the *inside*.**

DHEA Hormone Cream

To *solution* to loss of vital organ function involves accelerating the *outflow* of waste from the soft tissues, blood, and lymph, and *feeding* the bio-electric body powerful *right-spin* food hormone precursors. (A *precursor* is something that precedes something else.)

For example, we eat carrots to obtain *beta carotene* which is a natural plant food precursor to vitamin A. Dioscoria Macho Stachya is also a plant hormone precursor. The body converts it into DHEA *(dehydroepiandrosterone)* which is the body's Mother or "master" hormone.

The problem, however, is to get Dioscoria through the GI tract and into the blood. It is the **delivery system** that is responsible for getting the active ingredients absorbed. Once absorbed, the body converts them into DHEA and eventually into estrogen, progesterone, insulin, testosterone, and thyroxine just to name a few.

Dioscoria—also known as the Mexican wild yam— has NO side effects. People who are lucky enough to obtain the "good stuff" will testify to its effectiveness in regulating hormonal swings. It also acts as a natural mood elevator. Response time is FAST—hours to days!

Hormone *precursor* creme is used topically (skin) to supplement progesterone production and moderate estrogen dominance which is behind women's hormonal swings from PMS to menopause. The creme is also very effective as a wrinkle cream (for men or women) because it has the ability to stimulate and rebuild the elastic, reticular, and collagenous fibers deep in the skin. It works particularly well when used with glycolic acid skin cream and racemic clay creme.

Hormone *precursor* cream is absorbed through surface fat, and helps anyone who suffers with PMS or menopausal problems. There are several brands of **natural** precursor tablets and creams on the market. Many are loaded with *fillers* and of *low potency*, and a waste of money. The precursor I use incorporates an ancient Chinese herb called *N. Peiwuweitzu* to protect the liver from waste that comes into circulation as hormones are balanced and metabolic rate increases (see Source Index).

Eating Habits • Pavlov's Dog

Poor eating habits include eating in high stress or unpleasant circumstances. Sitting down to a *quiet* meal and allowing enough time for casual, pleasant conversation is *vital* to good health. Unfortunately, few people eat this way anymore. Fast track meals are now the rule and mealtime circumstances rarely resemble the ideal. People eat too fast, barely chewing, and guzzle something **cold** in situations of noise, stress, and confusion. Dietary planning should include *environment* as well *what* is going to be eaten.

The effects of "hit & run eating" on health are DEADLY even if you eat the very best food.

Pavlov did his experiments on dogs. Dogs are known for their ability to *gobble* their food. People, however, are not dogs. We do not have the powerful digestive enzymes and short digestive tract of a carnivore. Please understand, digestion is stressful to the body even if the food is good. So when the dinner bell rings, prepare yourself so your body will do more than just salivate. A meal should be a *celebration* of physical, mental, and spiritual forces.

Digestion requires the body to expend energy before it can get more energy in return. Bio-junk food has nothing to offer and produces an energy deficit and undigested food.

Undigested food *converts* to left-spin energy. In a constipated, anaerobic dominant gut and colon, undigested food converts into **gas** and **deadly** toxic by-products that give rise to degenerative dis-ease. **Bad habits create cumulative effects and a lifestyle that is difficult to change.**

Gas

Gas—particularly *foul* gas—is a GOOD indicator of an

out of balance condition in the vital organs and digestive tract. The fouler the gas, the more we should be concerned that things are NOT right. Foul or excessive gas is a sign of systemic (whole body) overload and should be considered ABNORMAL!

Spoiled animal flesh (carrion) is *necrotic* flesh. Meat is dead flesh, but it is not necrotic. In a constipated, airless environment, meat, fish, fowl, and cheese become the equivalent of carrion and produce highly toxic by-products and foul gas. High stress mealtime environments encourage **anaerobic** conditions and accentuates the production of foul *intestinal gas*. An anaerobic environment is a cancer environment! **The evening breeze between your knees should NOT smell like cheese!**

Otto Warburg, twice Nobel Laureate, was awarded the Nobel Prize in 1931—over sixty years ago— for discovering the *cause* of cancer. He said,

"Cancer has one prime cause...and that is the replacement of oxygen [aerobic] respiration of body cells by anaerobic cell respiration."

Dr. Max Gerson, who we mentioned earlier, went on to determine the role of sodium (main ingredient of table salt) in cancer. Both Warburg and Gerson agreed that the growth of cancer cells is initiated in a "low oxygen," high free radical environment. **Cancer does not exist in an oxygen-rich environment!** Aerobic activity follow by self-massage of the lymphatic system caters to healthy cellular respiration.

Table Salt

It is *impossible* to avoid sodium because it is ubiquitous. It is in almost all prepared foods, and it is certainly in municipal water supplies. If you crave salt, you suffer from "salt syndrome." This condition is remedied with ionic sea minerals and BEV water. A body that craves salt is a body that is deficient in minerals and toxic. The answer to carvings is a complete detoxification program which includes flushing the stones from your liver.

Table salt must NOT be used to meet salt cravings. It must be avoided because it is **deadly** to the body's cells and to the bacteria (mitochondria) that produce our energy. Thirst after meals indicates the body is *under* hydrated and/or the food was *over* salted. Table salt is a very powerful negative energy field that should be avoided.

The Water Molecule

The primary function of water is to act as a solvent and

a source of hydrogen and oxygen molecules.

Water carries *energy* INTO our tissues and cells. It **should** carry toxic *end products* of metabolism OUT of the body. When we drink water that is dead and biologically unfriendly to the body—distilled water, for example—we DENY the body the ability to move waste out of the system which leads to conditions of **excess** and the so called "deficiency" conditions that result from excesses. **Water is "THE" primary ingredient in body fluids.**

In order for water to effectively work as a solvent in the body, the H_2O molecule must possess an energy *signature* that will allow it to bond to waste energy fields and remove them.

Resonant frequency of biologically healthy water is 7.8 hertz, or Mother Earth frequency. To achieve that frequency, water must be extremely PURE and have a energy *footprint* related to restructuring of both the hydrogen and molecular bond angles within the water molecule itself.

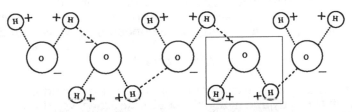

Look at shape of these "bent" or "polar" water molecules. Notice the two hydrogen atoms on each molecule are off to one side giving each molecule a lopsided appearance. Note the way the molecules bond with each other and the location of the (+) (-) charges. The square box contains one water molecule. The oxygen atom has a (–) charge, the two hydrogens a (+) charge. The heavy dotted line in the lower right corner of the box going from the hydrogen in the box to the oxygen to the right of the box is a **hydrogen** bond that connects one molecule to the other. The lines inside the box going from the hydrogens to the oxygen are **molecular** bonds within the water molecule itself.

Water stores it's energy in its bonds in direct relationship to the resonant frequency of the molecule(s). The purer the water, the stronger the bonds. It is the bonding angles and hertz rate that separates BEV water from other processed waters. Purity alone is NOT enough where it's at. There is yet another factor that has to do with electron saturation and pH. We will develop those important points in future chapters.

Why BEV Water

BEV water is the most biologically friendly water in the world . It's made in your own home with common tap water. Most water processing units on the market are concerned with removal of 90% of toxic wastes. BEV water approaches 99.5% removal. It is it energy *footprint* and *signature* that makes it so biologically active and makes it unique in the world of water.

BEV water molecules are highly charged and structured for living systems. BEV water is **different** than common distilled or filtered waters. BEV water is extremely reactive. By "reactive" we mean it acts like a *magnet* due its strong *right-spin* electrical charge and resonant frequency. A vibration chain or pendulum can be used to confirm BEV water's spin and charge intensity. The best test, of course, is to feel it in your body.

Other waters—like tap, reverse osmosis, deionized, and distilled—do not possess the characteristics of BEV water. BEV water is the best water for hydrating the tissues and energizing the cells and removing wastes from the body. Many wonderful things happen to people who drink this strange and wonderful water. BEV water is both a 3rd and 4th dimension energy substance. (We will develop these concepts as we go along.)

Live Food

Biologically friendly food also has a tremendous influence on the body and aging. Fresh, home grown vegetables and fruits is the best and least expensive choice.

If you do not have a yard, or space is limited, grow vegetables in pots, plastic buckets and so on. It is amazing how much fresh food can be grown this way. Even more amazing is how good it tastes and its effects on the bio-electric body!

Consider joining an organic gardening club. Many of them offer garden space for rent where the soil is rich and mellow from gardens before you. Or, hire someone to grow food for you and your family. Many older people have the time and would love to grow food for hire. These people are usually gardening pros and love to help others. Pay them well, gardening is hard work. They need the money and you need the food.

Gardening involves hard *load-bearing* work and is a good way to keep fit. Hard work is good for the body. I suggest a long handled spading fork instead of a tiller. Hand tools are inexpensive, they always start, and they don't burn gas.

For people who cannot garden, fresh live food can be purchased at health food stores and co-ops. Local organic or biodynamic farmers are an excellent choice and some even deliver or have drop points in cities. There are other alternatives for staples. Organic grains, beans, and flours can be found in stores, coops, or ordered in bulk from sources like G.G. Grains. [Call Kent Margeson @ 1-800-747-2467 or (719) 633-3793.]

Composting • Gardening

If you are going to get into gardening, you will want to learn how to compost organic matter. Proper composting technique *controls* the break-down process so you end up with a high energy product. Aerobic conditions create *right-spin* energy compost.

Aerobic compost catalyses healthy energy reactions in garden soil. Controlled breakdown of grass clippings, weeds, leaves, manure, and the like will not generate foul odors **unless** the pile becomes *anaerobic*. An anaerobic condition is what produces foul gas in the compost pile and the human gut!

Always use a good bacteria starter to get the pile going. Compost is MORE than old dead things that have turned brown. It is the living waste of friendly organisms and a real miracle. Several wonderful books on biodynamic composting are available (see Source Index).

Besides the food, gardening is superb therapy for the body and mind. It will simplify your life and focus your energies on healthful living habits. Once you become hooked on gardening, you will be a gardener forever! **Biologically friendly food—and water—is your *passport* to agelessness!**

Devitalized food is so common in most people's diet that some form of supplementation is needed. *Juice capsules* and *tablets* are an excellent source of organic fruit and vegetable energy. They have a high energy *footprint* and are second only to fresh or home grown organic produce. There is NO question that they are superior to the poisoned, left-spin fruits and vegetables found in super markets (see Source Index).

To become *Young Again!*

- Eat organic food
- Use juice tabs & capsules
- Avoid sodium
- Use ionic sea minerals
- Do aerobic exercising
- Avoid liquids with meals
- Eat some RAW vegetables
- Avoid all bio-junk food
- Drink plenty of BEV water
- Get plenty of sleep
- Avoid cold drinks with food
- Eat real food
- *"Chew your liquids and chew your solids until they are liquid!"*

It's what you do 90% of the time that counts. Aging reversal requires focus and commitment because the body is

OLD and *SLOW* and you are not young—YET! Follow the points we have outlined so far and absorb and apply the information in the balance of this book, and you will become *Young Again!*

PREVIEW: *Our next chapter explains WHY people snack and WHY they become fat, and WHAT happens to your body when you eat too much or too often!*

Harmonic Silver Water

Few injuries equal the trauma and pain burn patients suffer—both from the actual burns, and from the treatment and practices of allopathic medicine.

From a medical angle, the issue is infection. From a social angle, the issue is scar tissue formation. Infection and scars are energy issues that are fought and decided on a playing field of pure, Fourth Dimension energy.

To relieve pain and avoid scar formation—even in the case of 3rd degree burns—every household should have *harmonic silver water* on hand for unexpected emergencies.

Harmonixed silver water has a signature & energy footprint that is body friendly. When misted onto burned tissue or taken orally, the *energy* signature of the solution is **transferred** to the body. Healing progresses without incidence of scar formation and pain is muted. True healing is the product of energy **resonance** and **transference.** (BEV water promotes healing on the same principles.)

Refer to the pictures of Glen Roundtree on page 276. Glen is living *proof* that *harmonized* silver water works! He emerged from the trauma of third degree facial burns without scars. However, his arms and hands scarred where allopathic doctors treated him "their" way. Glen is a walking miracle! To quote his mother (in the aftermath of the accident), *"It was painful for me to look upon him!"*

Harmonic silver water has hundreds of health applications. Its monatomic structure is to colloidal silver, what sand is to boulders. Its size allows it to enter and exit the cells and promote healing without fear of heavy metal buildup. It is a one of a kind product (see Source Index).

The 90/10 Rule Of Life

Live your life so that you do things 90% correct and enjoy the other 10% to the fullest—and without guilt.

9

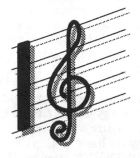

Satiety Blues

"Everything in Moderation."
Diane DeFelice

Fullness beyond desire! A primal drive fulfilled! Who can conjure a better feeling than a full stomach after a superb meal? Surely, food is one of the true pleasures of life. Aroma! Appearance! Taste! These are the things for which we live! Yet, in our drive to fulfill a basic physiologic need, we sow the seeds of old age and death.

Food requires a certain amount of time for complete digestion. When we eat too much food or too soon after a previous meal, the body suffers *overload* shock. Shock of any type puts stress on the vital organs (liver, thyroid, adrenals, kidneys, parathyroid, pancreas, pituitary, and testes). Dietary shock deserves our attention because it accelerates aging.

Snacks & Food Related Stress

People love to snack. They snack because they are hungry or because it is the thing to do—part habit, part social custom. The *experts* tell us it is good to eat every few hours. They tell us small meals taken more often are less stressful to the system and better for our health. They tell us small meals taken often maintain blood sugar levels and keep us on an even keel. They even tell us that multiple small meals increase productivity.

Unfortunately, the experts are WRONG! These things are NOT true. They NEVER were true. Let's stop and analyze what happens to the body when we eat too much or too often, which includes snacking. Snacks are simply small meals!

Food creates stress because it involves digestion. Digestion creates stress by drawing on the body's energy reserves. Food energy molecules must be broken down, transported, and reassembled into usable energy forms. Substances that do not promote health must be dumped or stored.

When we eat, we must borrow from our energy reserve account. It takes energy to get the process going, and if the energy generated from food does not repay the loan, we suffer an energy deficit that is reflected in loss of health and vitality in the vital organs.

The vital organs have *limited* capacity and resilience. They require rest BETWEEN meals. When they are denied adequate and regular rest, they come under severe stress. Eating between meals and eating more often than every four hours causes the organs and glands to LOSE their resiliency.

Food related stress results in organ *burn-out.* Burn-out means LOSS of unction. The organs age together. Initially, however, one succumbs, then others follow suit. The effect compounds itself in chain reaction style. This scenario can occur even if the food is positive energy and nutritious. *Quality, quantity,* and *frequency* are the controlling factors.

If snacks and meals are composed of *left-spin* substances, organ stress is greatly increased. When combined with meals that are spaced too close together, the body is left with NO alternative but to shift into OVERDRIVE in an attempt to use, neutralize, dump, or store food energy fields.

Food imposed stress creates an "involuntary" series of reactions in the body because the body has NO choice but to process what it has been given—even to its own detriment. The body acts as much out of duty as need when it is fed too much, too often, or when it is forced to process bio-junk food.

Snacking and bio-junk food create a vicious cycle that denies the vital organs needed rest and become stressed. As waste builds up, the hormones get out of sync. Enzymes become fewer and weaker, toxicity increases, and the organs atrophy. **Stress is energy seeking an outlet. Energy is never lost, it merely changes form.**

Trophy & Diabetes

Food related stress brings about *trophy* in the vital organs. *Trophy* means change related to nutrition. If we apply the prefix *hyper* or *hypo,* we are referring to a change in physiologic activity that is above or below the norm. Both hyper and hypo conditions lead to organ burn out or dysfunction.

For instance, *hypoglycemia* refers to a condition commonly known as *low blood sugar*. Dissected, the word means *hypo*-a low activity condition. *glyc*-sweet. *emia*-pertaining to the blood.

The body's organ system is *interdependent*, and whatever affects one gland affects all of them. Health conditions are **always** multiple in nature. Dis-ease is NEVER singular.

Dis-eases are SECONDARY conditions, and this includes degenerative dis-eases. Secondary conditions reflect an energy imbalance and presence of **excesses** in the system.

Deficiency Dis-eases & Conditions

We hear a lot about deficiency dis-eases and deficiency conditions, but there is NO such thing. The entire concept is but a carry over from the early days of allopathic medicine and the influence of Justus von Liebig's infamous agricultural theory called the *"Law of the minimum."*

Justus von Liebig developed his theory around 1830. He is regarded as the father of the synthetic fertilizer industry, and the destructive practices of present day agriculture. His law says, "the nutrient that is in the **minimum** controls." To him, soil was nothing but dirt. He believed that there are only three *essential* nutrients salts needed by plants—nitrogen, phosphorous, and potassium commonly referred to as NPK.

Pasteur and von Liebig were contemporaries, and like Pasteur's infamous Germ Theory of Disease, medical science adopted von Liebig's erroneous theory on nutrition. Schools of nutrition continue to perpetuate von Liebig's "law of the minimum" when they promote the idea that deficiencies are the cause of dis-eases and ill sub-clinical illness.

Science and nutritionists are wrong in this regard. Disease is exactly the *opposite* of what is popularly believed and taught. Dis-ease is nothing but the manifestation of conditions of **EXCESS** within the system. Excesses always manifest themselves as deficiencies. Excesses are energy field imbalances that *alter* health at the subtle energy level.

"Deficiency" conditions appear when excesses of toxic energy EXCEED the body's ability to deal with them.

For example, medical science teaches that the diabetic suffers from a shortage of the hormone *insulin*. They go on to further classify the diabetic as either glucose intolerance or insulin resistant. In actuality, the diabetic suffers from **excess** toxic waste energy fields in the tissues and fluids. The diabetic's body, however, "keeps" sugars circulating in the blood to BUFFER excess toxicity in the system. In other words, we have an energy problem related to OTHER **excesses** in the system. **The diabetic can be returned to normal without insulin.**

Sugar is a carbon based molecule. Without carbon, you cannot have the basic sugar molecule $C_6H_{12}O_6$. Carbon is a BUFFER and moderates all life on planet Earth. To understand more about carbon's role, I highly recommend Leonard Ridzon's fascinating books, The Carbon Connection and The Carbon Cycle. (See Source Index).

Diabetes in children has little relationship to adult diabetes except in name only. We now KNOW that Type I diabetes is **directly** related to DPT and polio vaccines where the "live" or "attenuated" viruses **mutate** and cause the child's immune system to attack itself (more later).

Fifty million people suffer with diabetes. Science's failure to understand diabetes at the subtle energy level will continue the suffering. Independent action, without the blessings of higher approved authority, is a prerequisite for anyone wishing to rid themselves of this curse.

Let's review. There is no such thing as a deficiency dis-ease, but there is such a thing as the accumulation of EXCESS toxic energy. Moreover, we do not grow old and die from degenerative dis-ease. Rather, aging is a cumulative *condition* and death the confirmation of **"excesses beyond control."** We die when EXCESS negative energies neutralize positive energies resulting in energy synchronization.

Glands & Gyroscopes

The vital organs (glands) function like gyroscopes on a ship. They keep us *even-keeled* by overcoming shifts in the bio-electric body's energy balance. They keep us in optimum health if we do not "sabotage" them with incessant snacking, bio-junk food, unfriendly water, and the presence of EXCESS waste.

We should NOT allow how we *feel* to determine our decisions on health. Remember, long before the SIGNS of dis-ease become visible, negative energy forces are hard at work in the subtle energy level. The proof is all the sick and dying people, who "felt" just fine—*yesterday!*

The "lag" between onset of dis-ease, manifestation of SIGNS, and diagnosis by the doctor is about 20 years!

Mental Hype • Body Abuse

Hype is taking its toll the world over. People have become skilled in the awesome power of mind over body and drug over mind. They use both to **drive** and **whip** the bio-electric body. And when asked how they feel, people usually respond "great!" At the same time, over 80% of the US population suffers from sub-clinical illness.

Hype is the waste product of an unbalanced person. It goes with unrealistic mental euphoria. Hype can be used to drive the body *beyond* its ability to physically respond. Snacks, bio-junk food, and food supplements are also forms of hype.

If we use hype to WHIP and DRIVE the bio-electric body, we enter the "twilight zone" of Time—a Time warp—where aging occurs and the passing of Time accelerates.

Symptoms of hype-driven dis-ease are not so plainly visible, but the SIGNS are easy to see. They have their origin in the 4th Dimension world of ENERGY!

Eventually, dis-ease shatters *hype's* hold on us! But until that time comes, we live out of our energy reserves.

Dis-ease is the *manifestation* of stress. Dis-ease is a confirmation of aging. Dis-ease is the *manifestation* of Fourth Dimension Time in man's Third Dimension world. Aging and dis-ease are the result of our failure to square our energy account. Death is energy bankruptcy! *Hype* is modern man's Achilles' Heel because it involves unrealistic positive thinking and an unbalanced lifestyle. **When we avoid hype and live the simple life, aging and the passing of Time comes to a halt.**

Food Digestion Tables

The following tables indicate the amount of time required for different foods to **leave** the stomach. Only *basic* foods are listed. A couple of common bio-junk foods are listed because these substances are prevalent in our society—coffee and white bread, for instance.

Please keep in mind that this information applies to the *normal, healthy* stomach without stress or known problems like enzyme and HCL (hydrochloric acid) shortfalls, ulcers, etc. Also note the very small amounts of food used in these examples (1/2 ounce). Large amounts of food take longer to digest. If more food is eaten too soon, undigested food is *forced* into the small intestine and colon where toxic, anaerobic conditions control the aging process and the passing of biologic Time accelerates.

One-half to Two Hours

Pure Water	Light Wine
Tea	Milk
Coffee	Bouillon
Beer	Soft eggs

Two to Three Hours

Coffee w/cream	Cocoa w/milk
Asparagus (steamed)	Potatoes (mashed)
Fish (broiled)	White bread
Oysters (broiled)	Butter
Eggs (scrambled, fried, hard boiled)	

Three to Four Hours

Chicken (broiled)	Bread (whole grain)
Carrots (steamed)	Spinach (boiled)
Cucumber (raw)	Apple (raw)
Beef (roasted)	Salmon (broiled)
Tuna	Ham
Lentils (boiled)	Beans (boiled)
Green beans (steamed)	Lettuce (raw)

Dietary habits chronicle aging!

A Story About Satiety

Dr. Carey Reams told a story that took place during the years he and his wife were raising their large family. As the story goes, the neighbors and their children were over for dinner . When the food bowls were placed on the table, the neighbors made an effort to hide their surprise as their eyes were drawn to the modest size of the various bowls of corn, peas, mashed potatoes, gravy, meat and desserts.

Expecting just such a response, Reams—in his characteristic style—laughed and predicted that there would be food left over. As you might guess, this is exactly what happened. Everyone had a wonderful meal, a great time, and departed with their gut plum-full!

I tell this story to draw your attention to the *satiety* enjoyed by all with a limited amount of food. What happened at the Reams' home is exactly the OPPOSITE of what occurs at tables today when we stuff ourselves.

Reams' food was alive—chuck-full of enzymes and loaded with bio-active minerals and vitamins. Today's food is DEAD and EMPTY. It provides minimal *energy* for the body and requires people to stuff themselves in order to *feel* full because positive energy forces are absent. Most commercially produced foods are *left-spin* energy substances. The body cannot use negative energy and must neutralize it or store it as FAT!

Did you catch those last four words—stores it as FAT? I hope so, because what we are discussing and piecing together, line by line, chapter by chapter, is going to shed light on the obesity problems that are plaguing 75% of Americans.

We could surmise that what really took place at the

Reams' dinner table was that everyone was courteous and took only small portions of food and all left the table hungry—faking it all the way. But Reams was not a liar. He told the story to make the point that good food, bio-active food, food with a right-spin energy *footprint* is very nourishing! You can believe that everyone at that table left *full and gratified BEYOND desire* which is the correct definition of the word *satiety.*

Few people experience real satiety these days. Instead, they know only the pseudo version. *Pseudo* satiety is experienced when the stomach is full, but the body is not nourished. In other words, we quit eating because we run out of space—NOT because we are nutritionally satisfied. **America is a nation of overweight people whose nutritional needs go unfulfilled.**

People leave the table hungry, yet too full to eat more! It is impossible to satisfy the body's energy needs with empty, left-spin energy foods that are devoid of life giving nutrients!

It is very important that everyone learn to use a pendulum and vibration chain so they can measure food energy fields and lots of other things, too (see Source Index).

The Appetite

Appetite is a combination of *physical need* and *mental desire.* It is controlled by the satiety and hunger centers in the hypothalamus of the brain. It has long been established that the hunger center is ALWAYS active unless it is *inhibited.* The body uses two inhibitory mechanisms to regulate hunger: a **physically** full stomach, and a **nutritionally** satisfied body.

The hunger center is a cluster of nerve cells. It generates sensations that are a combination of physical need and mental desire. Snacking is a combination of BOTH. Most people meet their body's call for nutritional *energy* (true hunger) with EMPTY calories (physical hype) and cognitive satisfaction (mental hype). These are a deadly combination!

When we are **nourished,** the "I'm hungry" *satiety* center sends a message to the *hunger* center that its needs have been met. This causes the system to shut down and we lose our desire to eat. Real satiety is **nourishment** beyond desire!

False satiety is different, but the mechanics are similar. It is based on a FULL stomach. It is "bogus satiety!" When the stomach is full OR when our nutrient energy needs have been met, the satiety center sends a message to the hunger center and we lose our desire for more food. This is a *negative inhibition system* because one system controls the other. A negative inhibition system works flawlessly UNLESS we *sabotage* it with snacking and bio-junk food!

I'm Hungry Again

Later—after the stomach partially empties—the hungry person's body DEMANDS more nourishment, the appetite returns with a vengeance, and the cycle begins over again.

Hungry people in a bio-junk food society gain weight when they fail to meet their body's energy needs. Real hunger is one reason *why* people gain weight. The presence of *excess* toxicity is another. Hormonal imbalances are yet another. Add lack of aerobic exercise and *load bearing* work to the above scenario and the result is spelled **obesity!** These are the reasons *why* overweight people can't lose weight.

Natural **weight control involves feeding the bio-electric body, meeting its hormonal needs, and DETOXIFICATION of the tissues, blood, and lymph.**

The body's nervous system is divided into the central and peripheral systems. The stomach is controlled by the peripheral system which is divided into the sympathetic and parasympathetic systems. We have control over the sympathetic nervous system. It is controlled by our *mental* thoughts. We have NO control over the parasympathetic nervous system. It is involuntary. Both systems carry nerve impulses to and from the stomach.

Load-Bearing Work

Load bearing work is just that—load-bearing! People do not do enough of it. Society has come to view **physical work** as a curse—something to be avoided at all costs! Only poor or uneducated people do this kind of work! They are wrong; the body must be worked! Since people hate the word "work," maybe we should call it **load-bearing** *exercise* which better fits the sports bent of society. Unfortunately, for most people this kind of activity takes place on the couch in front of the boob tube. So let's compromise and call it **load-bearing** *activity!*

The body responds to load-bearing activity by building new tissues and repairing old ones. This kind of activity is called *anabolism.* When the body is "worked" on a regular basis, rejuvenation accelerates. Aerobic exercise, weight training, and garden work are just a few examples of load-bearing activity to which the body responds with new vigor.

The body completely replaces the bones, connective tissues, and fluids about every 7 years. Lifestyle and habit dictate whether your new body is better or weaker.

As people age, they lose their ability and desire to do physical activity. Part of this phenomenon is the physical inability to perform; part is a lack of desire. A sedentary lifestyle destroys the body and precipitates loss of bone and muscle mass—as well as loss of mobility. **The less mobile and more sedentary we are, the faster we age.**

You can perpetuate the rejuvenatory process and keep a youthful body by doing LOAD BEARING activity, keeping your body detoxified, maintaining hormonal balance, and insisting on food and water with a high energy *footprint.*

The Dowager's Hump

The dowager's hump is a classic SIGN of total systemic degeneration of the bones and connective tissues. This is the humped-back, bent-over appearance seen among older people. This SIGN is becoming common among younger people.

If you could look at the older person's skeleton (see page 100), you would see that their spinal column and related connective tissues have *shrunk*. Notice, the person has lost *inches* from their maximum height—which they achieved at their **anabolic peak**. These lost inches occur mostly in the spinal column through deterioration of the vertebrae, tendons, ligaments, and discs between the vertebrae. As this occurs, the rib cage settles until it RESTS on the pelvis (hip). **This process can take up to forty years to occur.**

Settling of the spine and rib cage distorts the visceral organs. A prolapsed (kinked) colon is very common. The organs are forced OUT of position and are PACKED closer together. This is WHY older people have so many problems with their bowels. Settling of the spine eventually results in a protruding belly and the *humped* appearance. **The process begins the moment we begin the slide down the catabolic side of the aging pyramid into old age.**

Dowager is an old English word that described a widow who held property from her deceased husband's estate, AND who had the imposing appearance of a humped back and shoulders. Hence—a "dowager's hump." The condition was predominately seen among the wealthy. The poor usually died too soon in life to get the hump. The wealthy dowager did not do any load bearing work, It was avoided because physical work belonged to the domain of the poor.

The story of the dowager carries an IMPORTANT lesson for people who want to avoid degeneration and who would like to stay young and vibrant.

"Hanging" is a simple procedure that can s-t-r-e-t-c-h the spine and joints and promote blood and lymph flow. Hang from a bar, a rafter, or a tree limb day and evening. Start slow (a few seconds if you are older) and increase each day. *Hanging* involves getting your feet off the ground, closing your eyes and relaxing the spinal muscles. Try to work up to several minutes each time you hang. This procedure allow blood and lymph flow in and around the spinal column so rejuvenation can occur. As always, detoxification is very important. In this case, the use of enhanced PAC's, and hormone precursors is crucial.

Osteoporosis • The Dowager's Hump • Calcium

Women are being stampeded into taking large amounts of elemental calcium compounds. These include calcium carbonate (oyster shell), calcium citrate, calcium gluconate, and calcium magnesium tablets just to name a few. These *expert* opinions to the contrary, these substances should be avoided. They do NOT belong in the human body. Use only minerals that have passed through the carbon cycle.

Medicine's theories behind calcium *madness* has to do with *post*menopausal women who tend to develop osteoporosis. This condition is defined as the loss of minerals from the bones accompanied by loss of bone mass (density), with resulting honeycomb effect that follows in the wake of bone mineral loss.

Calcium's primary job—both in the body and in the soil—is to act as a buffer of toxic waste energy fields. In osteoporotic people, their system is TOXIC and the body is forced to steal minerals from the bones in order to "buffer" toxic wastes in the blood and lymphatic fluids.

Medicine *foolishly* promotes calcium supplements in order to *prevent* or *treat* osteoporosis. Science acts as if *hypocalcemia* (low blood calcium) is a threat to the population. It is not! Osteoporotic people and postmenopausal women usually have normal to HIGH calcium levels in their blood (hypercalcemia). These people don't need additional calcium. Instead, they need to clean up and detoxify their bodies.

The best way I know of to detoxify the system is to combine colon therapy, enhanced PAC's, Yucca extract, and self-massage of the lymphatic system. It is very helpful to use natural hormone precursors to address hormonal imbalances and meet the body's needs until the vital organs can get going again. In the meantime, the body's needs are met.

If your *present* height is LESS than it was at your anabolic *peak*, you need to take ACTION today!

Rouleau-Dowager Hump *Connection*

Deterioration of the bones and connective tissues is serious business—and it plagues millions of people. It is an EFFECT that is closely linked to the formation of the dowager's hump. Poor circulation and excess toxicity is at the root of the problem along with Rouleau.

Pronounced *roo -low*, the condition is a forerunner of hundreds of degenerative conditions. Rouleau is commonly referred to as "sticky" blood. When the red blood corpuscles clump together, they cannot access the fine capillaries of the body. Translated, this means less oxygen and nutrients get to the cells, and less carbon dioxide and waste exits the cells. The *log jam* effect of clumped cells in the blood causes deterioration of the connective tissues (the bones are connective tissues).

When Rouleau is present in the blood (see pictures on page 136), it means that toxic waste energy fields are present and causing the corpuscles to stick together in clumps. Clumping of the red blood *corpuscles* (a corpuscle is a red blood cell without a nucleus) prevents them from accessing the fine capillaries of the body which only them to enter single file. Rouleau is particularly damaging to the organs of the head, in particular the posterior eye, ears, and scalp.

Sea mineral ions are of immense benefit in dealing with Rouleau. They should be included in the diet for their value and for their beneficial effect on Rouleau.

Five drops of *concentrated* sea minerals in every glass of water (BEV works best) is all that is needed to clean up the system. Used on a daily basis, the benefits are astounding. The pictures on page 136 were taken on a Nikon Opithat microscope with a 100 watt lamp and a Naessens condenser. Magnification is 15,000 times.

Rouleau appears 5-20 years BEFORE the doctor can render a diagnosis of a life threatening condition.

Summary

Becoming *Young Again!* is a one step at a time project—in REVERSE! Once you understand the relationship between satiety, dis-ease, obesity, toxicity, water intake, exercise, and nourishment, all that is required is action. So go to work!

PREVIEW: *Our next chapter looks at the world of "shadows" and commonly held beliefs. Jesus and the Great Pyramid of Cheops have much in common as you will see.*

Occam's Razor. The idea that things do not have to be proved beyond proof. *"What can be done with fewer assumptions is done in vain with more."* Medical science could learn from William of Occam, c.1285-1349.

A Book Worth Reading

Your Body's Many Cries For WATER was written by Dr. F. Batmanghelidj who made his discoveries as an Iranian prisoner after the fall of the Shah.

Dr. Batmanghelidj discovered that water cures a multitude of dis-ease conditions. He found that chronic under hydration results in rheumatoid arthritis, allergies, chronic fatigue, allergies, asthma, angina, and hypertension. He discovered that these are not dis-eases, but SIGNS and signals from a under hydrated body. Hydration stress is very real.

Dr. Batmanghelidj says "advanced" cultures are *trained* to ignore thirst signals. That we are *taught* to substitute coffee, soft drinks, tea, and alcoholic beverages for water. He says people take water for granted because it is inexpensive and available. He adds that it is NOT possible to meet the body's hydration needs with liquid substitutes that contain water.

Dr. Batmanghelidj's findings are astounding and his research is impeccable. Yet, he is shunned and his work totally ignored by the American medical "establishment!" They don't want a society of healthy people.

The doctor's answers are simple and his therapies are effective. The implications of his discoveries are far reaching and very RESULTS oriented. Dr. Batmanghelidj is a Wizard. We owe him our thanks. His wonderful book is highly recommended (see Source Index).

P.S. Iran's water comes directly from mountain sources. Seeing the results Dr. Batmanghelidj was able to get with good tap water, imagine the health benefits that would accrue from drinking BEV "restructured" water?

Hormones

Women are estrogen dominant. Men are androgen dominant. Women go through menopause. Men go through andropause. In between these extremes, BOTH sexes must attend to their hormonal needs if they want to stay young and enjoy good health.

Use of *natural* hormone precursors to offset imbalances and excesses is safe and smart!

10

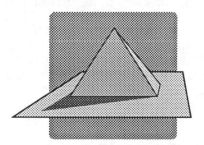

Shadow Land

"Most people would rather swallow lies than truth, especially if the liar has authority and the dis-information is soothing, like a fine liqueur."
Charles Walters

As Pontius Pilate passed by the side of Jesus at His trial, it was reported that he asked the great teacher: "What is Truth?" The Roman propounded a timely question that went unanswered, at least from the lips of Jesus. Pilate posed his question to Jesus, not as an interrogatory, but a statement about the Christ.

Socrates maintained that Truth could neither be proved nor disproved. Rather, it formed the basis of our beliefs by the reality of its existence. The Great Pyramid of Cheops is a present day TRUTH. It cannot be denied because it is there.

Earlier we posed the question, "Why do people like experts and expert opinions?" We also inquired, "How could anyone trust their most prized asset, their health, to the throw of medicine's dice?"

The answer to both questions is that the individual is relieved of personal responsibility when the decision process is given over to the experts. Forfeiture of responsibility gives an excuse and someone to blame if things go sour. Unfortunately, blaming others will NOT keep you young—or alive!

The "Expert" Syndrome

Medical science all too often tells us to do exactly the *opposite* of what we should do. Today, it treats its theories as gospel. Tomorrow, it casts them aside for new ones. In the process, it issues the proclamation, "magic bullet!"

An unsuspecting public buys into theories that were never true in the first place—like fluoridation of water and toothpaste, the cholesterol theory, and the Germ Theory of Disease. We are trained to turn off our good sense and rely on the *experts* in medicine, government and industry—who are "experts" at manipulating us.

Mass Delusions

In 1850 MacKay wrote, *Extraordinary Mass Delusions and the Madness of Crowds.* In it, he showed how unbelievably gullible we are, and that the more desperate the circumstances, the greater is our propensity to make unsound decisions *in mass*—usually with the help of the *experts.* **People go crazy in mass, but they return to their senses one at a time.**

People seek the health care *experts* because they hope to solve their health problems. They don't know where else to turn. They're in trouble and they need a fix.

If people would learn to **read** to their body's SIGNS and **listen** to the body's SYMPTOMS, they could prevent health problems and save a lot of pain, suffering, and money.

Without an endless supply of money—**especially medical insurance**—the experts go looking for *greener* pastures. Sick people can only escape medicine's claws under two conditions. When they run out of money, or when they're dead!

Medical decisions should NEVER be made on the basis of "who" is paying the bill. The better your medical insurance, the wider door to vault will open. The experts understand dollars—especially BIG dollars!

By definition, an expert is someone from more than fifty miles away. Our fascination with experts convinces me that this is the SAME phenomenon that makes the Law of Bureaucracy work flawlessly. This law has NO exceptions. It says: ***"Regardless of the intended result, exactly the opposite will result."***

We CANNOT rely on the experts. It is the experts who have taught us to *doubt* our intuitions and ignore good sense. The experts practice tunnel vision, that is why they are called experts. **We live in a world of shadows—where most of what we see and hear only *looks like* the truth.**

Remember: The more something is believed to be true—and the greater the number of people who believe it to be so—the greater are the odds that it is NOT true.

Allopathic medicine is in trouble. So are people who rely on it to save them from their poor decisions and bad lifestyles. Medicine's model is based on the Germ Theory of Disease. It, in turn, is based on the Scientific Method.

Consider the difference between conventional medicine's approach and vibrational medicine's approach to solving the hearing problem for the deaf.

At the age of fifteen, Dr. Patrick Flanagan invented the neurophone—a device to help the deaf hear. Flanagan sensed that the brain is a hologram and that it has different areas that are capable of performing **multiple** OR **duplicate** functions. Consequently, Flanagan used the integument (skin) as a pathway to the brain and to serve a duplicate function. The deaf person's "brain" could now hear.

Flanagan solved the hearing problem through visualization vs. surgical intervention. The brain is **not** hard wired as taught in the medical schools. The body can **regenerate** new brain cells. We **do** have the ability to grow new limbs, bones, dendrites, nerve fibers, skin, and connective tissues. Flanagan had **vision.** He understood the Creator's handiwork.

Cause & Effect

Earlier, we referred to something called single factor analysis, which translates: For every effect there is **single** cause; for every disease there is a **single** pathogen that is responsible. This kind of academic tunnel vision has gotten us into a lot of trouble. It is unrealistic because it is NOT true. Whenever we attempt to force the facts to fit a pet theory, TRUTH becomes secondary, *legitimate* science suffers, and trouble results. Such is the case with the hallowed "scientific method."

Charles Walters summed-up the problems inherent in the *scientific method* when he stated, *"Most of what is generally called the scientific system is not science at all, but merely a procedural aspect that calls for setting up experiments that eliminate other possibilities, or it deals with making instruments that enable the investigator to find what he/she is looking for. There is a second scientific method that, although unwritten, has far greater impact on scientists and their findings. This is the reality of project funding, "peer" review, and the publishing of scientific papers."*

Walters went on to say, *"The backbone of the scientific system has to do with asking the right questions, and a scientist can only ask the right questions after his/her life has absorbed the experiences that lead to a vision of the Creator's handiwork, hence the right question.   ...discovery is accomplished by the mind and soul of the whole person and cannot be reduced to a mechanical scientific (by-the-numbers) procedure. It stands to reason that you can't get the answers if you don't know the questions."*

The Double Helix

It was this second process that caused James D. Watson, one of the discoverers of the DNA molecule to rock the scientific world when he disclosed the behind-the-scenes power plays, jealously, and fights for funding in his book, *The Double Helix*. Watson also offered an antidote—the observation that scientific discovery involves human thought and vision *more* than test tubes, procedures, and microscopes.

Germ Theory Of Disease

The Germ Theory of Disease (GTD) is tremendously important to the aging process because it influences the way we perceive dis-ease. It so completely colors our thought processes, that we are blind to the subtleties and cumulative effects of bad living habits and poor choice of lifestyle. Because medicine does **not** recognize understand that the battle for life and health vs. death and dis-ease is fought, won or lost on a playing field that has absolutely **nothing** to do with the GTD, they are like blind men with fat egos stumbling in the dark— fearful of anyone who spreads the light of TRUTH.

We cannot rely on medicine and science to solve our problems because they don't know what the problem is. They don't understand the phenomenon of life at the subtle energy level, nor the manifestation of dis-ease. The proof for this statement is contained in the following fact.

Experts suffer from the same problems as the rest of the population. They grow old. They succumb to the same dis-eases. Their "magic bullets" do NOT save them!

The GTD is a theory, yet medical science treats it as holy writ. It is the cornerstone of the archaic medical model under which medicine labors. It is a stone around its neck!The GTD is so *accepted* that 99.99999% of the medical community own "stock" in it and live by it. Perhaps you do too. All conventional medical modalities—from diagnosis to treatment— is based on this **false** theoretical dis-ease model.

The model says we are nothing but a bundle of chemicals, proteins, fats, water, nucleic acids, flesh and blood. It says that dis-ease results when the body is "invaded" by a bug and this causes us to come down sick. It says that dis-ease erupts out of *nowhere!* These things are not true. Loyalty to the model stands in the way of change.

Regardless of medicine's bullheadedness, we are moving into an era where the reality of the 3rd dimension *physical* body and the 4th dimension *electric* body are beginning to be recognized and brought together for total healing.

A healthy bio-electric body is a synthesis of energy fields vibrating in *concert* with Mother Earth.

Things Are Changing

Lancet and the New England Journal of Medicine are now writing "pro" alternative care articles. This is a 180⁰ shift in position from the past eighty (80) years. They are positioning POWER so they can maintain **control** of the transition from allopathic to vibrational medicine. The driving force behind this change is big money—specifically the pharmaceuticals.

The movie, *The Medicine Man* is a *futuristic* movie. It was aired for a reason. It officially signaled the shift away from bogus organic chemistry and allopathic medicine to more natural modalities. Herbal based medicine is growing at exponential rates. Understanding herbs is the key to the future.

It's no accident that our present medical and economic system is being systematically dismantled. Consider, in 1994 40% of the people in the United States sought help through some form of *alternative* medicine. People are waking up and realizing that conventional medicine cannot meet their needs.

At the same time, *bogus* health journals and newsletters are making their debut. Natural healing is "the" thing to be into these days. Conventional doctors are authoring books and issuing newsletters that "trumpet" their charade. Few physicians can think outside the confines of their discipline. Their credentials are in the way. Most will have to be retrained.

Our present "health care" system will be in shambles for many years to come. **Do whatever you must to avoid getting caught up in it.**

The experts can ignore TRUTH, but they cannot deny it, for TRUTH is there—like the Great Pyramid of Cheops—etched in stone and timeless. Becoming *Young Again!* involves the recognition and application of TRUTH.

PREVIEW: *Our next chapter looks at HOW water functions in the bio-electric body. It is a foundation chapter in reversing the aging process. Elixir Of The Ageless provides answers to questions seldom asked.*

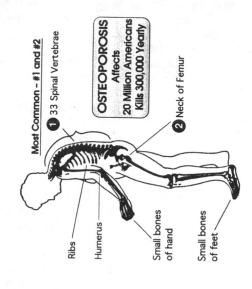

Most Common – #1 and #2

1 33 Spinal Vertebrae

OSTEOPOROSIS
Affects
20 Million Americans
Kills 300,000 Yearly

2 Neck of Femur

Ribs

Humerus

Small bones
of hand

Small bones
of feet

**LOCATIONS IN THE BODY
WHERE PAIN AND MISERY HIT HARDEST**

Age
55 years

Age
65 years

Age
75 years

Compression fractures of thoracic vertebrae lead to loss of height and progressive thoracic kyphosis (dowager's hump). Lower ribs eventually rest on iliac crests, and downward pressure on viscera causes abdominal distention

Progressive Spinal Deformation In Osteoporosis

11

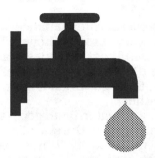

Elixir Of The Ageless

*"In health and in sickness, pure water is one of
the choicest blessings. It is the beverage given by
God to quench the thirst of man and animal, and
to cleanse the poisons from our system."*

Byrne

At birth, the human body is over 90% water. By age 3,
average body hydration level is 75% water. Adult hydration
levels can dip to 65% in men and 52% in women. At death,
hydration level can drop another 5-10%. Fat holds 55% water
and muscle 75%. The brain from 75-85%. These figures have
meaning because the impact the aging process. They partially
explain *why* we age, and they **hint** at what we can do about it.

The *bio-electric* body requires water to function. When
we are water deficient it is called *neglect*. When we drink
contaminated water, it is called *abuse*. Most people's bodies
suffer from both abuse and neglect. The *bio-electric* body can
bounce back from abuse and neglect, but it can't do it without
the help of *biologically friendly* water!

Water has many faces; some wet, some dry, some
heavy, some structured. Water has different names. There is
distilled water, reverse osmosis water, deionized water, carbon
block and ceramic filtered water, hard water, soft water, tap
water, ionized water, Grander water, Ludwig water, Ange

water, Pi water, Egg water, Miracle water, Willard water, Micro water, saline water, electrostatic water, and BEV water. Like food, some waters are pure and wholesome, while others are the harbinger of dis-ease and death.

Water dictates health and vitality. Water is "the" controlling dietary factor in the aging reversal process.

Water Questions

Travelers sometimes experience water that is so dry that they can hardly get wet in the shower. They also experience water that is very *wet!* What qualities makes a substance as simple as water so different? Is it the well from which it was drawn, or the earth through which it migrated that makes the difference? Is it neither?

Why does some water taste good and some not? Why does some water quench the thirst while another water satisfies so poorly that we avoid it? Why do some religions erect shrines around *certain* waters? Why are certain water holes around the world called *health* spas? Why is water used in the rite of baptism?

Why do plants grow better when it rains than when we irrigate? Is all rain water the same? Why is water used as the transport medium for fluorine and chlorine? Why is water used as the carrier for pesticides and herbicides? Why do we ad poisons to drinking water? Why do people like to camp near lakes and rivers? Lastly, what does water have to do with reversing the aging process?

Water In The Body

There are TWO fluids in the body —blood and lymph— and water is the foundation of both of them. We need water to sweat, bleed, blow our nose, breathe, menstruate, spit, cough, and defecate. Without water the mucous membranes that line our air passages and gastrointestinal tract cannot function. All four excretory corridors—SKIN, LUNGS, KIDNEYS, and BOWELS—rely on water!

Water is the ONLY dietary substance over which we can exercise *complete* and *total* control.

BEV Water

"Choice" of drinking water is the single most important health decision a person can make. Water interfaces every system in the body at the most fundamental level of existence.

My choice in drinking water is called BEV water. I drink

it because it is the healthiest drinking water known. It is made by a proprietary process that gives the word WATER new meaning. In addition, the BEV process *transcends* conventional concepts of water purity.

Experts like to talk about "pure" water, but they can't agree on exactly what *pure* water is. Chemists will tell you distilled water is pure water, but it's not so. Distilled water is purer than tap water, but it's not *pure*—and it's not healthy!

Pure water molecules are void of ALL substances except one oxygen and two hydrogen atoms. Pure water should also be free of the vibrational frequencies that were imposed on it by the contaminants it once contained.

BEV water is extremely pure water, plus its structure and memory have been enhanced and cleared. BEV water is a right-spin energy substance that acts like a liquid magnet when it is turned loose in the body.

Please refer to the water molecule diagram on page 79. Notice the hydrogen bonds connecting the H_2O molecule in the box to the adjoining molecules outside the box. These are *hydrogen* bonds, and they cause water molecules to **stick** together. The effect is referred to as **cohesion.** The stronger the hydrogen bonds, the more cohesive will be the water. The more cohesive the water, the more ENERGY it possesses, and the better people feel when they drink it. BEV water is VERY **cohesive!** This quality gives it a very high energy *footprint.*

Water with a high energy *footprint* likes to **coat** things. The phenomenon is called **adhesion.** Again, the stronger the hydrogen bonds, the greater will be its adhesive qualities, and the greater will be the water's effect on the body. *Adhesion* and *cohesion* make water "feel" wet. BEV water is VERY **adhesive** and VERY **wet.** These qualities are a reflection of BEV water's high energy *signature.*

Cohesion and *adhesion* are a reflection of the **strength** of the hydrogen bonds *between* the water molecules. BUT THERE IS MORE! These qualities are further enhanced by the **ANGLE** of the hydrogen and *molecular* bonds within and between water molecules. Please refer to the drawing on page 79 and note that each hydrogen atom is connected to an oxygen atom at an **angle.** So called "normal" bond angle is 104.5°. The BEV process enhances the energy footprint and signature of water by manipulating the **angles** *within* and *between* the water molecules. All of these thing give BEV water **life!**

Water that contains inorganic minerals, toxic chemicals, viruses, bacteria, radioactivity, etc. has POOR cohesion and adhesion, WEAK hydrogen and molecular bonds, and INFERIOR bond angles. Traditional water processing units are **primitive** in comparison to the BEV proprietary process which

removes all pollutants from water, **erases the** vibratory memory of pollutants, **alters** bond angles, and **strengthen** bond angles. I am describing what people refer to when they say, *"This water feels different in my mouth and body!"*
Pollutants that hitch a ride on water's energy, alter the bond angles and weaken water's *magnetic* footprint and diminish its *electrical* signature. The end effect is that the water has LESS energy to donate the body, and the LESS ability to transport wastes out of the system. **BEV water is very friendly to the human body!**
BEV water cannot be left exposed to the air or transported through metal or plastic pipes. It so alive that it will "pull" contaminants from the atmosphere which causes it to lose its energy! Moreover, BEV water must be stored in the tank in which it is made, in glass bottles, or in non-reactive polycarbonate containers.
It is not unusual for people who drink BEV water to reverse years of sinus problems. People who drink it have more energy. Bowel habits change. Metabolic wastes are carried OUT of the system. **Non water drinkers become water lovers!**
Tap, distilled, and conventional reverse osmosis waters are NOT good for the body. They contain little free energy. They have impurities attached to their molecules. The body must restructure them BEFORE it can use them. You cannot reclaim your health with these waters. If you insist on drinking them, at least add some sea water ions to help yourself.

Skin • Sweat • Lungs

The skin is the primary mechanical barrier to infection from bacteria. Skin becomes stressed if we fail to drink enough water. Skin that is exposed to water borne pollutants when bathing becomes stressed, and, in time, will lose its healthy appearance. Biologically **UN**friendly water attacks the connective tissues weakening the skin from the inside.
Failure to drink enough water, denies the body the opportunity to shed its wastes through sweat. When we sweat, we secrete water + toxic waste energy fields.
The ability to freely sweat is a good SIGN. Skin that does not freely sweat becomes stressed from the toxic wastes buildup in the surface tissues. **Excess** waste **forces** the body to dispose of its wastes via the kidneys, lungs and bowel—which are usually overloaded already. Wastes that cannot be exported from the body are stored in FAT the body *manufactures* for this purpose. Failure to drink enough water greatly accelerates the aging process. Low hydration levels cripple the respiratory system, diminish blood and lymph fluid volumes,

compromise the bloods ability to carry oxygen, and raise blood pressure and pulse.

Water & The Lungs

The lungs also rid the body of waste energy fields. The lungs are VERY dependent on mucous secretions to protect these delicate tissues from airborne contaminants. Mucous production is dependent on water intake. Low hydration levels in the tissues cause the mucous membranes that line our mouth, throat, respiratory, and GI tracts to come under severe stress. Mucous lubricates the nasal passages and airways. It transports airborne wastes OUT of the body. Mucous coats and protects lining of the stomach and small intestines. Conditions like colitis, diverticulitis, and irritable bowel syndrome have some of their roots in limited mucous secretion. Many health conditions vanish as water intake increases. The value of BEV water in the self treatment of dis-ease should be obvious. Read *Your Body's Many Cries For Water* (see Source Index).

More "Cries" For Water

The term **hypo**volemia comes to mind. It means low fluid (blood and lymph) volume in the body. People who are sick, immobile, or bed ridden often suffer from hypovolemia because they do not drink enough water. Men who suffer from sexual impotence are under hydrated and toxic—and their hormones are unbalanced due to **excesses** in the system.

Fluids like milk, juice, SOFT DRINKS, and beer are **liquid** foods. And while there is no question these foods contain water, the water they contain stresses the system. As with distilled and traditional reverse osmosis waters, the body must dismantle and restructure liquid foods in order to use it.

BEV water does NOT stress the system or cause the body to waste vital energy. Traditionally purified waters must be manipulated before the body can use them.

Under hydration is a problem of epidemic proportions for much of the population and particularly among the old and sick. The elderly are notorious for not drinking enough water, and their health problems are a direct reflections of it. Drug usage, lack of exercise, a poor diet, and negative thought patterns tell the rest of the story.

Illness • Colon Therapy

Sick and elderly people respond quickly to copious amounts of BEV water with liquid sea minerals. Tap water should be avoided because it is contaminated with pollutants, and because it resonates at **unhealthy** frequencies.

Colon therapy is enhanced by the use of biologically friendly water. Bile flow is dependent on water. Liver stones will form and indigestion problems develop without enough water. Arthritis, fibromyalgia, gout, myasthenia gravis, system lupis, and dozens of other conditions all respond to BEV water.

Colon problems manifest and multiply in people who fail to drink enough water. Colon therapy is one of the BEST things a person can do to regain their health and stay on top. Unfortunately, colonics are thoroughly un-American. People dislike them because they sound strange and are a *pain in the butt.* Nevertheless, they work!

Both fat AND skinny people hold large amounts of mucoid, fecal matter in their colon. People say, *"Oh! I don't need colon therapy! I go two or three times a day!"* **Regularity is a WORTHLESS means to determine the presence of colon lining buildup. Build up begins as early as 8 years old and gets worsens with time.**

When the most popular cowboy in movie history died (his name was John W...), over seventy (70) pounds of **mucoid matter** was removed from his colon upon autopsy. The odor was *beyond* description! The great actor's transverse colon—the part that hangs over the belt line—was almost **twelve inches** in diameter! The lumen (opening) through which his waste flowed was only one inch in diameter! The difference was mucus, old fecal matter, toxins, and accumulated drugs. A "healthy" colon should be about two inches in TOTAL diameter.

When you see someone's belly hanging over the belt line, you are seeing some fat and a VERY engorged, and prolapsed (sagging) colon. Consider it a red flag condition.

Colonic In A Bottle

Colon therapy is wonderful blessing for those people who are willing to do it. For those who are not willing to do colon therapy, Yucca extract, Kombucha tea, and enhanced PAC's are very effective. Put the two approaches together and the starts rewinding itself immediately. The soft tissues (muscles & ligaments, and tendons) regain their resiliency. The liver defats. Bile flow accelerates. The hair starts growing again. Aches and pains melt away. In my case, my dark brown eyes became half green! **Wonder what I was full of?**

Deep Breathing • Aerobic Exercise

Deep breathing and aerobic exercise lead to vibrant

health. These therapies are a simple and effective way to avoid or treat hundreds of health conditions. They increase oxygen levels in the blood and tissues, and they accelerate the flow of toxic energy from the lungs. Deep breathing also builds mental focus and sense of well being.

Weak lungs cannot process enough oxygen, nor can they serve to release toxic energies into the atmosphere. They are prone to infection and scar tissue formation. A weak respiratory system backgrounds most dis-ease conditions. Rouleau(sticky blood) goes part and parcel with limited lung capacity and function. **Deep breathing is a cost free and effective way to improve anyone's health.**

Soft Drinks

Soft drink consumption in industrial societies is epidemic, and the problems that spring from their use is similar to the effects of alcohol usage.

Soft drinks upset the body's calcium:phosphorous ratio. They are LOADED with phosphoric acid, sodium, and aluminum ions (from the can). They raise hell with the kidneys and unbalance body pH. The sugar in soft drinks steals the body's mineral ions. The aspartame they contain destroys the liver. **It takes 32 glasses of highly charged alkaline ionized water to buffer the effects of just one can of soda** (more on ionized water on page 220). The nick name *"soda pop"* derives from the high amounts of sodium soft drinks contain.

Soft drinks have become a socially acceptable beverage because they are considered to be safe to drink. (They're not!)We see them differently than cigarettes, coffee, and alcohol because their effects are experienced over very long periods of time—NEVER in direct connection to their consumption. Soft drink junkies are addicts as much as any smoker, coffee hound, drug user, or alcoholic.

The list of conditions that spin off of soft drink consumption and addiction is **staggering!** A complete detoxification and a liver flush program ends cravings and addictions.

Energy Production & Water

Water is rich in oxygen and the body uses it in internal respiration at the cellular level. The mitochondria in our cells use it to burn our glucose sugars. This is a flame less process—a catalytic, enzymatic type of process where hydrogen electrons are the energy shuttles that feed the *electron transport system* that controls cellular oxidation and the production of ATP.

BEV water is rich in active oxygen and hydrogen atoms.

BEV purity and biological activity gives it the ability to bond to and transport large amounts of sea water ions. When BEV water is used to make Mikrowater (see page 220), the therapeutic applications of BEV + Mikro is mind boggling.

Ionized Water

Ionized water has become a big deal in Japan where over 10,000,000 use it. Now, that BEV technology is inexpensive and available, the potential for creating **SUPER ionized Mikrowater** has taken a quantum leap and become reality.

To make SUPER Mikrowater, first you make some BEV water with BEV processing equipment using water from your tap. As the water is made, it is transferred into a special polycarbonate holding tank for storage (ionic sea minerals are mixed with the finished BEV water that is in storage). SUPER Mikrowater is made by further processing the ion charged BEV water in the Mikrowater unit.

The ionizing unit takes the mix of BEV water and sea minerals and splits the molecules and atoms into TWO completely NEW and totally different products.

Acid & Alkaline Water

Conventional Mikrowater units dispense acid water @ pH 4-7 and alkaline water @ pH 8-10. The pH of **Medical grade** SUPER ionized Mikrowater can be driven down to pH 2 and *saturated it with* hydrogen ions that are *highly oxidized.*

Acid water is used to promote beautiful skin, to heal wounds and connective tissue infections, and promote a youthful appearance. I have a video of a Japanese man with gangrene in the leg that was so far advanced that surgery was eminent. When the man's leg was submersed in **medical grade** ionized acid water, AND *at the same time* he drank **Medical Grade** Mikrowater, complete and TOTAL healing took place! And this was **before** we had the ability to create SUPER ionized Mikrowater using BEV and sea ions as the basis.

Alkaline ionized water is the exact **opposite** of acid ionized water. Where acid water is highly *oxidized,* alkaline water is highly *reduced.* Translated, this means the alkaline and acid mineral ions are divided as electron saturation is increased or decreased as measured by *reduction.*

Reduction is an chemistry term. It is a type of reaction in which a substance **GAINS** electrons and its positive valence is decreased! Alkaline SUPER Mikrowater has NEVER been available in the West until now. With the marriage of BEV water and Mikrowater, incredible healings can take place at accelerated rates right in your own home. The pH of **medical grade** SUPER Mikrowater can be as high as pH 11.5 for people with dis-eases like diabetes, cancer, fibromyalgia, myasthenia gravis, systemic lupis, nervous disorders, and cerebral palsy. NOTE: The water does NOT cure any of these conditions. It gives back control of the body's "terrain" to its rightful owner—YOU!

Let there be no mistake. If I had a degenerative disorder of any kind, I would take my life under my total and complete control, stop destroying my liver with medications, begin the process of detoxification and rejuvenation, and show the doctors and the scoffers that the experts don't know what they are talking about. Instead of getting mad, I would teach them a lesson by outlining every last one of them!

SUPER "alkaline" Mikrowater neutralizes acid wastes in the body, while heavy saturation of electrons in solution promotes rapid healing. The marriage of BEV + Mikrowater gives new meaning to the word "therapeutic."

Fatigue & Water

Fatigue is a SIGN that the body has accumulated **excess** acids in the system. It is a SIGN that our supply of electrons the mitochondria use to create the high energy molecule ATP is low. When we *overdo*, when we experience muscle *soreness*, when the body is in a **TOXIC** state, acids build up in the system. Lactate formation occurs when there is a **shortfall** of available oxygen at the cellular level. This state leads to **incomplete** oxidation of blood glucose sugars. Lactate is the salt of lactic acid and the waste byproduct of **fermentation** at the cellular level. Lactate—like carbon monoxide from automobiles—derives from **incomplete** combustion. Lactate formation is nature's way of forcing us to get rest so the body can recycle its acid **wastes** before they overload the system.

The new Far Infrared saunas from Japan rejuvenate the body by neutralizing acid wastes in the tissues and speeding metabolism (see pages 159, and 366).

Alkaline ionized SUPER Mikrowater accelerates the rejuvenatory cycle so we tire less easily and heal faster. **It is VERY important that the reader understands that tap water should NOT be used to make ionized Micro Water.**

Tap water is a problem in the USA. Toxic free well water is no more. Municipal water is loaded with poisons. When tap water is used to make **acid** ionized SUPER Mikrowater, toxic wastes like fluorides, heavy metals, and chlor*amines* concentrate to *unsafe* levels. To avoid this, BEV water is used as the basis for making ionized water. SUPER ionized Mikrowater is the most recent advance in the creation of **therapeutic** water that is used to treat degenerative illness and dis-ease.

To improve your health, drink BEV water with sea mineral ions. To experience the next quantum leap in the evolution of water and healing, install a SUPER ionized Mikrowater processor to go with your BEV unit.

Urine

Urine is the metabolic waste product of the kidneys. An examination of urine produces clues as to what is happening in the body. pH is an extremely important indicator. An alkaline (above 7.0), indicates one set of circumstances. An acid pH (below 7.0), means something altogether different.

Most people's urine pH is below 6.0. According to a nurse friend of mine, 90% of the people she checks have a pH between 5.0 - 5.5, which she says is "normal." If her patients are indicative of the rest of the population, she is prophesying a nation of people whose health is in serious jeopardy. I asked her to check my urine, the result was pH 7.2. This is good!

Low urine pH is a RED FLAG for cancer. Cancer manifests itself when urine pH drops to 4.5. Blood and saliva pH along with the resistivity of these fluids must also be factored into the physician's diagnosis in order for urine pH to be have conclusive value.

In general, low pH is bad news and flags a body that is in a life and death struggle at the cellular level. Low pH signals degenerative dis-ease in both the formative and advanced stages. Treatment of an acid condition calls for systemic detoxification, SUPER ionized Mikrowater, therapeutic fasting, Yucca extract and enhanced PAC's.

Water pH • Sodium

Most tap water is between pH 7-9, highly oxidized, and toxic. Tap water may be 'safe' to drink, but it's NOT good for you. Alkaline water should be pure and highly reduced.

For each number you move up or down the pH scale, the acidity or alkalinity is one-hundred times greater or weaker. At a pH of 8.5, tap water is one-hundred and fifty times more alkaline than tap water at pH 7.0. It takes a LOT of dissolved minerals to raise water from its natural pH of 6.0-7.2 to 8 or 9. Lime (calcium carbonate) raises pH. Sodium raises pH. Aluminum raises pH. Cities use all of the above, but especially sodium hydroxide (lye) to manipulate pH. Sodium hydroxide is **extremely** alkaline, and the sodium (symbol Na) is poison to the cells. People who are fighting cancer, must NOT drink tap water. People who don't want to fight it should do the same.

Remember, water can be a carrier molecule at any pH. When you see water with a pH above 7.2, you can bet it has a train load of inorganic minerals and chemical passengers attached to its molecules. The more passengers water transports, the less "free" energy that is available to the body. The more waste shuttled into the body in drinking water, the less waste that can be carried OUT. Water pollutants have a left-spin and a negatively impact the bio-electric body.

Casts & Albumin In Urine

Casts are sometimes found in urine. They are aptly named. Casts are deposits of mineral salts (like the ones in drinking water), hyaline, and plasma proteins (albumin) that have taken on the shape of the kidney's tubules.

The tubules collect urine and any wastes it may contain. Casts are a RED flag! They're indicative of: pH imbalance, degeneration, under hydration, and excess mineral salts.

Albumin is a blood and lymph *plasma* protein. It does NOT belong in the urine. Its presence may indicate a urinary infection. Unless there is an infection, albumin's presence in the urine means it is slipping past the kidney's nephrons (blood filters). Albumin in the urine means aging is accelerating.

Urine tells a story. If you drink plenty of water it should be straw colored between meals, and bright yellow after meals. The doctor often want a urine sample from the first urination of the day, which is dark, strong, and cloudy. If you fail to drink enough water, urine becomes dark and strong. If too much table salt is consumed, you will urinate less and retain excess waste. If you sweat heavily and don't offset fluid and electrolyte loss, urine becomes dark and strong and urination may become painful.

Go on a three day lemon juice fast and the first urination on the second day will be **extremely** dark. When collected in a small bottle and set on a shelf, it will form dark brown diamond shaped CRYSTALS! These crystals represent plasma protein waste byproducts like uric acid.

Kidneys & Aging

The blood is filtered by the kidney's nephrons at the rate of 250 gallons a day, or 1000 quarts every 24 hours. If kidney function is weak, **excess** waste will accumulate in the system and will eventually get a diagnosis from the doctor.

Waste build up in the system as a result of compromised kidney function underwrites every single degenerative dis-ease known. Restoration of kidney function can be accomplished through detoxification using Yucca extract, Kombucha tea, enhanced PAC's, Rene's tea, and BEV water. Rebounding and self-massage of the lymphatic are most helpful.

The Bowel

When we are young, people experience regular bowel movements because muscle tone in the visceral organs (organs of the abdominal cavity) is good. Adequate and regular exercise is an important part of most kid's lives. As we grow older, the story changes—and so does our health.

Visit a doctor who thinks "basic," and one of the first questions he will ask is, *"when did you last have a bowel movement?"* Your answer tells a story.

The word *bowel* comes from the French and Latin. It means, *sausage* (intestines resemble sausage). Next time the doctor asks the same question, your response should be, "I moved my sausage ......yesterday, a week ago, etc."

Freud said we are possessed by defecation in our early years of development. He called it the Anal Stage. Gandhi was once described as a man who had been over potty trained. It is reported that daily he asked each of his wives if they had moved their bowels that day.

Even Lawrence Welk had a thing with constipation. He always pushed a laxative on his show. The laxative company had a smart marketing team. They knew that people over forty is the perfect audience to target! Today, the target audience would be people 5 years and up!

Bowel and colon problems have their origin in a weak liver . A healthy liver is the key to a healthy colon. Flush your liver stones, and you're bile will flow

Water Therapy

Water has other uses besides drinking and bathing. It can be used to break fevers, relieve constipation, cleanse the colon, **AND stimulate the flow of bile from the liver.**

The first thing my mother would do when us children were sick was to give us an enema and empty the lower bowel. We hated it, but the results could not be denied.

In 1983, I pushed myself too hard and became very ill with the flu. My temperature hit 106° F. I was in serious trouble. At two in the morning, all I could think of was to crawl into the bathtub and turn on the cold water. It didn't help! In desperation, I gave myself a colon irrigation and emptied my bowel. Within 15 minutes the fever dropped to 100° degrees F. I used no medication of any kind, and I recovered quickly.

Hemorrhoids • Constipation • Prostate

Hemorrhoids and constipation are first cousins. So are colitis and diverticulitis. Each sets up house for the other and together they make a *miserable* team. Constipation always precedes the other three. It can be prevented and treated with colon therapy, BEV water, Yucca extract, and PAC's.

Water keeps the stool moist and soft. Lack of water results in hard dry stools. Dietary fiber attracts and holds water, which acts as a lubricant during defecation. Fiber also acts as an intestinal broom.

People say hemorrhoids are caused from sitting on cold tree stumps, hard chairs and the like, but these things are NOT true. Truck drivers swear they result from poor seats, vibration and road bounce. These things are NOT true either.

If you ask a hundred medical doctors what causes hemorrhoids, constipation, and the like, rare is the one who will mention the word WATER!

If you are constipated, drink three or four glasses of water and HOLD IT! Do not urinate even if you think you are going to wet your pants! **Frequent urination robs you of your bowel movements and cause you to grow old.**

A full bladder puts *pressure* on the colon, stimulates peristalsis (rhythmic movement of the intestines), and causes gas and cramps that result in a bowel movement.

Other natural remedies for colon problems include eating meals on schedule, eating plenty of raw vegetables, apples, dried prunes, drinking lots of Kombucha tea, and using fruit and vegetable juices in capsule or tablet form.

Try and drink one 8 ounce cup of water per hour. A steady flow of water and foods with speed food transit time from the mouth to the toilet.

50% of men over forty-five years old have prostate problems because they are obese, don't drink enough water, eat a poor diet, have hormonal imbalances, and are constipated. Insufficient water brings on constipation which causes the to swell and push against the prostate. This condition allows bacteria **to migrate** from the colon into the prostate and produce the inflamed, swollen condition called *prostatitis.*

A swollen prostate constricts the urinary tube and slows urination. Older men are known for "dribbling" their urine because their prostate won't allow the urine to pass. In other words, they can't make water!

When a man is young, all he thinks about is making love. In his middle years, all he thinks about is making money. When he becomes OLD, all he thinks about is making water!

The use of Saw Palmetto, hormone precursors, zinc picolinate, flax oil, and **Far Infrared** products can eliminate many a prostate problem. Men with prostate problems should also use Yucca extract, enhanced PAC's, and do colon therapy.

The Goal

Reversing the aging process involves paying attention to the BASICS while you replace *old* bad habits with *new* good habits. Doing nothing means you will grow old and suffer miserably along the way. Taking action today, means that tomorrow you will become *Young Again!*

PREVIEW: *In our next chapter you will learn how to save thousands of dollars in dental bills, and how to feel good!*

Dump Those Stones!

The single biggest issue in returning a person to vibrant health are is the presence of stones in the liver.

Liver stones BLOCK bile flow out of the liver, causing bile to back up and poison all body systems. Bile wastes settle in the joints and connective tissues creating arthritis. They erupt from the skin as pimples and psoriasis. They create **excesses** in the system and bring on conditions like prostatitis, PMS, gout, and cancer.

Liver stones are really gall stones. They form in the liver and range in size from B-B's to large marbles. Occasionally, they dislodge from the liver and collect in the gallbladder. Now they are gall stones. Their accumulation will eventually block the bile duct and require emergency surgical intervention. A liver flush is simpler and safer.

All people—including children—have stones in their liver. The way to get them out of the liver and body is to do a "liver flush."

Preparations include the use of Yucca extract and PAC's to loosen and dispose of toxic wastes from the system and to prevent their reabsorption as they make their way down the intestines. These things also prepare the body for the flush procedure. Three days before the flush takes place, a special formulation is used to soften the stones to the consistency of soft putty so they will **painlessly** pass out of the body.

Everyone has stones in their liver, and the older you are the more you have. Count on it! My 79 year old friend, Pearl, painlessly passed 152 stones! She will receive her wish for good health! (See Source Index).

12

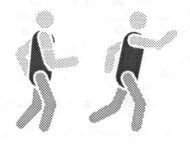

I Feel Good

"Stress is like a chicken. It knows where to roost!"
John Thomas

We describe the way we feel in terms of black and white. "I feel good!" "I'm sick!" People don't like shades of *gray* when it comes to the way they feel.

If we substitute the word *aerobic* for good, and *anaerobic* for sick, our descriptions shift from black and white to *gray*. Our words no longer *appear* to carry the same meaning, but they do help us to better understand WHY we feel *good* or *sick*.

Breathing • Respiration

When we are **aerobic,** we are "with air." When we are anaerobic, we are **"without air."** Both of these states of being are influenced by the way we breathe.

Shallow breathing encourages the accumulation of wastes in the tissues and accelerated aging, while deep breathing causes the body to shed its wastes and rejuvenate itself.

Shallow breathing promotes an oxygen starved body, windedness, low energy, and poor focus. Deep breathing promotes an oxygen rich tissues, unlabored breathing under stress, high energy, and steely focus.

Exercise and strenuous activity promotes deep breathing, and if the body is encouraged to build endurance, it can be pushed fast enough and long enough until it reaches the "aerobic" state.

Breathing *(respiration)* takes place on two levels: external and internal. **External respiration** is sort of a mechanical process that occurs in the lungs, while **internal respiration** is more esoteric and less mechanical, and takes place in the cells.

The exchange of carbon dioxide (CO_2) and oxygen (O) in the lungs is called *external respiration*. The exchange of CO_2 and O PLUS the burning of glucose sugars and the production of the energy molecule ATP is called *internal respiration, and it occurs at the cellular level.*

Clinical vs. Subclinical

Aging is seen in the mirror, but it occurs at the cellular level and BELOW. By *below*, I mean at the "subtle energy level" of our existence which is in dimensions beyond the Third Dimension level in which we act out our lives.

The doctor uses Third Dimension SIGNS to diagnose dis-ease. SIGNS *clinical.* Symptoms are *not* observable or measurable, so they are referred to as **subclinical**.

When we are clinically ill, we are usually under doctor's care, in the bed, or maybe even in the hospital. **Clinical illness is official!** When you are "clinical" you are in trouble! To repeat, clinical medical conditions display SIGNS that the doctor can measure and use in the diagnose dis-ease. This is important!

Subclinical illness occurs in the occult (hidden/masked) stage of dis-ease. It manifests itself at the *subtle energy level* of our existence. It is a **gray** state of being, often described as "feeling a little off." People tend to ignore these *off* feelings, hoping they will go away. Instead, they eventually take form in our Third Dimension world in the form of serious illnesses which is called **CLINICAL** illness—the kind that is rewarded with an official diagnosis form the doctor, like cancer etc.

Most people live out their lives at the **SUBCLINICAL** level, which is the twilight zone **between** true health and official dis-ease—a world where **abnormal** is accepted as normal. We think and talk about the way we feel in terms of black and white, but we LIVE out our lives in shades of *gray!*

Microbes

Aerobic and *anaerobic* states of being dictate health and dis-ease. The *aerobic* state is a right-spin condition, while the anaerobic state is a lift-spin condition. These "states" of energy existence determine what **type** and **stage** of microbe (bacteria, virus, or fungi) that will **develop, inhabit**, and **PROSPER** in the body of man, animal, and plant.

Pathogenic **microbes LIKE an anaerobic environment. They are blamed as the cause of dis-ease, but they do NOT cause dis-ease. Instead, they are only actors fulfilling the roles that YOU & I dictate to them as a result of our chosen lifestyle and habits.**

If we dissect the word pathogenic we get: *path*-suffering, disease. *gen*-producing, giving rise to. *ic*-pertaining to.

When a condition is described as pathogenic, it is a "diagnosed" condition that displays certain **agreed upon** SIGNS. This makes it a CLINICAL condition.

Pathogenic conditions are described as *morbid* conditions, hence, the term *morbidity* as used in life insurance company morbidity tables to predict death rates among a population. A *pathologist* is a specialist in *pathology:* which is the study of the nature of disease, its causes, processes, effects, alterations of tissue structure and function.

Microbes

Microbes change form according to THEIR environment and OUR state of health. Thus, the terms polymorphic or pleomorphism. A body with a right-spin energy *footprint* supports aerobes that help us maintain peak health. Aerobes are non-pathogenic microbes that like an oxygen rich environment. If our energy *footprint* becomes left-spin and anaerobic, aerobes change form and become **an**aerobes (microbes that demand *oxygen free* environments), or facultative **an**aerobes (microbes that can tolerate oxygen, but don't require it). Pathogenic microbes are "once friendly" organisms that turn against us with a vengeance. They include viruses and fungi, and all of them—friendly or otherwise—exist in the blood of man, animal, and plant. We carry in our blood the SEEDS of our own destruction. *"The sins of the father shall be with us to the tenth generation [and beyond]."*

A constipated colon is an **an**aerobic arena that was formerly *aerobic*. The following polymorphic microbes are common in the human body. Staphylococcus is an aerobe that is involved in skin infections. Clostridium is a facultative anaerobe that produces **entero**toxins (*entero:* related to toxins of intestinal origin) that are responsible for deadly botulism. E. coli is a colon bacteria that is crucial to good health, can turn and kill easily.

The job of pathogenic life forms is to ATTACK the organism (YOU & ME) when we are weak and under stress and remove us from the face of the Earth. This is why people who exercise enjoy better health. Exercise delivers air and nutrients to the cells, and removes metabolic wastes and CO_2 via the lymph and blood to the liver, lungs, and kidneys for disposal.

Cavities • Dental Plaque

Cavities and periodontal conditions like gingivitis, pyorrhea, and bleeding gums are the result of microbial activity in the mouth. The bacteria that create cavities secrete a protective substance that shields them from air (oxygen) while they dissolve the enamel on the teeth. These facultative bacteria **create** the environment they need to do their dirty work. They can *only* do in a low pH saliva environment. *(Periodontal conditions are easily treated with a bio-magnetic dental irrigator in your own home See Source Index.)*

Low pH saliva, blood, or urine is indicative of a body under stress. pH outside the norm **translates** to a life of sub clinical illness or clinical dis-ease.

When the hygienist removes dental "plaque" from the teeth, it alters the bacteria's *anaerobic* environment—but it does NOT stop new plaque from forming again. In time, you must return and have your teeth cleaned again. Some hygienists and dentists coat the teeth with plastic to discourage the bacteria from taking root on the teeth. This is helpful, but it does NOT solve the problem and it costs plenty. Coating the teeth with plastic is the dentist's version of *palliation.*

Smart dental hygiene PREVENTS plaque formation in the first place. No plaque, means no decay. Plaque, gingivitis, bleeding gums, and pyorrhea are EASILY prevented and easy to self-treat with a simple, inexpensive device called a **bio-magnetic dental irrigator** (see page 204 & Source Index).

Instead of spending $75-150 dollars twice a year to have your teeth cleaned, why not equip your home with a *bio-magnetic irrigator* and wash your problems down the drain? This inexpensive dental device can save a family a fortune in dental bills. All you need is tap or BEV water to go with it.

You can even use the dental irrigator to clean your dog's teeth—that is, with the animal's own cleaning tip, of course. Veterinarians charge $100 and more to clean an animal's teeth. **A bio-magnetic irrigator is the best thing in dental care since the tooth brush!** Here is how the device works and why every family should have one.

Magneto-Hydro Dynamics

Plaque is a negative energy field. The coating the bacteria secrete to protect themselves has a negative (-) electrical charge on its surface. The hydrogens in the water molecule have a positive (+) charge.

Magneto-hydro-dynamics (MHD) is the *process* used in bio-magnetic irrigation. MHD uses an electromagnet to free up the hydrogen ions (H^+) in the water molecules so they will strike the negatively charged (-) surface of the plaque. Positive charged H^+ protons oxidize the plaque's negative charged protective coat by **stealing** electrons from it—a process referred to as oxidation. As the plaque loses its protective shield, it—and your gum problems—are washed down the drain! **Instead of** mechanical devices that *scrub* the teeth, or common devices that squirt water at the teeth with NO results, a bio-magnetic irrigator works! It can't injure the gums, and won't cause them to recede. It's therapeutic effects will STOP the gums from bleeding, and prevents further deterioration.

The process just described is an electrical event not unlike the rusting of iron or disappearance of aluminum window screens in a salty, ocean air environment. We live out our lives in the physical world, but life and health is decided at the subtle energy level of our existence—a level that is invisible!

Magneto-hydro-dynamics is a blend of vibrational medicine and technology. The process is acclaimed worldwide. The reason you have probably not heard of it is that the dental industry will suffer a huge loss of revenue once people wake up and realize that they can enjoy FEWER dental problems and save a lot of money with a bio-magnetic irrigator in their home.

Use a bio-magnetic irrigator and you will not detect the smell of decay when you floss. The bio-magnetic irrigator is vibrational medicine's answer to dental problems!

Birds Of A Feather "FLOCK" Together

Dis-ease is an expression of negative energy dominance! Contrary to conventional thought, LIKE energy attracts LIKE energy. The sick body tends to become MORE sick unless positive is action is taken to "create" a healthy environment and break the dis-ease cycle!

Low vitality is a negative energy state. Negative energy *activates* viruses and pathogenic bacteria that "FEED" on these energy fields. A toxic body CANNOT experience rejuvenation unless left-spin energy fields are neutralized or flushed from the system. Detoxification and rejuvenation is where it's at!

In a polluted body, positive energy fields are hijacked and used to support and promote dis-ease!

"YOUR" body's bio-electric *terrain* ultimately determines the EFFECT an energy field will produce. The terrain,

NOT the microbes, determines **when, where,** and **how** dis-ease will manifests itself in **"YOUR"** life. Tune-in to your *bio-electric* body and your bio-electric clock will rewind itself while you enjoy *limitless* energy and a young body.

Stress & Attitude

Place a person under mental or physical stress and dis-ease will **explode** onto the scene—not because of the presence of microbes and "bugs," but because stress is an energy condition that caters to the NEEDS of pathogenic life forms. In other words, **stress seeks an outlet**—and it takes the course of least resistance to express itself. It is easier for stress to attack an old injury or settle into an area of the body with a weakness, than it is for it to "create" a new health problem. It should come as NO surprise that conditions like hepatitis, chronic fatigue syndrome, mononucleosis, arthritis, myasthenia gravis, systemic lupis, fibromyalgia (just to name a few), can come out of seemingly nowhere. **Your thoughts and attitude can "create" dis-ease in YOUR life! Don't forget it!**

Dis-ease usually appears in the wake of circumstances that are high stress. We seem to deal with stress when we are under fire, but when the heat is off, dis-ease or illness strikes.

The point is this: body, mind, and spirit are irrevocably linked. Thoughts and attitude are a **potent** force in dealing with dis-ease and the maintenance of good health. A good attitude, however, cannot overcome the problems created by a toxic, under hydrated body.

Under Siege: *Fever*

"I'm sick!" There are two kinds of conditions, local and systemic. An infected finger is a localized condition. But a systemic condition places the WHOLE body under siege, causing it to *revolt!* Systemic conditions bring on things like vomiting, runny bowels, phlegm, chills, fever, and horrid gas.

Fever that accompanies dis-ease is the body's reaction to the presence of a morbid condition and should NOT be considered bad. Contrary to popular belief, fever is good and serves a useful purpose. Fever is an EFFECT of an accelerated metabolic rate. Fever is a condition of **hyper** *thermogenesis* (*thermo:* heat producing; *gen:* origin of; *sis:* condition).

Mucous that accompanies colds and flu the VEHICLE that carries toxic wastes from the body. This is the body's way of surviving. Illness erupts when toxicity levels EXCEED the body's ability to maintain homeostasis. Dis-ease is an out-of-body energy condition.

If it is not allowed to go above 105° degrees, fever does

a wonderful job of denaturing and destroying bacterial and viral proteins. It kills them and neutralizes their negative influence on the bio-electric body. *(Far Infrared saunas, body wraps, and seat cushions help in a similar fashion.)*

Fever destroys bacterial and viral breeding grounds — particularly in the colon (large intestine) and appendix. Fever is the body's way of ridding itself of dangerous left-spin energy conditions. If a fever rises too high, (above 106° F, however, it can denature enzyme proteins in the brain and can be deadly.

Medicine and society have held strange views about the nature of fever over the years. For example, at the time of the American Revolution, people associated body lice with health. When fever got too high, the lice would leave and the person usually died. People and medicine BOTH invoked single factor analysis and came to associate the presence of lice with health. Lice=life. No lice=death. Obviously, this is wrong, but it's a good example of the problems incorrect thinking produces.

Denatured Proteins

If you drop the contents of a raw egg into boiling water, you will see the egg's proteins change form. The egg will become firm and solid. The heat denatures the egg's protein enzymes, alters their form, and causes the egg to become hard. This is what a *febrile* (fever producing) condition does to bacteria—it destroys them by altering their protein enzymes and structure. Alter an organism's proteins, and the organism dies. **Healthful living requires constant vigilance of any energy form that negatively impacts our protein enzymes.**

Muscle Tone

When we become overheated—as in heat stroke or when we have a high fever—protein enzymes are altered and we bed rest is required. Fever weakens our protein enzymes and overdrafts the ionic minerals that are responsible for maintaining **muscle tone.** Muscle tone gives us the ability to stand, hold up our head, or maintain a position. Without tone, we would function like a jellyfish.

The muscles that control the vital organs receive their orders through the *involuntary* parasympathetic nervous system. Loss of tone in the vital organs places the *bio-electric* body under severe stress. The best solution when fever strikes is colon therapy. Colon therapy includes colonics and enemas. **It is direct, physical intervention designed to ALTER the bio-electric terrain.** A clean colon restores tone to the vital organs by creating a low stress environment in the bio-electric body.

Medications

Antibiotics, aspirin and other forms of **chemotherapy** (chemical therapy) alter body function and accelerate aging. Their use is detrimental to the long-term maintenance of balanced body metabolism. Despite the *apparent* positive results they produce in the short term, their long term side effects will eventually be seen in the mirror.

Drugs are prescribed, but they are not safe. ALL drugs have **known** side effects. They are prescribed on the same basis that is used to justify the chlorination of public water supplies, or the spraying of our crops with poisons. If the benefit outweighs the risk, the drug is prescribed.

What is NOT mentioned is the long term effects of drugs on the vital organs and glands. Older people—particularly those in nursing homes—take as many as FIFTY (50) pills a day. The side effects of these left-spin substances is beyond comprehension. Drugs are *disastrous* to the bio-electric body and the **LIVER** in particular.

New drugs are pushed by the pharmaceutical companies to replace those whose patents have expired. These new drugs are MORE expensive and each new generation of "new" drugs carries ever increasing risk. We have been taught to differentiate between "prescribed" drugs and illegal drugs like cocaine, LSD, etc. There is little difference between them.

"How To Stay Healthy Until It Is Time To Die"

Personal survival demands we learn to live our lives in harmony with nature so we have NO need for *legalized* drugs.

Do you know anyone who has suffered horribly from the side effects of drug therapy, or maybe someone who walked into the hospital or clinic for testing and was carried out—feet first? If you apply the lessons in this book, you can avoid falling prey to the *vulturous* medical system.

Drugs are drugs! They diminish liver function and burden the kidneys. They do violence to the kidney's nephrons (the filter units that clean the blood). They destroy the liver's hepatocytes (the functional cells process the tens of thousands of *bio*chemical reactions that keep us alive and healthy.

A body suffering from dis-ease is a body under siege, and drugs only force the vital organs to do double duty as they destroy organ function.

Vibrational medicine and the natural approach avoids chemical drugs, instead opting to use homeopathic remedies (resonating energy fields), **food** based energy supplements that don't stress the system, and natural modalities like colon therapy, therapeutic touch, magnetics, qi gong, tai chi, massage, lymphatic self-massage, rebounding, BEV water, fresh air, and herbs, just to name a few.

Colon Therapy

An enema is the short and quick version of a colonic, which is similar to a DEEP enema. A properly executed colonic will cleanse the rectum descending, transverse, and ascending colon, plus break loose the mucoid waste in the cecum that often interferes with the ileocecal valve (the cecum is the fist-sized pouch from which the appendix hangs—see page 46). A good colonic that reaches the ileocecal valve penetrates 6 feet into the body.

The small intestine ends and the large intestine (colon) begins at the cecum. Undigested food and wastes enter the colon by way of the *ileocecal* valve that separates the two. **People with cancer usually have their ileocecal valve "locked" in the open position.**

One of the primary goals of colon therapy is to shed the colon lining and mucoid material that often blocks the ileocecal valve and prevents it from closing. *When Yucca extract is used along with enhanced PAC's, shedding of the colon lining becomes faster and easier.*

The second and equally important goal of colon therapy is to stimulate peristaltic activity and cause the liver and gall bladder to dump bile. The "stirring" action of a colonic may cause temporary upset due to poisons that are loosened and brought into circulation. The use enhanced PAC's, has remedied this former problem.

An enema is NOT a substitute for a colonic. Enemas purge only the lower foot or two of the bowel. However, their effectiveness should not be underestimated. Every person should own a five dollar enema bag and take it with them whenever they go out of town or traveling. Water, the bag, and a motel bathroom are all that is needed to save a visit to the hospital, or Montezuma's revenge.

Colon equipment is more expensive, but it lasts a lifetime. (I've had mine for 15 years!) It is easy to use and nicer than lying on a towel covered floor and having to get up and down to fill the bag which only holds a quart of fluid, and **hoping** you make it to the toilet before you release your bowel.

It's nice to do your own "colonics" in the privacy of your own home. Clinics often charge one-hundred dollars or more per visit—IF you can find someone willing to do it. At home, you have the benefit of using BEV water, Kombucha tea, Rene's Tea or coffee—yes, coffee!—as the cleansing solution.

Colon therapy is a remedy that has PROVEN itself over and over again. It speeds the rejuvenation process. Everyone should equip their home with colon equipment because colonics are better than any pill and the equipment lasts a lifetime. In the case of severe illness, colonic equipment can save your life. Colon therapy may be un-American, but I am here to testify that it is the most effective way to buy back those lost years and maintain a hold on vibrant health. Do them regularly, and you will **SHOUT,** "I feel good!" as you become *Young Again!*

PREVIEW: *Our next chapter deals with the HIV virus and its progeny, AIDS. There is an important connection between "weeds" and viruses.*

Dogs • Cats • Horses

Animals are no different than people. They suffer from the same physiological problems that humans do and their bodies respond and rejuvenate similarly.

Arthritis in pets results from toxic waste buildup in the joints and connective tissues. Diabetes is the end product of hormonal imbalances and toxic excesses. Hair loss, mange, skin conditions, etc. indicate failure of the liver to dispose of excess wastes. Distemper is a viral condition similar to AIDS, mononucleosis, hepatitis, and a dozen other blood related conditions. Obesity represents metabolic slow down of the entire system.

Pets respond quickly to PAC's, Yucca extract, and Klammath alga in their diet. They should also be given liquid ionic sea minerals in their water. Rene's tea (for virus infections) is administered by intravenous drip with the help of your veterinarian. Squirt Yucca down the throat with an eye dropper. Give one squirt per day for small dogs, two squirts for medium sized dogs, four squirts for large sized dogs. Your pets will love you.

Out Of Country

If you travel out of country, go prepared. Take along enhanced homeopathic remedies for viruses, bacteria, Ricketia (spider and insect bites), plague, acute stress (physical or emotional), and systemic organ and glandular supports for your bio-electric body.

Enhanced homeopathic remedies are good insurance, so don't leave home without them!

Statistics & Palliation

It's difficult to discuss "health" with people who have been schooled in the scientific method. It's not that they are anti-health—they are not. Rather, their world is built upon medical statistics and studies. Theirs is a world of numbers—numbers that prove something is or isn't so. The *passwords* into their world are "statistics show" and "scientific proof."

Medical science sees health and dis-ease in terms of single problems that demand single answers based on "findings." Medical science demands that "health" people play their statistical games or suffer the ridicule of "no scientific proof."

Anyone with a lick of sense knows that you must take care of yourself or good health falters and dis-ease results. "Health" minded people know that if you eat nourishing food, drink plenty of pure water, get enough exercise and rest, entertain positive thoughts, keep your bowels clean, and do the things we have discussed, you will enjoy excellent health. **Our PROOF is *healthy* human beings living in accordance with nature's laws.**

Medical science sees "health" as a numbers "game." Their games keep the public confused by dazzling them with skewed studies and statistical gymnastics. **Their PROOF is millions of subclinically sick people who *bear witness* to medicine's "findings."**

Palliation lends itself to the numbers game called "statistics." *Palliation* (see glossary) is a powerful tool of *manipulation* in the hands of medical science. *Palliation* allows science to state its case in the short run and make health claims with total impunity.

Medical science **knows** the risks that accompany drug usage. However, drugs provide credibility and "scientific proof." Without these tools of manipulation, medical science would lose its strangle hold on the people and the endless cash flow that derives therefrom.

Health minded people do not live in fear of medical science's statistics and studies. Rather, we ignore them. For us, they are moot.

We pursue peak health and vitality and we try our best to live according to nature's way. Nature rewards our efforts with peak health instead of subclinical statistics.

We measure results in years YOUNG!

Bio-Electric Vincent

B.E.V. (BEV) stands for Bio-electric Vincent in honor of Professor Louis-Claude Vincent who developed the theoretical standards for the most biologically friendly water known for the human body. BEV water has the following qualities and characteristics.

BEV water is a good source of oxygen for efficient metabolism in the human body. Its HIGH energy molecules deliver potent right-spin energy to the cells.

BEV water is a naturally potent biological solvent of body wastes and toxins. It carries them OUT of the body while serving as both a food and energy source.

BEV water molecules do not allow passengers like hard minerals, trihalomethanes, bacteria, viruses, chlorine, chloramines, fluorides, or toxic chemical wastes to piggyback their way into the bio-electric body.

BEV water is <u>VERY</u> aggressive. It acts like a liquid magnet by attracting wastes to itself.

BEV water keeps the body's cells properly hydrated and resonating at healthy frequencies.

BEV water is made from common tap water in your own home. Quality is monitored with a conductivity meter.

BEV water processing units do not require electricity to work. There are no elements to clean. The system requires minimal maintenance.

BEV water provides health minded people with the means to control their "terrain." Controlling the terrain is crucial to rejuvenation.

BEV water is body friendly and enjoyable to drink.

BEV water is the ultimate liquid food. Other drinking waters simply do not compare (see source Index).

Beating Alzheimers

Beating Alzheimer's is a book worth reading for people who are dealing with this dreaded condition.

Over 20,000,000 people are **diagnosed** Alzheimers dis-ease. It is **projected** that over 50,000,000 people will have the condition by year 2,000.

If you would like to learn how to avoid this curse for yourself or your loved ones, I suggest you read this book today—and implement it tomorrow (see Source Index).

13

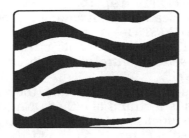

Viruses & Weeds

"There is no difference between plant and animal."
Dr. Guenther Enderlein, 1898

Medical science knows little about viruses. The average person knows almost nothing about them. Most folks think a virus is like a bacterium—a "bug" that you somehow "catch!"

The doctor will tell you that antibiotics hold no power against viruses. If you are sick with a viral infection you are told to stay warm and drink lots of fluids.

The *informed* person will follow this advice. They will also drink copious amounts of BEV water, use colon therapy, and take a hot bath with a cup of Epsom salt, a tablespoon of ginger, a pint of hydrogen peroxide, and on the way to bed take a shot of whiskey. **The informed person does not wait to be told to clean the bowel and flush the body of its poisons.**

In college, little time is spent discussing viruses. They are poorly understood by the student, and probably by the instructors, too. NOTHING is taught about how to deal with them on a practical level.

Viruses Today

We hear a lot about AIDS, influenza, herpes, Hepatitis B, Chronic Fatigue Syndrome, Epstein-Barr Syndrome, and mononucleosis. These are *here and now* viral conditions.

The best cure for any type of viral condition is prevention. Short of a clean healthy life style, we MUST focus on the **conditions** under which viruses prosper. We need to understand the connection between these "fringe" life forms and the aging process. We need to develop an *energy* perspective.

The virus is an anomaly, a paradox, and a slave master. It's the point man of nature's garbage crew. A virus is NOT a life form, but it is not dead either. It cannot reproduce on its own, but it is OPPORTUNISTIC—as are bacteria and fungi. In other words, when WE create a suitable environment, the virus springs to life by *seizing* control of the cellular machinery at the subtle energy level.

Viruses are energy fields and they have an energy *footprint*. A virus is a strand of either DNA (deoxyribonucleic acid) or RNA (ribonucleic acid) that is protected by a protein capsule (energy shield), but this is an incomplete picture.

Viruses exist in the *grey* area between living and non-living things and cannot reproduce or perform normal life functions on their own. Viruses are *entirely* dependent on energy generated INSIDE the cells of the target host's body.

Viruses are classified based on their composition (DNA or RNA), origin, mode of transportation, reproduction methods, and where they first manifest themselves in the host.

Viruses are so small that it takes an electron microscope to view them. Because they are ubiquitous, there is NO avoiding them. In a healthy body, viruses do not pose a threat to the host because the "terrain" is not suitable for viral growth. Consequently, viruses *cannot* access the host's cellular machinery. This applies to animals and plants alike.

However, when we are under mental or physical stress, we disrupt our energy fields and we turn off our protective shields. The immune system is one of those shields.

The immune system can overcome viral activation and it can restore homeostasis, but only IF we provide the environment that supports rejuvenation.

Viruses—like their cousins bacteria and fungi— have a job to do. Their job is to rid the Earth of weak life forms—be it plant, animal, or human!

HIV & AIDS

HIV (human immuno deficiency virus) is the virus that is associated with AIDS (Auto Immune Deficiency Syndrome). HIV uses an enzyme called *reverse transcriptase* that allows it to work in *reverse*. This is why HIV is called a **retrovirus** (*retro* means after the fact, in reverse). As the HIV virus mutates, it is given other names like HTLV 1, HTLV ll, HTLV lll, etc. HTLV stands for human T-cell **lymphotrophic** virus.

Dissected, the word *lymphotrophic* looks like this: **lymph**-the watery, clear fluid in the blood minus the blood corpuscles (think of the clear fluid that oozes when a wound is healing). **troph**-a change or a turning; **ic**-pertaining to. A lymphotrophic virus then, causes a *change* in certain cells within the lymph fluid.

The T-Cells

HIV has an affinity for our T-(helper) cells, which are lymphocytes, and originate in the *thymus. Cyte* means cell. So a lymphocyte is a cell in the lymph fluid. In this case, we are speaking of the T-cells. Viruses wage war in the plasma proteins of the "lymph" BEFORE the war spills over into the blood, which explains why some blood samples test negative.

An energy shift from positive to negative in the *lymphatic fluids* produces a similar shift in our health. A weak immune system is the equivalent of Captain Kirk dropping the star ship Enterprise's defense shields. Bio-junk food—including things like soy and canola oils—weaken the immune system and alter T-cell function. A weak immune system is an open door to dis-ease.

AIDS Not A Virus

AIDS is not a virus. It is a *syndrome* of secondary conditions brought on by the HIV virus infecting and weakening our immune system (T-cells). HIV is an adenovirus (*aden*-a cavity as in the lungs or chest). This class of viruses is OPPORTUNISTIC and usually results in death from infections of the chest cavity, as in *pneumonia.* You do not die from AIDS, but from secondary complications like pneumonia. Actually, you die when cellular oxidation at the mitochondrial level cannot produce enough right-spin energy to keep you alive. In other words, we die from the inability to neutralize, buffer, and overcome the build-up of TOXIC waste energy negative forces that synchronize our bio-electric grid.

Once the HIV virus manifests itself, a "syndrome" of conditions called AIDS develops. Contrary to popular belief, AIDS is not a dis-ease of homosexual origin. Little of what the public has been told about AIDS by the "experts" is true. Much of the information about AIDS and other "new" dis-eases is "disinformation" purposely disseminated to keep the public confused. **ONLY a correct understanding of body physiology and energy management will end medical science's strangle hold on mankind.**

Sabotage

Retroviruses, like HIV, enter and sabotage the cell's genetic information base (DNA or RNA) and then use the cell's ENERGY to take-control and reproduce its self. This is not what nature intended for life on Earth. On the other hand, the virus' job is to kill and rid the Earth of weak organisms! Viruses proliferate in a toxic body, which explains why colon therapy is so important to reversing the aging process.

Viral proliferation in the body is *confirmation* that things are not right. It should cause every THINKING person to deduce that the environment must be *"au fait"* (favorable) or viruses would not be proliferating.

The problem is the "status" of the *bio-electric* body— NOT the presence of pathogenic life forms. Viruses only attack people who are polluted; people who eat DEAD, poisoned food. They attack people who are malnourished, constipated, and anaerobic. They attack people who do not get enough aerobic exercise and fresh air, or who fail to drink enough biologically "friendly" water, like BEV.

Pathogenic life forms (viruses, bacteria, yeasts, and fungi) act like invading armies when "opportunistic" circumstances develop. However, they are not invaders at all. Rather, they are indigenous to our blood.

Blood NOT Sterile

Contrary to medical teachings, the blood is NOT a sterile medium. Medical science has fostered this mistruth in the face of irrefutable evidence to the contrary. Anyone interested in verifying this should read *Hidden Killers* and *The Prosecution and Trial Of Gaston Nassens* (see Source Index).

All life contains the seeds of its own destruction within its own fluids. That is why Dr. Enderlein said, "There is NO difference between plants and animals." He understood that when the terrain of man, animal, or plant loses its energy "balance," the bacteria, viruses, and fungi **automatically** begin a dis-ease cycle that involves the metamorphosis of new, and different pathogenic life forms from **WITHIN** the fluids of the organism itself.

The pharmaceutical companies and the medical system will lose billions of dollars if this simple TRUTH ever becomes widely known. **Recognition that the blood is NOT sterile is tantamount to open refutation of the Germ Theory of Disease.**

Pride and greed prevent medical science from refuting its false theories. Millions of people have suffered and died needlessly. Millions more will follow. Life was meant to be a celebration, not a requiem. The choice is yours.

Cell Electrical Charge

Strong, positively charged cells and tissues are not affected by viruses. Tissues that are waste stressed and anaerobic are attacked by viruses because they have low electrical vitality and poor resistance. Cells and tissues that are compromised have weak enzyme function and insufficient oxygen. It is under these conditions that viruses take over the cell's machinery and reproduce themselves.

Viruses *steal* the body's energy and use it to multiply and form cancers. Cancer tumors and masses are HUGE fields of *negative* energy that control all metabolism within their sphere of influence. **Cancer viruses proliferate in a body that is anaerobic AND whose cells are loaded with sodium.**

An *anaerobic* body is an OLD body. Old bodies RESIST becoming *Young Again!* Dis-eases are energy wars and the bullets they shoot are negative energy bullets. Cancer plays by its own set of rules. Conventional medicine's "magic bullets" are worthless in this arena. The PROOF is all the dead and dying people! The solution is a healthy lifestyle and immediate detoxification of the tissues and fluids. **Ignore conventional medical wisdom and you will live a long and happy life.**

Useful Oxygen Forms

Hydrogen peroxide (H_2O_2) and ozone (triatomic oxygen, or O_3) are useful products. Their effectiveness is related to the amount of oxygen that is available for therapeutic healing and their unstable molecular structure. Instability allows them to give up their oxygen atoms freely. Oxygen is a highly magnetic element, which accounts for the "bent" or "polar" shape of the water (H_2O) molecule (see page 79).

Oxygen therapy has some effect on cancer **masses,** but little effect on **tumors.** Skilled healers sometimes inject H_2O_2 or O_3 directly into cancer masses with good results. Given intravenously (in the veins), or by infusion in the rectum or vagina, these therapies can be highly effective. Oxygen works best when it is **combined** with other modalities.

One VERY promising—and safe—oxygen modality calls for inexpensive equipment that produces medical ozone (O_3). An ozone generator detoxifies the air and helps people with respiratory problems to breathe easier and have more energy. Emphysema patients respond almost immediately. Phlegm and mucus ceases to be a problem.

Therapeutic ozone destroys pathogenic molds, fungi, yeasts, and viruses. Cigarette odor is completely neutralized. An ozone generator is a good investment against winter illness and can save a family thousands of dollars in medical bills.

Recent advances have produced ozone equipment that is inexpensive and easy to use. Ozone is made from the same air that we breathe. A good ozone machine also works as an ion generator that cleans the air of dust and carpets of life forms so they can be vacuumed away. Self cleaning units are the simplest and best (see Source Index).

Exercise & Viruses

Aerobic exercise is extremely important in the fight against viral related dis-eases. Exercise increases lymph and blood fluid circulation and raises plasma and cellular oxygen levels. It also revitalizes the organs and glands while it speeds detoxification of the system. **People who exercise regularly suffer fewer viral infections and enjoy better health.**

Much has been written on the benefits of aerobic exercise. Recently , however, the press is parroting the idea that we don't really need aerobic exercise. A recent article read, *"The benefits of aerobic exercise have been overstated. People can get all the exercise they need cleaning the house, or walking out to dump the trash."*

Nothing could be further from the truth! This is a "disinformation" campaign at the expense of the public. If people buy into the NO aerobic exercise line, they will suffer needlessly and grow OLD! At the same time, exercise experts are now parroting the benefits of "hyper" aerobic exercise. Do not listen to them. Instead, seek *moderation* and *balance* in your exercise life. **Hyper anything translates: *abuse!***

Good circulation is a prerequisite to good health. Blood and lymph movement negates waste build-up in the system and creates a hostile environment for pathogenic life forms.

There are many brands of aerobic exercise equipment on the market. Find a good one and use it daily.

Rebounding

A rebounder is a mini trampoline. It is THE most important piece of health equipment you can own because it can move massive amounts of lymph fluid. A rebounder is approximately thirty six inches in diameter and stands about six inches off the floor. The correct way to use a rebounder is to stand flat footed on the mat, begin gently swinging the arms **together** from front to rear, and then add a very slight bounce with the body. Do this for five minutes morning and evening.

Rebounding prevents stagnation of wastes, particularly in the legs and head. Water follows the waste and edema (excess fluids in the tissues) follows.

Rebounding is a vital step in the regeneration of hair, hearing, normal eyesight, and attractive skin. Considering that the head receives 40% of the blood leaving the heart, it's easy to understand why the very fine capillaries of the scalp, eyes, and ears become clogged and SIGNS of old age—balding, loss of hair color, wrinkles, poor hearing, and visual problems—appear. Dietary intake of soy and canola oils clog the capillaries slow fluid movement.

Rebounding should be immediately followed with special self-massage techniques to force lymphatic wastes into the blood so the liver can flush them via bile secretions. Yucca extract, PAC's, and fresh lemon help the most in this area.

Viruses & Food Molds

Have you noticed the vegetables and fruit being sold in the grocery stores are growing strange molds? Molds that cause food to rot almost before you can get it home and eaten? Molds and viruses tell a story.

According to Leonard Ridzon, molds are the lowest level of parasitic growth. Mold color determines the toxicity level of the substance it is consuming. White molds grow on the least toxic substances. Red mold grows on the most toxic substances. Grey, black and green molds are in between. Fuzzy, smooth, and shiny molds tell a similar story.

The agricultural *experts* have been in charge of our food supply for a very long time. They have convinced the farmer to use hard chemical fertilizers, pesticides, and herbicides. All of these potent left-spin energy substances affect mold growth and the energy footprint of the food we consume.

The *experts* have upset nature's balance, and in so doing have brought marginal health and dis-ease upon us all. We are aging faster because we are eating "expert" food that does not nourish us. Instead, it poisons us! These are the same *experts* whom Rachel Carson vilified in her 1959 blockbuster book, *Silent Spring*. This book is must reading if you would like to better understand the nature of the dilemma we face. Silent Spring is more pertinent today than when it first appeared (see Source Index).

Fresh fruit has little flavor. Mineral levels in our foods are low. Dis-ease proliferates. The *experts* tell the farmers to use chemicals to ward off the bugs and weeds. The more they throw at the bugs and the weeds, the stronger they come back!

Nature will NOT be mocked, and mankind is paying the price.

Weeds & Aging

Look at the weeds. They are proliferating at astounding rates in the face of voluminous amounts of herbicides. Each year, the weeds return bigger. They are mutating. They have a job to do. They are getting ready.

Leonard Ridzon is a farmer. He is close to the Earth. He is a living Wizard and the most original thinker I know. He is also the author of the books, *The Carbon Connection* and *The Carbon Cycle*. Both are must reading (see Source Index).

Ridzon has recorded ragweed over forty feet tall! Weeds are to the soil what pathogenic life forms are to the body. They attack and take over. They appear to be the problem, but they are only reacting to changes in the terrain—the soil and air in this case. Their job is to protect Mother Earth and to reclaim abused soil and air with the help of the microbes. It is the weed's job to **absorb** the negative energy fields in our polluted atmosphere and put them in the soil where the microbes can get at them and detoxify them.

Weeds are not plants out of place. The proliferation of noxious weeds is no more an accident than the molds on our fruits and vegetables or the viruses in our body. They are SIGNS. Signs give rise to the diagnosis of dis-ease. Dis-ease unchecked amounts to a death warrant. Dis-ease at the sub-clinical level means a population of weak and sick people.

Answers

Asking a question implies that there is an answer. But without the *right* questions you will NOT get the right answers. There are plenty of correct answers to the questions we have raised thus but you will not find them in the press, scientific literature, or college texts. You will only find the pieces—and incomplete answers. Science asks piecemeal questions—usually the wrong questions—and pontificates piecemeal answers.

If you want to regain control over your health, you must invoke your good sense, seek your own answers, and put into practice the things you are learning from this book. Without the willingness to take action, knowledge is worthless!

Overview

When we create and use poisons against the Earth we wage war. When we use herbicides to kill plants that God put on this earth for a purpose and dare to call them noxious weeds, we wage war. When we foul our air, we wage war. We are at war with every living thing on this planet including ourselves and we are paying the price.

It was a blessing that Rachel Carson, author of *Silent Spring*, died a few years after her book was released. She came from *within* science's camp, and science turned on her—like a pack of coyotes—and proclaimed her a witch. They continue to burn her at the stake for the truth she dared to speak. They are still trying to burn her TRUTH from our consciousness, but TRUTH does not go away. Like the Great Pyramid, it is there!

Anyone with a lick of uncommon good sense knows that things are not right. The hole in the ozone layer is no accident. The hurricanes are not accidents. The floods, crop circles, and crop disasters are not accidents. These things are the direct result of science and money turned to EVIL purposes—and all of the inhabitants of the Earth are paying the price.

Mother Earth Is Vomiting

Mother Earth is deathly sick! She is vomiting Her guts out. She is fighting back the only way She knows how—with viruses and bacteria, abnormal weather patterns, floods, and weeds. She will overcome.

The abnormal pressure created by negative energy forces causes the Ozone Layer to periodically open and close. In this way, deadly energy fields are released into space before every living thing on the planet dies!

Industrialization as we know it incompatible with Earth. Man made energy fields alter life at the *subtle* energy level of our existence. They produce mutations in our children. And Earth and Her inhabitants are CRY OUT—"Dear God, we're sick!"

A Word from the Author... The aging process has many pieces. Camouflaged pieces. Odd pieces. Pieces found in odd places. Pieces that fit together so precisely that when we come to understand *HOW* we become old, it may *appear* to be over simplification.

Not so. TRUTH is simple. That is why *few* people are able to "see" the path—**especially** the "experts" in the fields of science, nutrition, and medicine. It is a straight and narrow path that leads to a place where dis-ease and old age are not. Seek that path and you will become *Young Again!*

PREVIEW: *The next chapter deals with the transfer of energy. Laying on of hands. Microwave ovens. Carpal Tunnel Syndrome, radiation, and irradiation of food.*

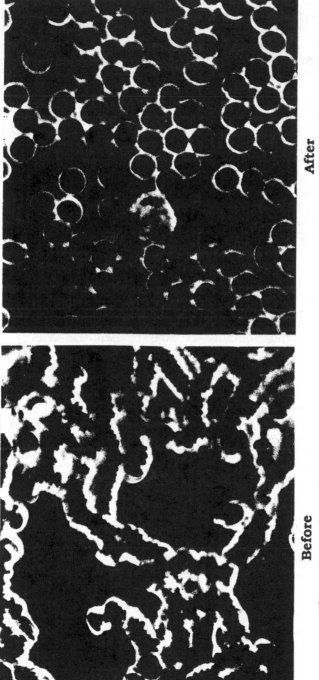

After

Before

Elimination of ***Rouleau*** from *live* blood one hour after drinking water with liquid ionic sea minerals. "Sticky" blood looks like rolls of pennies stacked together. The effect is due to negative energy wastes in the blood. Healthy blood does not stick together and is free to access the fine capillaries of the body and deliver oxygen and nutrients and remove toxic wastes. Photos are of "live" red blood corpuscles (red blood cells without a nucleus). Magnets and magnetic products produce a similar effect on body fluids which accounts for their therapeutic effects. Taken on a Nikon Optithat microscope with a 100 watt lamp and a Naessens condenser at 15,000 magnification.

Drinking Water Comparison

BEV Water: Biologically friendly to body; extremely pure water (up to 99.5% contaminant removal); removes parasites, viruses, bacteria, heavy metals, radioactivity, toxic organic chemicals; no microbial growth; self-cleans toxic wastes; superb flavor; feels "silky" in mouth; energizes body; uses principle of *resonance* to raise H_2O frequency; and principle of *transference* to increase body's activity level; hydrogen and molecular bond angle restructuring; cost per gallon approximately 5-10 cents.

Distilled Water: Biologically dead water; partial purification; water unfriendly to body; concentrates toxic, volatile gases (PCB[s], THM[s], TCE[s], chlorines, chloramines); microbe growth problems; very expensive to operate (uses electricity); very slow; requires continuous maintenance; flat taste; zero energy frequency; diminishes body vibratory rate; zero carbon exposure time; cost per gallon approximately 50-80 cents; parts replacement cost high.

Reverse Osmosis: Partial purification (75-90%); quality and flavor better than distilled water; incomplete removal of bacteria, viruses, and parasites; does not provide BEV restructuring; okay taste; *resonance* and *transference* zero to poor; limited carbon exposure time; cost per gallon approximately 15-20 cents; membrane replacement cost high; wide variation in quality; requires additional stages.

Carbon Block: Purification poor; not self-cleaning; glues in block react with water; serious problems of microbial growth; good removal of toxic organics; fair carbon exposure time; cost per gallon approximately 15-40 cents; replacement cost low, occurrence often.

Ceramic Cartridge: Purification usually good; fair taste; no self cleaning; buildup of microbial and toxic wastes; cartridge subject to fracture and leakage; expensive to replace, occurrence often; no BEV restructuring; low energy water; no resonance, no energy transference to body; cost per gallon 25-50 cents.

Bottled Water: Questionable purity; expensive to use.

"Water is MORE than wet! Water is FOOD!

Fake Hormones

Radiomimetic chemicals are everywhere around us. Pesticides and herbicides are good examples—as are synthetic hormones from the doctor. Food additives and preservatives are radiomimetic. Air and water are loaded with them. People are full of them.

Radiomimetic chemicals *mimic* nuclear radiation. They initiate uncontrolled chemical reactions by stealing electrons from healthy tissues and producing free radicals.

DDT is a good example of a radiomimetic free radical chemical. In a woman's body, DDT is converted into estrogen-like substances that mimic estrogens and raise holy hell in the body. Soy oil and foods do likewise.

In the past, it was difficult to rid the body of unwanted chemical energy fields. Today, we have enhanced PAC's, Yucca extract, and enhanced homeopathic remedies that can expel radiomimetic chemicals—plus viruses, bacteria, and heavy metals—from the body. Systemic detoxification is fundamental to good health.

180° Off Course

We are told to stay out of the sun because it causes cancer, that soy bean oil, soy products, and canola oil are good for us, to take aspirin, that liquid foods are acceptable substitutes for water, that science's version of a balanced diet is good for us, that routine work from house cleaning to dumping the trash is as good as aerobic exercise, not to eat butter, to avoid eggs, that there is no difference between "synthesized" vitamins and those created by Nature in our food, that tobacco and second hand smoke are causing the proliferation of lung cancer, that alcohol in moderation is good for us, to take "calcium" to solve the problems of osteoporosis, that red meat is bad for us, that chicken is good for us, to eat fish in lieu of both, that healthy "processed" food are as good as fresh food, that dis-ease finds its roots in the Germ Theory of Disease, and that genetics controls all.

None of these things are true. Follow the expert's advice and you will grow old fast and die early. All of the above is *disinformation* and *misinformation* emanating from the halls of science, medicine, and the media.

If you want proof that what I am saying is **true**, and what *they* are saying is **false**, look at all the sick and dying people—**including the "experts" themselves!**

14

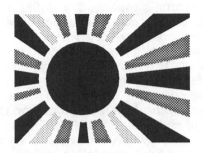

One Day At A Time

"The highest [energy] form of hostile organisms are fungi that are always present in the tissues of a corpse, and often in the tissues of sick patients."
Dr. Guenther Enderlein 1916

We live in a physical world, and we perceive dis-ease to be a "physical" process because we can *see* and *feel* and *measure* dis-ease's EFFECT on our "physical" body.

We know that the bio-electric body is a *composite* body—part physical, part electric. We also know that dis-ease is the manifestation of "conflicting" energy fields where left-spin is the DOMINANT energy circumstance.

The conflict between energy fields occurs in the "invisible" world—a world that we do NOT see even though it is there. The process we call aging also takes place in this "invisible" world. It occurs one day at a time.

Laying On Of Hands

A example of *positive* energy flow between the visible and invisible worlds is the practice of "laying on of hands." Most religions have a version of their own.

Laying on of hands is an example of the power of prayer. It is a *hybrid* practice that bridges the visible and the invisible. It involves the *transfer* of positive energy from a *healthy* person to the body of a sick person. It is a practice that demands tremendous focus.

The event does not always produce the desired change in the sick person. Laying on of hands is NOT a science, but a religious **modality** that has substance and meaning. It involves the transfer of ENERGY!

Often, nothing happens. The suffering person experiences no change in their condition. Lack of results sometimes elicits skepticism and mockery when the event should be recognized for what it is; people with good intentions trying to help an ailing fellow traveler. Few participants understand the electrical phenomena involved, but they devoutly care about their friend or loved one.

Laying on of hands is a phenomenon that involves the **manipulation** of electrical ENERGY. The principles involved are no different than those used when dowsing for water, or using a pendulum to determine left vs. right-spin substances—except that it takes place in a religious environment. All of these practices involve energy and intense "focus." Positive results are called *miracles*. We do not fully understand the forces of the *invisible* world.

In the religious arena, people accept healing at face value and without explanation because the end result is beneficial to them. We must also come to accept the benefits that derive from the manipulation of *bio-electric* ENERGY, because it, too, is beneficial to us.

If healing could be produced by way of a black box with flashing lights, no one would question it. We need the same objectivity when we discuss energy phenomena, because they involve energy manipulation, positive thinking, and focus. When we combine mental focus with physical touch—as in laying on of hands—good things happen whether it be in church, a hospital, or in the presence of a healer.

Therapeutic Touch

The Nursing Process makes use the phenomenon known as *therapeutic touch.* This involves the use of *touch* when caring for the sick—like laying on of hands. It is not always effective, but is effective enough that it is taught in nursing schools and used in daily practice by caring health practitioners.

At birth, touch is our most highly developed sense. Babies acknowledge the touch of another human being. When touch is combined with genuine care, the practitioner can "open" congested energy areas in the body and redirect electrical energy for purposes of healing.

First, the nurse assesses the person's energy state using *gut* instinct and the "reading" of energy auras. The nurse then promotes healing in the patient by opening up body meridians so *Chi* energy can flow. Chi is the energy of life. Therapeutic Touch brings results and heals people. Think of someone in whose presence you feel loved and whose touch—a hand, a hug—can make you feel safe, healed, free of your fears. Therapeutic touch is similar. In order for healing to take place, however, both parties must "tune in" to each other.

We are talking about the use of ENERGY manipulation in healing. Science pronounces it quackery. Nevertheless, it is of practical value to vibrational medicine. Therapeutic touch, dowsing, laying on of hands, measuring energy fields with a pendulum or vibration chain, magnetic therapy, and muscle testing are all energy-related practices.

Reversing the aging process involves the manipulation of ENERGY for its therapeutic effects.

Energy Abuse

The proliferation of *negative* electrical energy pollution is a serious problem. It is a FORCE that has subtle effects and disastrous consequences on the aging process.

Consider the microwave oven. It is very popular throughout the USA and the industrialized world. I remember when it first appeared on the scene. A lot of fluff and excitement accompanied its introduction to an unsuspecting public. It was touted as *the* answer for the mother on the run and the conservation of energy. We were even told of its "health" benefits!

Oh, how I remember the power companies making their case for the marvelous benefits of *microwave age* cooking. Where I lived, they even assigned an "expert" to assist people in the transition from the old way of cooking to the new. Microwave recipes appeared in the *food tips* bulletin that accompanied the power bill.

Few People Questioned

Few people questioned the idea of the microwave oven—except the usual "cranks," and everyone already knew they were nuts. Objections were ignored.

Microwave ovens initially made their way into the schools and other government run operations in the name of *efficiency*. They also began appearing in restaurants across the country. Owners and cooks alike loved them because they were so *people-friendly*. They insured that the food and plates would be piping hot when served. Preparation became easier, too.

Today, you are considered in the stone age if you do not

own and use a microwave oven. These *electrical* appliances are now considered a necessity for people on the run. People love them because they equate nourishment with a hot meal.

Unfortunately, microwave cooked food is neither alive nor life supporting. It should be avoided because its effects are NEGATIVE. The use of a microwave oven is something over which we have TOTAL control—if we choose to exercise it.

Effects Of The Microwave

Microwave ovens are a source of potent left-spin energy. They are dangerous from the standpoint of leakage. They are dangerous from the standpoint of the electromagnetic field they create. They are DEADLY to your nutritional health!

Microwave energy destroys food enzymes by altering their molecular structure. These devices produce an energy frequency that is *anti-life*. It is incompatible with living things, and it is in conflict with good health. When healthy organisms are subjected to these freak energy frequencies, they become *sub-clinically* ill and suffer with symptoms often described as "syndromes."

Food enzymes are combinations of proteins, vitamins, and minerals in an active molecular form. They grant permission for life. In their natural state, enzymes are right-spin energy. The body uses them to build and repair tissue (anabolism). But when microwaves "zap" these living molecules, they become altered and useless to the bio-electric body. When biochemical reactions fail to occur, we age by default. Scrambled enzymes promote aging and death. Their effect is *catabolic!*

Two Seconds

Food cooked in a microwave oven for as little as two seconds takes on the pall of death. When eaten, the body is forced to process these **freak** energy molecules. Freak energy fields must be *neutralized* before the body can get on with the business of life and health which we call *anabolism.*

All microwave ovens are susceptible to energy leakage despite opinions to the contrary from the "experts." Microwave energy is *invisible* and it alters the bio-electric body in the *invisible* realm. It does violence to adults and children who are in the same *room* where one is operating, and the food is toxic to those who eat those *zapped* food molecules.

Microwaved Blood

Microwave ENERGY destroys the structure of the water

molecule—turning a life giving food into an antagonist. It *denatures* the enzymes in blood. Blood is 90% water. Can you guess what it does to human blood plasma proteins?

It was reported that in a hospital in Oklahoma, a nurse used a microwave oven to warm blood. When the blood was given to the patient—he died! Blood is a *living* substance. As little as two seconds in a microwave is all it takes to KILL it. I doubt any "expert" will use microwaved blood to prove this statement wrong!

Police • Carpal Tunnel Syndrome

Lawsuits have been filed throughout the country by policemen who used RADAR guns for traffic control. No one told them about the cancer causing effects of *microwave* energy fields. Eye cataracts and joint problems result from, and are antagonized by, microwave radiation. Microwave created de-generative dis-ease has MANY faces. Microwaves alter the *bio-electric* body in the invisible realm—quietly and slowly.

Do not expect the courts to protect people from microwave devices. Doing so means biting the hand of powerful interests. Faceless experts with adequate credentials can always be brought forth to testify that there is "no scientific evidence!"

Carpal Tunnel Syndrome (CTS) is a big problem for tens of thousands of people. Repetitive activity is often blamed as the controlling factor. Yet, whenever microwave radiation is present the problem is greatly exaggerated. That is why CTS is especially prevalent among supermarket checkers and computer operators—people that are exposed to small but continuous amounts of microwave energy.

Microwaves aggravate nerve fibers and connective tissues (ligaments, tendons, muscles). Some people are affected more than others. Some suffer other "syndromes" that have yet to be given a name. We are concerned with the LONG TERM effects of microwave energy on aging.

Computer Terminals

We hear little about computer induced health problems—except for eye strain. But have you noticed how you feel after several hours in front of one? Tired! Maybe drained is a better word. Have you noticed the number of computer operators who have carpal tunnel syndrome and immune system problems? Did you know that you can protect your immune system by wearing a Super Magnet over the thymus gland?

Super Magnets protect you from alternating energy fields. These special neodymium magnets are imported from

China and are 12,000 gauss strong. Super Magnets are "permanent" fields of DC energy that neutralize the insidious effects of 110 volt radiation coming from fluorescent lights, TV, and computer terminals. Special screen filters help with glare and screen radiation, **but they do NOT alter the energy field itself!** Ergonomic keyboards are not the answer.

Like microwave radiation, not everyone experiences problems from exposure to alternating current energy fields—at least not in the beginning. For most people, the effects are *subtle* and *slow* to manifest. When the bio-electric body can't take any more, SIGNS of dis-ease magically appear out of nowhere and the doctor provides the diagnosis.

Symptoms of electromagnetic pollution are usually *subclinical*. Degeneration occurs quietly and slowly—under cover—until dis-ease announces itself. In the meantime the vital organs begin to die.

[I am wearing a Super Magnet to protect my vital organs and immune system while I process these words. I sleep on a magnetic mattress and use a magnetic pillow. Women use Super Magnets to lesson pain during their periods by taping them over the ovaries (front and rear). Cancer patients use them effectively. People who suffer with sinus problems and head colds place BLOCK Magnets under their pillow to break up congestion (see Source Index)].

FOOD: Radiation & *Irradiation*

The word "radiation" can be used as a verb or an adjective. It paints the picture of energy radiating outward from a central point—like light from a light bulb, but it also describes energy as a "substance."

Fission energy is *radiation* that comes from nuclear devices or their radioactive wastes. This type of fission energy does violence to living tissues and grossly affects the aging process.

People are afraid of fission (nuclear) energy for good reason. Fission energy *ionizes* living molecules. Another word for ionization is *scramble*. *Scrambling* of living molecules makes life impossible and it accelerates aging.

Irradiation is another term being touted in the media. It too can be a verb or an adjective. It describes the "act" of applying *ionizing* radiation to living things. It also infers that energy is a "substance." In the case of food irradiation, negative ionizing energy is used to scramble food energy molecules and makes them worthless. Eat enough ionized food and you will grow old and die early. Radioactive isotopes and waste products from the nuclear industry are the source of the *fission* energy that is used to "irradiate" America's food supply.

The word "irradiation" is a *bastard* term. It has little meaning and it confuses people who are not wise in the ways of crafty wordsmiths. It is a *quasi-scientific* term used to disguise a lie and distort TRUTH.

Irradiation focuses on the "act" involved, rather than on the "effect" the act produces. People think nuclear when they hear "radiation." When they hear "irradiation" they don't know what to think. In the eyes of the public, *irradiation* does NOT mean the same thing as *radiation*. The word irradiation is neither black nor white. Rather, it is *grey!*

The wise person avoids microwave radiation, refuses to eat "freak" food, and avoids subjecting their body to the effects of 110 volt alternating current energy radiating from computer terminals and fluorescent lights. There are several ways to neutralize the effects of negative energy radiation. One of the best is to wear a Super Magnet over your thymus and heart. Other methods are discussed in detail in the book *Vibrations* (see Source Index). Every person should take a **defensive** posture against aberrant radiation fields.

Food that is "irradiated" has NOTHING to offer the *bio-electric* body. Instead, it steals and neutralizes our vital force. When we eat it, the loss is a COMPOUND loss!

Radiation • Irradiation • Genetically Engineered Food

The term "genetically engineered" is a **new** synonym for irradiation. It is acceptable to the public because it sounds scientific and does not hint of "radiation." In future chapters on hair loss, balding, and blindness, you will see that genetically engineered food is no different than irradiated food. Both are "FREAK" energy fields.

The "experts" talk of the wonders of food preservation using *irradiation.* "They" talk of bacterial contamination of food and water from microbes like E. coli 0158.H7 and Cryptosporidium and scare us with bogie man stories. What they forget to mention are the *real* reasons behind the desire to irradiate America's food. They *know* that chemically grown food has poor shelf life and must be "treated" in order to keep it from spoiling in storage and on the shelves. They want to give it a **"forever"** shelf life. People who eat irradiated and bio-junk foods experience the industrial version of "forever."

Irradiated food has a 'forever' shelf life. Its *living* enzyme molecules have been destroyed. The bugs and microbes will NOT eat food whose molecules have been *scrambled.* They can "read" the energy signals given off by left spinning foodstuffs. They are smarter than people. They follow their instincts.

Don't buy irradiated food. Don't eat microwaved food. Learn HOW to use a pendulum and vibration chain to check the spin of the food you buy and to *predict* the effect it will have on your bio-electric body BEFORE you eat it! Every person must learn to develop this skill. Your life depends on it!

Measuring Energy Fields

It is easy to verify the presence of stray energy fields. The following method measures *SOME* negative energy frequencies, but there are many.

To check, connect a radio to a long extension cord and locate a spot on the dial *between* two stations that is *silent.* Next, turn-up the volume to maximum. Lastly, with the radio held in front of you, approach your computer monitor, TV or whatever. When the radio begins to buzz, you have entered that device's *electrical field of influence.* Remember, you are only measuring SOME of the stray radio frequencies. The same effect can also be observed coming from a common electric razor. Our concern is the *length* of time spent in the negative energy force field as well as the *strength* of the field.

When using any electrical device like a computer, stay beyond its field of influence and wear a Super Magnet. The EFFECTS of these anti-life energy forces are very subtle—like the effects of microwave ovens on food molecules. They don't kill you, but they do rob you of your LONG TERM health and vitality. The connective tissues and joints are affected in the early years. Serious problems express themselves *later!*

A two inch thick slab of LEAD can prevent the penetration of nuclear radiation, but it **cannot** block electromagnetic energy fields. *Never* use an electric blanket. If you are cold, solve the problem with aerobic exercise, rebounding, and don't forget to use DHEA hormonal precursors in BOTH tablet and creme form. They work! (more later).

Medicine & Radiation

Radiation therapy and *radioactive chemo*therapy used in the treatment of cancer are devastating to the body. The public has been "sold" on their value by allopathic medicine's propaganda. People get confused and fail to differentiate between diagnostic X-rays and the deadly *misapplication* of nuclear radiation. Radiation is not a "therapy" because it is anti life and "palliative" (treatment of signs and symptoms without cure of the underlying dis-ease), at best. The public has been trained to focus on "hope" instead being told of the violence that is done to their tissues with *ionizing* radiation. The public is being TRAINED to welcome irradiation of their food supply, instead of being told of the plethora of symptomatic illnesses, dis-ease, and death that will surely follow.

Ask The Experts

If the things we are discussing regarding microwave radiation, irradiated food, and genetic engineering are true, why are the *experts* not telling you about it?

The answer is because these areas of risk are NOT being funded for study by the *experts*. The corporate and government GRANT SYSTEM is not about to study anything that might quash the two biggest monopolies in history: electrical power generation and allopathic medicine. **It is up to you to protect yourself.**

Ignorance doesn't count and it most certainly will not keep you young. Aging is the TOTAL of all the *negative* influences in your life. You become young the opposite way that you become old. You become *Young Again!* one day at a time.

PREVIEW: *Our next chapter looks at wrinkled skin—WHY it occurs and WHAT you can do about it. It also discusses body odor as it relates to aging.*

Sex Drive

Loss of sex drive indicates deterioration and atrophy of the internal vital organs. The problem is systemic and goes *beyond* just sexual malaise.

Loss of sexual interest is indicative of malfunction in the ovaries and testicles, prostate and uterus, thyroid, adrenals, thymus, pancreas, and liver.

Secondary conditions like obesity, diabetes, skin disorders, thinning (and balding) hair, unhealthy nails and hair, yeast infections, bowel disorders, loss of muscle mass, and wrinkles are first cousins to loss of sex drive.

There is no question that hormonal imbalances are involved in waning sex drive. There is no question that systemic toxicity is central to all of the above.

To reclaim lost sex drive, one must systematically go about reversing the process that brought about the loss in the first place.

The older you are, the longer the metamorphosis will take to complete. Patience, focus, good mental attitude, and the **willingness** to do whatever is required are prerequisites that precede the return of sexual interest.

Understanding Diabetes

Diabetes plagues millions of people in industrial societies. Yet, in third world countries where people are on native diets, the incidence of diabetes is very low.

Medical science blames genetics for the dramatic increase in diabetes. They are wrong. The problem is fourfold, and genetics is NOT one of them.

Diabetes is the product of dietary **excesses,** loss of the gallbladder, hormonal imbalances, and auto immune problems resulting from immunizations.

Diabetes is **proof** of metabolic slowdown and hormone imbalances. Slow down of DHEA production begins at age 24, followed by a drop in progesterone and testosterone levels. As hormone production slows, metabolism slows, and **excess** waste accumulates in the system.

Type II diabetes is the most common type. It occurs between ages 35 and 55. **These are the years** when women and men *begin* their descent into menopause and andropause. Womens hair thins, and mens hair falls out. Both pile on the fat. Vision problems manifest. Skin texture changes. Sex drive wanes. Muscles turn to flab.

In Type I diabetes (AKA as juvenile diabetes) is a *severe* condition where the child's immune system attacks the pancreas cells responsible for insulin production. It is an *"autoimmune"* condition brought on by the introduction of a **SUPER antigen** into the body. A superantigen is a foreign protein that makes the immune system go crazy.

DPT (diphtheria, pertussis, tetanus) and polio vaccines contain **SUPER antigens** and greatly **increase** the probability that diabetes and hearing deficiencies will develop. It is estimated that up to **75%** of Type 1 diabetes is brought on by the introduction of *mutant* SUPER antigens.

Associated Press recently confirmed that *attenuated* strains of the polio virus *"can and do mutate once inside the body!"* And so do hepatitis B, DPT, and flu vaccines! Vaccines cannot be trusted!

Also, surgical removal of the gall bladder is a 99% guarantee that diabetes will develop within 20 years— **unless** the person takes protective measures against it.

Iatrogenic impairment is another risk (*iatro*-medicine induced dis-ease. *gen*-creation of. *ic*-pertaining to.). So are nosocomial or hospital related infections.

Avoid and treat diabetes through lifestyle changes, use of ETVC, detoxification, hormone precursors, and vaccine*neutralization* (see Source Index).

Magnetics & Good Health

The health minded person can benefit from the use of therapeutic magnetic products.

Therapeutic magnets are stored energy. They work at the *subtle energy level*. When used in mattress pads, shoe inserts, or taped over injuries, they bring relief to suffering people.

I sleep on a magnetic mattress pad because it is simply wonderful! It is loaded with dozens of special magnets in alternating pole arrangements. It can be used on the floor or bed. Some folks prefer a magnetic mattress, instead of a pad. They come in all sizes.

Travelers can use a magnetic seat cushion to eliminate "jet lag" and its negative effects on the bio-electric body. Jet lag is the physical manifestation of electrical interference at the subtle energy level of our existence.

Arthritis sufferers get good results with therapeutic magnets. Combine magnetics with PAC⁵and Yucca extract, and arthritis becomes a past tense condition. Best of all, the dangers of drug related side effects are traded for rejuvenation and a healthy body.

In the 21st century, the use of *therapeutic* magnetism will become a recognized healing modality. There is no reason to wait. It's available today (see Source Index).

Prostatitis

Men who suffer with prostatitis or BPH (benign prostatic hyperplasia) can "solve" their problem through the use of magnetic, Far Infrared, and colon therapies, Saw Palmetto, zinc picolinate, *enhanced* PAC'ˢ, flax oil, hormone precursors, SUPER Mikrowater, and Yucca extract.

How well does this self-administered regime work? Very! Risk? None! Never let the *experts* perform a prostate stab or surgery just to **'have a look'** (see Source Index).

Bleeding Gums • Periodontal Dis-ease

Use a bio-magnetic dental irrigator to solve problems like gingivitis, bleeding gums, and other periodontal dis-eases. This simple appliance transforms water into a *powerful* substance that prevents plaque formation on the teeth and under the gums. No plaque, no problems!

The Healthy Colon
How To "Read" Your Stool

Floaters—stools that float in the toilet. Indicative of excessive fat intake and or inability to digest fats; a liver in trouble; systemic overload.

Stringers—stools that are stringy (narrow-fat-narrow-fat). Indicative of a congested colon, kinked colon, involuntary tightening of the muscles that serve the colon due to nervous tension, high stress, negative thinking.

Pelleted Stool—round pellets. Indicative of slow transit time from mouth to toilet, under-hydration, inadequate roughage, and/or lack of rhythmicity (see glossary).

Pale Colored Stools—Indicative of liver malfunction, viral infection (white stools are seen with hepatitis). Stools should be medium brown.

Bloody Stools—Indicative of hemorrhoids or ulcers, lack of exercise and roughage, colitis, under hydration, lack of rhythmicity, bacterial infection, stress.

Dark Colored Stools—Indicative of slow transit time, old blood from ulcer, colitis, under-hydration, dietary influence from eating dried prunes, raw beets, and greens.

Fat Headed Stools w/Tapered End—Indicative of "pooling" at rectum, under-hydration, ignoring nature's call, lack of roughage and exercise, incomplete evacuation.

Normal Stools—medium brown color, easy passage, little taper, blunt end, transit time within 24 hours.

Complete Stool Evacuation—characteristics of normal stool with nothing "held back." Bowel movement often ends with distinctive pocket of gas.

NOTE: Precede each meal with two prunes and end with an apple to provide a "break" in the stool train. Eat fresh spinach, chard, collards, kale, or comfrey greens daily to create a "gap" in the stool train and complete stool evacuations when the bowels move.

15

Grandma's Lye Soap

"Oh, little Herman and brother Therman,
Had an aversion to washing their ears.
Grandma scrubbed them with lye soap,
And they haven't heard a word in years."
                                    Dr. Roger Lent

The Integument (the skin) is the largest organ of the body in surface area. It includes the **hair** and **nails**, and it is one of FOUR exit portals for the elimination of toxic wastes.

Like its siblings—the bowel, kidneys and lungs—a functioning integument helps prevent the build-up of toxic wastes that would otherwise take the form of acne, psoriasis, wrinkles, skin ulcers, and boils—just to name a few. The skin is the body's first line of defense against dis-ease. When the skin becomes stressed, regardless of the underlying cause, dis-ease soon follows in the wake.

The skin functions much like the lungs. It breathes. It absorbs. **It releases wastes through perspiration, secretion of oil and fats, and the growth of hair and nails**. The blood and extracellular fluids *between* the cells provide the moisture given off as sweat. Sebaceous (oil producing) glands secrete oil and fat based toxins.

Wastes that cannot escape from the body become

trapped in the **dermis** (surface layers of skin) and **subcutaneous** tissues (below the dermis) eventually erupt as pimples, boils, psoriasis, or appear as wrinkles.

Wastes deposited in the connective tissues (collagen, elastic, and reticular fibers that make up the ligaments, tendons, and muscles), cause these tissues to harden and break down. In turn, the skin loses its pliability and shape. Sagging facial skin and sagging breasts are good examples of *breakdown* in the connective tissues. In the joints, the process gets labels like: arthritis, bursitis, and gout.

Collagen makes up about 30% of the body's proteins tissues. The protein matrix into which minerals are deposited to form our bones, is also made of collagen.

Wastes combine with body acids in chemical reactions that promote **calcification** of the soft tissues (calcification is displacement of soft tissues—including the tissues of the vital organs and glands—with mineral **salts** and crystalline deposits). Bone spurs represent abnormal calcification of the bones.

Aging occurs in the blood and fluids that circulate between the cells. These extracellular fluids become known as "lymph" once they are picked up by the lymph capillaries for return to the blood. **Extra**cellular fluid is not the same as **intra**cellular fluid, which resides inside the cells. We will discuss both in more detail later.

Hormonal Shifts & Slowdown

DHEA (de-epi-hydro-androsterone) is the mother hormone. The body it to create dozens of hormones—like insulin, testosterone, estrogen, etc. DHEA is produced by the adrenal glands, but production slows as we reach our anabolic peak, In other words, the descent into old age is directly related to the rate of slowdown in DHEA hormone production.

There is absolutely NO question that aging is directly related to slowdown in hormone production and hormonal imbalances. Anyone who wants to look and feel young MUST come to grips with the hormone issue. I use hormone precursors and "enhanced" PAC's because they work. *(I do colon therapy because it works. I drink Kombucha tea because I've seen what it can do for people. I eat good food (mostly home grown), drink BEV water, and get aerobic exercise because these addendums to my lifestyle provide me with proof that the thing I speak of in this book. R-E-S-U-L-T-S is okay with me!)*

Supplementation with hormone precursors is crucial to controlling the aging process. It goes hand in hand with detoxification, good food and water.

Skin & Wrinkles

Wrinkled skin, flaccid muscles, and loss of vitality are some of the effects of waste accumulation in the tissues and fluids. So is **calcification** and **atrophy** (tissue death; loss of function). In other words, the *functional* cells of the organs and glands are replaced by *nonfunctional* cells, resulting in **scar tissue** formation. These processes weaken the vital organs and renders them incapable of producing sufficient hormones, and enzymes to maintain peak health.

Wrinkled skin is the product of hormonal imbalances and waste accumulation in the underlying tissues.

Old skin, unhealthy hair, and arthritic joints are hardly signs of youth and vitality. They represent deterioration and slowdown in metabolic activity. Wrinkles bother people who want to look young. They are a SIGN of trouble. The beauty industry uses the "mud against the wall" approach by putting collagen in their products, but this is futile. Aging skin and hair are INTERNAL in origin. External approaches (the use of professional grade glycolic acid, racemic clay, and hormone creme) complement internal detoxification measures.

Movie Stars • Glycolic Acid • GH$_3$

As we age, outer skin layers build up and become tightly bonded. The skin becomes stiff and leathery on the face and neck. Cracking and bleeding occurs on the chafe points of the body as conditions worsen—especially with the elderly.

Movie stars resort to face lifts to remedy their wrinkles. They understand that a young face pulls better at the box office than does an old face. The stars also understand that the younger you look and feel, the longer you will be a movie star and be able to enjoy life. We should take our cues from them.

Society is strongly biased AGAINST the aged. People who look and feel young enjoy a big advantage!

Movie stars go to expensive dermatologists for face lifts. They have their wrinkles and skin treated from the OUTSIDE with sophisticated skin care products that contain **high quality** glycolic acid. Glycolic acid is the smallest of the five alpha hydroxy acids. Unfortunately, 99% of what is sold across the counter is the less effective 1-4 hydroxys that get poor results.

Glycolic acid combines with dry, outer skin layers (the stratum corneum) and causes dead skin to loosen, fluff, and slough so it will wash away. Glycolic acid stimulates the formation of NEW collagen in the dermal (true skin) layers. The dermis anchors the outer skin layers (epidermis) to the subcutaneous membranes giving it more tone and the ability to hold more moisture.

The second step to beautiful skin is to use racemic clay to draw out poisons from beneath the skin. The last step involves the use of hormone precursor creme to stimulate the formation of new collagen, elastic, and reticular fibers. Used in this order, the skin takes on a supple appearance. This approach helps people look young on the OUTSIDE while they go about rejuvenating their body on the inside via colon therapy and cellular rejuvenators like GH_3, hormone precursors, Kombucha tea, and *enhanced* PAC's.

Glycolic peels dead skin, racemic clay "draws" out toxic wastes, and hormone creme stimulates healthy skin.

Quality glycolic acid comes from natural products and is hard to find. Stores and beauty lines promote alpha hydroxys with concentrations as high as 30%! The issue is quality, NOT strength. Damaged skin is a common side effect of poor quality.

Racemic clay is a **one-of-a-kind** calcium montmorillionite earth that has many therapeutic uses. For the face, it is combined with aloe, glycerine, and water, and used in sequence (glycolic acid, clay masks and hormone precursor creme) for impressive results (see Source Index).

Urine & Your Face

The term **Acid** is a chemical term. An acid is a hydrogen donor. Natural vinegar contains natural acetic acid. Acids taste sour. Natural acids like those in raw apple cider vinegar and Kombucha tea rejuvenate the body. Read Patricia Bragg's *Apple Cider Vinegar Book* (as well as the Kombucha books from Austria) to learn how to use these amazing natural food products (listed in Source Index).

Natural acids are healing. Urine contains acids that beautify the skin. Scandinavian women are known for washing their face in their own fresh urine! Urine keeps the skin smooth and young because of its **uric acid** content. Urine is a powerful *therapeutic* if used properly. A tube of glycolic acid, some racemic clay, and a jar of hormone precursors are preferable to most people. *[To learn more about the use of urine for therapeutic purposes, read Your Own Perfect Medicine and learn what the medical people hope you will never discover (see Source Index)].*

Aging involves self-digestion (cannibalism) of the body's tissue proteins. "Auto" digestion is the body's way of meeting its *protein* needs. Weak kidney function can also cause a rise in blood uric acid levels.

Uric acid formation stems from deficiencies in vital organ function and dietary overload. Diet plays an important part in uric acid production. So does a shortfall in the production of digestive enzymes—especially in older people.

Detoxification accentuates enzyme production so digestion can return to normal. Older folks should use digestive enzymes. My favorite is "green" papaya which assists in the breakdown of proteins in the stomach. People who suffer with indigestion after a meal find relief in green papaya, yucca extract, and apple cider vinegar.

Rich Man's Dis-ease

People whose diets are overly rich in animal proteins often suffer with gout. Historically, gout was known as a rich man's dis-ease. The rich suffered with inflammation of the feet, toes and hands because they overloaded their systems with too much animal protein and fats. These stress the system and cause the **liver** to form STONES that slow or block bile flow. (Bile is a fat emulsifier and a vehicle for waste removal.)

Learn how to safely flush your liver of stones. Gallstones originate in the liver. Any person suffering with poor health— especially a degenerative condition—usually harbors hundreds of stones. The process is simple and painless, but does require preparation (see Source Index for more information).

Social pressure makes it difficult for wealthy people to maintain a healthy lifestyle. Alcohol, late evening meals, and fancy cuts of meat, often bring on gout. Eating HIGH on the hog is a carryover *cliche* from centuries past. Rich food overloads the body with **purines** (protein waste molecules from nitrogen rich meat, fish and fowl) and overworks the kidneys, causing a sharp rise in blood uric acid levels.

Poor dietary habits, hormonal imbalances, and toxic buildup exhaust the vital organs that produce our digestive enzymes. Alcohol shuts down the liver and prevents it from detoxifying the body of wastes like uric acid.

Excess uric acid in the blood and lymph combines with alkaline mineral bases like calcium and forms salt crystals. When waste crystals settle in the joints of the toes and extremities, they cause inflammation and sheer misery. Gout is a classic SIGN of old age. Medications DO NOT address the cause of gout! They treat only the symptoms! Palliation is the word that best describes science's approach to gout. Unfortunately, no one tells the patient that the medication destroys the liver. **Patients are more concerned about who is paying the bill (insurance), than with what is happening to their long term health. Dumb!**

In the past, gout was not a problem for middle class and poor people who traditionally did hard, physical, load-bearing work. A sedentary lifestyle belonged to the domain of the wealthy. Today, with the advent of the "service" society and the computer, sedentary life styles are epidemic. Wealth and opulence are no longer gout's domain. The middle class and poor now share the misery of gout.

Precipitates like uric acid crystals, gall, liver and kidney stones, and bone spurs are ABNORMAL. They are SIGNS of aging. The body does not handle *precipitates* well. It expresses its dissatisfaction with inflammation, swelling, and pain. In the case of stones, death occurs if they block a duct and are not removed. Stones BLOCK waste excretion from the liver and kidneys causing toxic overload (toxemia). Stone removal has become easier, but technology is a POOR alternative to prevention—even if you have good insurance. It is not difficult to dissolve kidney stones and flush liver and gall bladder stones if the person wants to be healed.

Waste and toxin problems are compounded by poor quality drinking water. Tap water is full of toxic "organic" chemicals and useless minerals in unbalanced form that have NOT gone through the carbon chain (more later). It is best to obtain your mineral nutrient needs from fresh, home grown food. I strongly recommend supplementation with ionic sea minerals (see Source Index).

[Grandma mixed and heated animal fats with lye (sodium hydroxide) and got lye soap through the process of **saponification.** *But when her soap was used in* **hard mineral tap water,** *she got soap scum in the tub. The scum comes from a reaction between the soap and the hard minerals in the water. This is called "precipitation." The scum settles-out or precipitates from the solution. Precipitation of dietary oils like soy and canola creates similar effects in the blood and lymph.]*

Clogged and hardened arteries (atherosclerosis and arteriosclerosis) are like the scum in grandma's tub. Plaques are a combination of chlorine, fluorine, chlor*amines,* oils and fats, body wastes, and indigenous minerals in the water.

Plaque formation in the arteries is a SIGN of impending trouble. It's also the product of a crummy lifestyle and poor choices. Soy and canola oils also play a crucial role in plaque formation and clogging of the fine blood capillaries. We will discuss these devilish oils in great details in future chapters.

Calcium & Fats

Despite medical opinions to the contrary, elemental mineral pill supplements taken for arthritis and osteoporosis are **worthless, at best!** They do, however, create new and different problems in the body. Doctors prescribe elemental calcium carbonate (oyster shell) and citric acid calcium compounds because it "thinks" calcium is deficient. Medicine tries to FORCE the body to accept these unbalanced elemental energy fields. Once in the body, however, they create more problems than they supposedly solve. They precipitate OUT of the body's fluids and help form plaque, bone spurs, and salts that clog our arteries. Avoid them!

Dietary oils and fats are very much involved in degenerative dis-ease and aging. Unfortunately, what the *experts* have told public about fats and oils for the past forty (40) years is in total error! Want proof? Look at all the dead and dying people (more on this in future chapters).

Body Odor

Body odor (BO) is a SIGN of a *polluted* body. It's the result of buildup and secretion of toxic wastes from the tissues, plus the action of bacteria that feed on those wastes. BO is more than socially offensive. It is the **shadow** of old age. When you smell BO, you are smelling aromatic molecules evaporating from the skin's surface.

We first become aware of body odor at puberty. It is usually related to hormonal activity and increased secretion of waste energy fields. BO is closely related to slow down in vital organ function (liver, adrenals, pancreas, ovaries/testes, thyroid, parathyroid, thymus, pituitary, and kidneys). The stronger the BO, the more potent are the toxic waste energy fields. **Strong BO is good reason for concern!**

You do NOT have to be old to have foul body odor. If you are old in body and young in years, you will have strong BO. If you are old in years and old in body, the odor will overpower the best of deodorants. A healthy, clean body has little, if any, BO.

Children have a good sense of smell. They are quick to detect toxins escaping from their grandpa's or grandma's body. They are smelling old age! The young smell sweet and fresh because they are YOUNG—usually in years; for sure in body. Body odor is ABNORMAL. It is symptomatic of internal aging, a sign of *catabolic* activity, and a good indicator of waste accumulation in the tissues and fluids. It is helpful to take note of older people's skin, color, pallor, and lack of vitality. These things paint an unfortunate and sorry picture. They can be avoided or treated with colon therapy, Yucca extract, BEV water, and enhanced PAC's.

People with potent BO can shower five times a day with grandma's lye soap, use the best of deodorants, and get zero results. BO "oozes" from the body as fast as it washed off. *The problem is internal, NEVER external.*

An energy shift to the left in the terrain of the

"invisible" body causes a similar shift to the left in the "visible" " body. We age from the inside out.

As the terrain of the body changes, so does the life forms that inhabit our "not sterile" blood (read *Hidden Killers*, see Source Index). Skin lesions like psoriasis, athletes foot, and impetigo appear on cue as wastes overload the system. These SIGNS of toxicity are best solved through detoxification.

Deodorants & Menstruation

The need for deodorant is a SIGN of internal aging. People who are young in body do not need deodorants.

Anti-perspirant deodorants should NEVER be used. They BLOCK the sweat glands, and cause a buildup of metabolic wastes in the lymphatic system. These deodorants contain toxic ALUMINUM ions that are involved in degenerative conditions like *Alzheimers.*

Note the areas of the body where sweat is heaviest. They are areas of high lymph node concentration—like the groin, armpits, neck, and head. The lymph is our "other" body fluid. It is of equal or greater importance than the blood. Cancer originates in the lymph system and it is impossible to rid a body of cancer if the lymphatic is sluggish or clogged.

BO and cancer are conditions of the lymphatic system. When we detox the body, BO and cancer go away.

Hormones—as well as toxic waste—affect body odor. A good example of hormonal influence on body odor is menstruation. When the female body is flushing itself, hormonal shifts accelerate the escape of aromatic molecules. Humans seldom detect these subtle changes, but animals like the bear can. They have attacked women who are menstruating.

Men experience a monthly hormonal shift in body odor and temperament, too. In men, the equivalent of menopause is called andropause (*andro*-refers to androgens which are **male** hormones. *pause*-cessation of).

Menopause and andropause are the product of atrophy and loss of function in all of the vital organs, but especially in the testicles and ovaries. They are correctly named "the change." Hormone precursors can moderate or even eliminate the hormonal shifts experienced by both sexes during the *change* and make life more enjoyable and less stressful.

At the turn of the century, menopause was called "the climactic" because it represented the PEAK in one's life and a SIGN of approaching old age. When **menopause** and **andropause** begin, aging of the internal organs has **ALREADY** taken place. These are "past tense" terms. Their effects can be eased or reversed if a person is truly committed to it. The body will UNDO and rebuild itself if it is given the opportunity. Only YOU can provide that opportunity!

Women (and men) are aging so fast that it is COMMON for them to experience "pre" menopausal and andropausal symptoms 15 years ahead of their time. The situation is easily remedied, but commitment and patience.

We get a "new" body every 2-7 years. It's up to each of us to decide whether our new body will be stronger or weaker than the one being replaced.

No Sweat

People sweat. Some people sweat profusely. Other people hardly sweat at all. Sweat is a good indicator of how efficiently the skin is functioning as a waste exit portal.

If you sweat heavily, it is a very good sign providing you keep the body adequately supplied with plenty of water and ionic minerals. If you do not sweat easily, you must ASSIST your body to do so.

I seldom sweat. My solution is to spend twenty minutes a day on an aerobic exerciser. This makes me sweat and the exercise promotes circulation of blood and lymph. Aerobic exercise equipment should be non-jarring to the joints. This kind of exercise is a fun and inexpensive way to move body fluids and create a high oxygen state of being.

If your skin does not function as a waste portal for your body, you must ASSIST it or suffer the consequences. The body was made to be worked and used. Failure to do so accelerates the aging process.

Far Infrared Saunas Are Here!

Steam baths and mineral hot springs are a wonderful ways to cleanse the system. So are hot tubs, but they have many limitations including space, lack of portability, electricity, bacteria, and cost. A Far Infra Red sauna from Japan, however, has **ALL** of the benefits of traditional cleansing methods with **NONE** of the problems. Water and electricity are not needed. This new technology rids the body of toxic "acid" wastes. It is these wastes that pave the way for cancer and a thousand other degenerative conditions (see page 366).

Skin: A Two Way Door

In Dr. Dan Skow's book *Mainline Farming for Century 21*, he mentions a question that was once asked in the medical literature. "Given two quarts of water that is contaminated with a volatile chemical at 7 parts per "billion," would it be better to bathe in it for fifteen minutes or to drink it?"

The experts answered, "Drink it because four times more chemicals will enter the body by taking a bath in it than from drinking it."

There is no question that we absorb large amounts of poisons via the skin. Yet, the mucous membranes that line the mouth, throat, and GI tract have a combined surface area that is 600 times greater than the skin AND they absorb more efficiently too. **The experts were wrong!** (Frankly, it was a dumb question because two quarts isn't enough water to bathe in anyway. Reader options should have included "neither.")

The skin is bidirectional. It vents and absorbs. Most people recognize that medications in the form of topicals are easily absorbed through the skin. But few realize the massive amounts of environmental poisons that access the body through the swinging door called *skin*, which includes the lining of the bronchioles and lungs.

[Please recall, the body breathes by way of the lungs (called external respiration) and by way of the cells (called internal respiration). The body relies heavily on the skin as a waste exit portal.]

Most man-made chemicals are toxic to living things. They react with body chemistry because they are negative, left-spin energy on the loose! Most face creams, make-ups, hair dyes, and aerosols are absorbed into the body via the skin and lungs. (Ask a former beautician if it is possible to become toxic through the skin and lungs.)

If chemical toxicity is severe enough, the body will break out in a rash, hives, or develop asthma like conditions. Sometimes death results. The body was not meant to deal with the barrage of poisons that bathe it daily. I strongly suggest that every person learn to use a pendulum and vibration chain to guide your choices and to be able to anticipate body response PRIOR to exposure. This is very simple, but effective technique.

The body has but three options when it comes to dealing with toxic chemicals. Flush them out of the system via the exit portals (bowel, kidneys, lungs, skin); isolate them in body fat; or deposit them in the basement membranes of the skin, arteries and joints—or all three!

Time Bombs

A body that is overloaded with toxic wastes, must opt for a combination of options two and three (above). Unfortunately, these tow options only postpone our day of reckoning. When that day arrives, you notice a lump in your breast, an abnormal pain deep in the bones, or bleeding occurs from the vagina or rectum. It is then that the doctor says, "YOU HAVE CANCER! We must operate immediately," or, "You must begin chemotherapy tomorrow!"

And all you can think about is "Why me? What did I do to deserve this? This is not possible. I'm NOT old enough to have cancer. Surely, the diagnosis is wrong."

BUT, you did have a hand in this story, didn't you? Don't bother with excuses. They don't count! Claims of ignorance won't ease the hell you face! Wouldn't it have been easier—and less expensive—to have learned HOW to take care of yourself so you would NEVER have to face cancer?

Imprint these thoughts in your memory and LIVE by them. Protect yourself through prevention. Neither government nor medicine can protect you. Control your health by "reading" your body's signs and symptoms. In matters of health, never blame others. You alone are responsible.

The "health care" industry is a financially healthy oxymoron. It protects its own health and economic interests. Learn to protect YOUR health and economic interests by taking care of yourself. Be willing to do whatever is called for in your drive for good health and longevity. **Becoming *Young Again!* is a matter of choice!**

PREVIEW: *Our next chapter is about "wildcats." It was one of the favorites of those who reviewed this book prior to publication.*

"Stupid is as stupid does! Take control of your life!"
John Thomas

Bio-Magnets

Bio-Magnets can be used for therapeutic healing and for protection. People suffering from arthritis, prostatitis, sore feet etc. who try Bio-Magnets attest to the effectiveness of magnetic therapy. They know it works!

Bio-Magnets are worn on the body, build into mattress pads, inserted in shoes, and applied to sore joints with wonderful results. Magnets can also be used to buffer stray voltage, and stimulate the immune system, and erase stress from the bio-electric body (see Source Index).

Kombucha Tea

The name *kombucha* refers to a *fungus-like* organism and its byproduct kombucha tea. The Kombucha "mushroom" looks like a waffle. It grows and floats in a nutrient solution of regular or herb tea and white sugar. **Kombucha is a LIVING chemical factory. It converts a left-spin energy field (sugar) into right-spin energy field. The reader is reminded that energy is never lost, it just changes form. Kombucha does to sugar energy what soil microbes do to toxic soil energy.**

No one knows where or when Kombucha originated. Its propagation dates back at least **3,000 years.** Its *therapeutic* properties have been revered in the Orient for centuries, but the West is just now learning about it. It's the "tea" that is used to rid the body of cancer, gout, arthritis, grow hair and return color, and treat other disorders. Its effectiveness is enhanced with *proanthocyanidins*.

Kombucha tea is easy to make, and the organism is easy to care for if you follow a few simple rules. Start with an **"uncontaminated"** mushroom. Avoid give away starter organisms because many are contaminated.

Kombucha tea contains hundreds of enzymes, hormones, and vitamins. The offspring can be used on skin infections, as a facial mask, on bald heads, and as a poultice to treat athlete's foot, to name a few applications. **My family loves Kombucha tea, and so do I. We make about six gallons a week. It tastes similar to hard apple cider. It is carbonated, but non alcoholic.**

The tea in *no way* resembles the original mix of left-spin ingredients, meaning tea and white sugar. The mushroom, or a baby, is used over to make more batches of tea, which takes about 10 days. The process is very simple.

Kombucha fulfills Hippocrates adage *"Let your food be your medicine and your medicine be your food."* Kombucha is a food and a natural therapeutic.

We now have good clinical information (two English books from Austria) about the beneficial effects that derive from drinking Kombucha. Clean, viable, mushroom starts are also available.

I highly recommend that every reader get into making and drinking Kombucha tea (see Source Index).

"I firmly believe that if the whole materia medica could be sunk to the bottom of the sea, it would be all the better for mankind, and all the worse for the fishes."
                                                Oliver Wendell Holmes

Colon Therapy Book

Fifty years of hands experience in colon therapy and forty colored pictures is what the tissue cleansing book is all about.

The colon book should be read by anyone who is serious about health and longevity. If you are new to the subject, or *uneasy* about the idea of colon therapy, this book will help you understand how to set up and do colonics. Colon therapy removes those Howdy Doody lines from the face and put spark back into the sick person.

Ileocecal Valve & Cancer

Six feet up from the anus is the beginning of the colon (large intestine) and the end of the small intestine, (the ileum). Between the large and small intestines is the ileocecal valve.

The ileocecal valve controls the movement of waste and nutrient absorption in the gut. In cases of cancer, the ileocecal valve is "jammed" open by mucoid matter. This causes the cancer victim to starve to death.

Colon therapy clears the ileocecal valve and returns it to normal function, while it rids the body of cancer by mechanically freeing the colon of its mucoid lining.

People as young as 15 years have colon lining. Anyone over 35 years is loaded. If you're 50 years and older, your problem is **beyond** description!

Spell Pycnogenol "Magnogenol"

Do you use pycnogenol? I do, but the one I use is spelled *Magnogenol* with emphasis on the "mag."

Pycnogenol is good stuff, but most products on the market are diluted and the user only gets a "hint" of the possibilities and benefits that derive from their use.

Magnogenol contains 3 pycnogenols plus an awesome complement of other ingredients. It is the most biologically active and cost effective PAC available.

Magnogenol is **both** "fat" and water soluble, which is one of the reasons it works so well. I know of no other fat soluble PAC. **All health conditions respond to its use.**

The benefits that derive from the use of *Magnogenol* are awesome (see Source Index)!

Aluminum Poisoning

Aluminum ions are extremely toxic to the body. Fluoride is used in the production of aluminum. Acidic foods and most waters that come in contact with aluminum cause a chemical reaction to occur. Avoid the use of aluminum cookware or foil.

Aluminum cookware becomes "pitted." The pits are evidence of ions that have gone INTO the food/water (BEV water is destroyed by aluminum). Aluminum cookware that is coated with "non stick" resins (teflon etc.) should also be avoided.

As long ago as 1920, Dr. Jethro Kloss documented the toxic affects of aluminum cookware in his book, *Back To Eden* (see Source Index).The aluminum industry and the American Medical Association reacted violently to Kloss' writings.

The GREATEST sources of dietary aluminum are tap water and soft drinks. **Cities use massive amounts of ALUM to treat drinking water.** Avoid tap water where possible. Never drink soft drinks because their effect on the body is just as damaging as *alcohol!*

Baking powder and foods with alum are loaded with aluminum. RARE is the baking powder without aluminum sulfate. Quick breads/pastries are loaded with aluminum (get aluminum free baking powder at health food stores). Alum is an approved food additive that is on the FDA's "gras" list (*gras* stands for "generally" recognized as safe). Do not depend on others to protect you and your family. Take responsibility for yourself.

In the body, aluminum ions react with toxic waste, attack the *nervous system* and helps provoke *degenerative* conditions like Alzheimers, myelinoma, neuropathy, cerebral palsy, fibromyalgia, myasthenia gravis, etc.

Aluminum detoxification is accomplished with BEV water, colon therapy, and super foods like Klammath algae and Harmonic pollen. (see Source Index).

Breast Cancer

Breast cancer has *NOTHING* to do with genetics, and everything to do with lifestyle. Change your lifestyle and you can avoid medicine's cut, slash, and burn tactics.

16

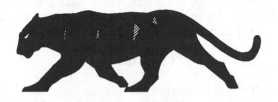

Wildcats

"The skin is to the body, what the soil is to the Earth."
John Thomas

The halogens are known as the "wildcats" of the earth's elements. They are gases, and chemically speaking, they are extremely reactive.

The term *halogen* can be dissected: *hals*-Greek for salt; *gen*-to produce. When a halogen combines with a metal—like the sodium in sodium chloride (table salt)—it forms a salt. When a halogen combines with hydrogen, it forms an acid, like the fluoride in **tooth paste.**

The halogens are IMPORTANT to the aging story.

When the halogens are part of a balanced mix of mineral ions—as in sea water or soil—they coexist in balanced form and do not pose a health problem.

But when man isolates the halogens and they are part of an *unbalanced* mix—as in chlorides and fluorides—they dramatically accelerate aging.

Consider common rock salt (halite) which is sodium chloride (table salt). Nature takes it OUT of circulation and puts it into storage in the earth. Man comes along, mines it, puts it on the dinner table, and defies nature's dietary laws.

Chlorine and fluorine are HALOGENS. They are also gases. When these gasses are dissolved in water, they change their nature by binding with the metal ions and contaminants in the water. Chlor**ine** becomes chlor**ide**. Fluor**ine** becomes fluor**ide**. They have become salts in solution.

The halogens are extremely unstable and chemically

active because they need only one electron in their outer valence shells. To counter their instability, man isolates and stores them as salt solids.

In LIVING systems, fluorine goes CRAZY once its chemical bonds are broken by hydrolysis (*hydro*-water. *lysis*-to cleave or break). It bonds to constituents in the blood and lymph and forms new, **unpredictable** compounds that are hostile to delicate life processes. For this reason alone, fluoridated water and tooth paste should be avoided!

Chlorine

Chlorine is a bactericidal. It indiscriminately kills bacteria. It's a very effective as a disinfectant (for instance, when we bleach our clothes during laundering). Chlorine is used to treat public water supplies. Chlorine is toxic to the liver.

Use of chlorine in public water supplies is justified on the basis of what medical science calls the "benefit : risk" ratio. Applied to the population, this means the benefit to the population as a whole outweighs and justifies the damage done to the general as a whole. *Please keep in mind that benefit:risk ratios keep the hospital stalls full!*

Chlorine's carcinogenic characteristics are well known, and are expressed in the body in many subtle ways. "Subtle" is the word, since no one dies from drinking chlorinated water.

For instance, chloroform is a byproduct of chlorinated drinking water. Chloroform is extremely toxic. It is a broad spectrum poison that indiscriminately kills both good and bad bacteria in the gut and tissues. Chloroform replaced ether as a general anesthetic in surgery rooms at the turn of the century. Both are deadly. Both have been replaced by other "less toxic" substances.

There is a strong relationship between chlorine's introduction and use in public water supplies (1908) and the statistical emergence of heart attacks and cardiovascular disease. The relationship is more than happenstance.

Prior to 1920, coronary heart disease was a statistically unknown in the United States.

Atherosclerosis (build-up of plaque in the arteries) is a chlorine-related condition. The logic of benefit to risk makes it a politically acceptable health problem. This is poor justification for the continued use of this killer.

Chlorine's initial popularity must be understood in the wake of the epidemic of waterborne dis-eases that ravaged the United States between 1910 and 1920—infecting or killing tens of thousands of people. In those days, there were few alternatives and sanitation was poor.

*No one wants to drink water that is contaminated with pathogenic bacteria. At the same time, those of us who are concerned with health and longevity **dare not** rely on officialdom to protect us. Most people in the USA rely on municipal water as their primary water source. More and more people are buying bottled water, which is better, but it is not the answer to the dilemma. The smart solution is to make BEV grade water in your own home with your own equipment.*

Due to outbreaks of E. coli and cryptosporidium bacteria in public water supplies across the USA, the Federal Government is pressuring municipalities and water districts to increase the use of toxic chemicals like the *chlor**amines***.

Chlor**amines** are extremely toxic to the liver. Water with chloramines must pass through a redox (reduction/oxidation) stage to dismantle these tough molecules BEFORE the water is safe for drinking and bathing. Common shower filters don't touch the chloramines. A good shower/bath filter has a 5 micron prefilter and a redox stage followed by carbon and be able to process up to 15,000 gallons (approximately 1500 showers! Common shower filters can't do these things.

When I travel, I carry a small wrench and one of these filters to avoid bathing in toxic water.

Sodium Hypo Chloride

Chlorine is dissolved into public water supplies from a salt block. A salt is more stable than a gas or a liquid. The reason chlorine is used in salt form has to do with "pH," which we will discuss momentarily.

From previous discussions, we know that a salt is a combination of a halogen (acid) and a metal (base). Water treatment protocol calls for the use of sodium hypo chloride. Sodium is an alkaline metal base and hypochloride is an extremely acid form of chlorine. Together they form a solid salt compound.

When the Jekyll and Hyde sodium hypochloride compound is dissolved in water, it separates. The chlorine kills the bacteria and the hydroxide raises the pH so the water will be palatable. The pH of most tap water is between pH 8-9, which is far too alkaline. Good tap water pH should be between pH 6.0 - 7.2. It should also be "free" of hard minerals and toxic chemical residues (pesticides, herbicides, etc.).

The presence of toxic residues and waste minerals results in water that is unhealthy to drink and biologically UNFRIENDLY to the body. Biologically friendly water contains no toxic residues and vibrates at healthy frequencies. The BEV process produces water molecules that are very friendly.

In the summer months, warm temperatures and high pH conditions require municipalities to use mercury to kill pathogenic bacteria (more in the mercury chapter).

Toxic chemicals enter the body **bonded** to *waste* mineral ions. In the body, acidic chlorine and fluorine bond with these toxic passengers and with body wastes and oils (like soy and canola). These newly formed toxins change the electrical charge in the blood and the balance shifts to the negative side as Rouleau appears. When Rouleau is seen under a dark field microscope, Rouleau it's a dead give away of dis-ease in the making.

Sodium and calcium are also players in the above scenario. High sodium levels in the blood show up as hypertension. The sodium eventually spills over into the interstitial fluid BETWEEN the cells, and upsets the sodium:potassium balance in the body. This sets the stage for cancer.

The body requires a **constant** supply of organic potassium. Fresh home grown, organic green leafy vegetables are the very best source of organic potassium. When dietary shortfalls occur, the body *steals* potassium from the cells and sodium invades and replaces it. Sodium invasion slows mitochondrial activity and causes an aerobic (with air) environment to become an anaerobic (without air) one. Aerobic (good) bacteria, like the mitochondria, cannot live in a high sodium environment. Viruses, on the other hand, *love* anaerobic, high sodium conditions, but cannot proliferate in a high oxygen (aerobic) environment.

Chlorinated tap water that is high in sodium tap water is weakening the entire population. There are better and safer alternatives, but powerful industrial interests support chlorination. Our situation today is not unlike the outbreaks of Childbirth Fever in Dr. Semmelweis' time. Chlorine, fluoride, and chlor*amines* are good for business.

Think of the money that would be saved if better and safer alternatives were used to process our drinking water. Consider the human misery that would be avoided. Why, even the water pipes in our homes would last for a hundred years! Ozone is used to treat water in Los Angeles and Germany, but it is very doubtful that chemical interests will ever allow widespread ozonation of public water systems. The problems is this: *Ozone cannot be patented!*

Fluoride

Fluoride is an American Institution, second only to hot dogs and apple pie. Americans have a love affair going with their sweetheart halogen, fluorine (fluoride is its salt form). The question is WHY? *(This book provides the answers for those who care to consider the issues. Maybe a few people who read it be saved before their bodies go past the point of no return. Avoid fluoridated tooth paste and fluoridated tap water at all costs!)*

Industry, medicine, dentistry, and the pharmaceutical companies have done a magnificent job of *brainwashing* Americans on the benefits of fluoride.

Fluorine is THE wildcat of the halogens. It is numero uno—number one—on the list of atomic elements for reactivity. God made sure fluoride was under lock and key by isolating it in underground water and mineral deposits. When man discovered fluoride's industrial uses, he opened a Pandora's Box.

Fluorine is toxic to all living things. Fluoride poisoning (fluorosis) of the tissues manifests itself as hundreds of symptoms. Because it is a "systemic" poison that takes *years* to show up, fluoride escapes blame. Medicine's challenge of "no scientific proof" is an effective cover for the industrial poisoning of America's population. **Fluoridated water is a crime!**

HARD (Teeth-Bones-Skin) HEADS

Fluoride hardens the teeth—and the head. The experts forget to mention its toxic side effects—negative effects that grossly outweigh any conjured benefit. Fluoride has a subduing effect. It "slows" the brain and makes us docile—and easier to manipulate. Fluoride is easily absorbed through the skin and mucous membranes of the mouth, respiratory system, and intestines. Fluoride is a perpetual money machine for the medical system, It creates a never ending line of sick people waiting to fill the hospital stalls so they can get their "magic bullet" cures.

Good medical insurance creates the illusion of security. Reliance on it causes people to forfeit personal responsibility for their health.

A certain toothpaste introduced in the late 1950's, received the endorsement of the American Dental Association. It uses fluoride in stannous form. Stannous fluoride is a tin-containing compound. Tin is a mineral and a metal. When you mix an acid (fluorine gas) with a metal ion (tin) you get a SALT—a crystal. We know that stannous fluoride is a salt because of the -ide on the end of the word. When you convert stannous fluoride—a waste product—from the status of waste to the status of a medically endorsed and publicly accepted pharmaceutical, you have really accomplished something. The profits to be made in a deal like this are immense.

Fluor**ine** is widely used in thousands of industrial processes. Fluor**ide** is the waste product. In the above example, fluoride is the waste product of the tin industry. Fluorine-containing compounds are VERY powerful left-spin energy fields with a signature and footprint that is anti life.

When fluoride **dis**associates, it becomes EXTREMELY unstable. It goes looking for something else to bond to—like our *protein enzymes*. It also bonds with the proteins in the bones and the minerals in the body and slow metabolism.

One of fluoride's favorite habits is to attack the collagen protein fibers that give the bones, skin, muscles, and ligaments their *resiliency*. Wrinkled skin is a good example of the side effects of fluoride. Wrinkles mean the skin is breaking down! (I talk to lots of people who are concerned about wrinkled skin. They don't like it. Yet, only one out of a thousand avoid fluoridated water and toothpaste. Hopefully the reader is plugging into what I am saying. Non fluoridated toothpaste is available and should be in every home (see Source Index).

If you dissolve a bone in an acid, the minerals will go into solution and leave a rubbery like substance that resembles a piece of spaghetti. This substance is the protein collagen matrix into which osteoblasts (bone cells) deposit minerals as the bones are formed.

The bones should NOT be hard and brittle. They should be rigid yet flexible. The little bit of "give" comes from the collagen matrix. Fluorine hardens the collagen matrix and causes the bones to become BRITTLE.

Over a period of years, people who use fluoridated water and toothpaste buildup **"excesses"** of fluoride and discover their bones have become brittle and their skin wrinkled. The *experts* blame osteoporosis, scleroderma, lupus, and exposure to the sun. Their latest trick is to call degenerative skin conditions "connective tissue syndrome." Broken bones AND weak joints are commonly seen among athletes and adolescents. Why? Something has changed. One of the somethings is the fluoride it the water, toothpaste, and in the cute little cup at school and in the dental hygienist's chair. **Fluoride is poisonous. It is also an extremely difficult molecule to remove from water. The BEV process does it!**

Medical science has endorsed the use of fluoride and is too stubborn and proud to admit its mistake. Consider what Sir Arthur Edington once said about the scientific mind.

"Verily, it is easier for a camel to pass through the eye of a needle, than for a scientific man to walk through an open door."

The public does not know that the famous fluoride study about natural fluoride in well water and the absence of dental caries (cavities) was bogus. What the experts fail to mention is that man-made *sodium* and *stannous* fluorides are

FAR more reactive and hostile to living tissues than is naturally occurring fluoride. "Living" systems are dynamic and unpredictable. People are unlike sterile, laboratory test tubes. Heat, pesticides, and noxious dietary oils are present in the body. **Fluorine REACTS with these things and ages us.**

Powerful interests in dentistry, medicine and the pharmaceutical houses influence public policy in regard to issues like fluoridation of drinking water supplies. The insidious *"grant system"* decides WHO gets public monies and WHAT projects science will study—money dictates!

These same powerful interests determine what is taught in the medical and dental school curriculums and see to it that text books are heavily biased. "Power" finds ways to foist its deadly waste products—like sodium and stannous fluoride— onto a trusting and unsuspecting public. The *expert* becomes a patsy and a rubber stamp. Degenerative conditions are assigned new labels to keep the public confused.

Synergy • Synthesis

Synergy is a term we need to understand. It refers to the "combined" action of two or more chemical agents. Synergy can be positive OR negative. Uncontrolled synergy can produce negative consequences for human beings.

Synthesis is a closely related term. It refers to the restructuring of molecules. A healthy, youthful body is the result of *anabolic synthesis* (positive *bio*chemical synergy). Organically grown food, BEV water, and "food" based supplements with a high energy footprints are examples of things that fuel positive synthesis.

Fluorides, chlorines, pesticides, mercury, toxic air, food dyes and additives, soy and canola oils, chlor*amines* and some forms of oxygen can "trigger" chain reactions in the body. If the immune, digestive, and hormonal systems are weak, these reactions go out of control and destroy tissues and cells, and produce toxic waste byproducts. It is impossible to avoid the effects of free radicals. They are ubiquitous.

Free Radicals • Antioxidants • Organic Food

Free radicals "trigger" uncontrolled oxidation of the cells and tissues. The actions of free radicals can be HAULTED by the use of potent **"antioxidants"** called Proanthocyanidins or PAC's. *Anti* oxidants STOP uncontrolled oxidation which is the addition of, or loss of electrons to/from stable cells. Uncontrolled oxidation is "catabolic" activity. **Free radicals cause us to "cannibalize" ourselves.**

Pesticides are an example of free radicals. They are man-made "organic" chemicals. The term is a misnomer. I call prefer to call them poisons!

Pesticides—are organic by definition. The word **organic** is used to describe them because these deadly molecules contain CARBON (atomic element #12). Carbon is the essence of life on Earth. It is immoral to use it to create anti-life substances and call them organic.

Crafty wordsmiths and bogus science jumble terms so their **poisons** will APPEAR to be to friendly to Earth and Her inhabitants. Confusion is the tool. *Unholy* profit is the goal. Sick people, animals, and plants are the result! This is why I keep reminding the reader to avoid and ignore the recommendations of "experts." **Their advice will seal your grave!**

When the term *organic* is applied to food, the implication is that it is "free" of all poisons and that the food was raised using natural fertilizers as opposed to commercial, NPK salt fertilizers. **Organic food is generally better than non-organic food, but it is no substitute for home grown food!**

Everyone should grow some fresh vegetables—be it in pots or a section of the yard. Even small amounts of "live" food have a powerful effect on health.

Doctors & Dentists

The entrenched scientific, medical, and pharmaceutical establishment is at odds with personal health and longevity. They have a vested interest in keeping things status quo so they can bilk the people of their money.

Many professional people suffer from **professional myopia.** Yet, we must remember that they are the product of their training. Also keep in mind that professional people are **"watched"** by their licensing boards. Those who step out of line or put the patient's best interest first are at odds with their fellow practitioners! Doctors and dentists who act on TRUTH must be very careful, and keep a very low public profile.

It's good to know the alternative health care professionals in your area. But remember, healthy people have little need for medical care.

Recently, I moved from a city that had over two-hundred dentists. All of them—except two—use fluoride and mercury amalgam. That's TWO out of two-hundred! The rest claim ignorance. They quote chapter and verse from the medical literature in their defense. They refuse to seek out alternative training and learn to care for people in a humane manner. Most REFUSE to think or act outside of the "accepted" protocols of their profession—even when they know better!

They are caught between profitability and control by the medical review boards. Their patients suffer accordingly.

Many medical insurance carriers refuse to insure people who work in dental offices because of the inordinately high incidence of sickness and dis-ease. The mercury and fluoride they use are Trojan Horses in their own camp—and they pay with their health and lives, just like their patients.

Mercury • Fluoride • BEV

Heavy metals—like mercury, cadmium, and lead are serious business. The BEV process bonds to and removes heavy metal ions, fluorides, and chloramines from the body. Klamath algae, Yucca extract, and PAC's help here too.

French professor and engineer Claude Louis Vincent is responsible for developing the theoretical framework of BEV. His work was further elucidated by Dr. Franz Morell of Germany. Dr. Dennis Higgins translated the theoretical work of Vincent and Morrell into practical reality.

The USA is experiencing a huge increase in neurological BRAIN conditions like Alzheimers, myelinoma, multiple sclerosis, and brain tumors—conditions that were unknown or seldom heard of forty years ago. There is a definite connection between fluoride usage and these degenerative conditions. Fluoride weakens the immune system and assists in the destruction of the *neurilemma* (the membrane sheath enveloping the nerve fibers).

Mining and smelting operations are notorious for pouring fluoride dusts into the air. Nothing will grow where these dusts have contaminated the air and soil (look at the landscape around mining operations in the USA). Third world countries suffer miserably from the uncontrolled use of industrial fluorides. The faces of the people are OLD!

Fluoride is a systemic poison. It is in conflict with the desire to become *Young Again!*

PREVIEW: In our next chapter, you will discover WHY sex hormone production shifts as the bio-electric body ages.

"If you think health is expensive, wait until you try disease!"
Merlyn Anderberg

Travel Package

When I travel, I take a magnetic seat cushion, shower filter, pollen, PAC's, ETVC, algae, and juice capsules. The filter protects & provides drinking water, the magnets stimulate, and the foods supplement my diet.

Think About It!

Did the cancer patient always have cancer? Was the diabetic always a diabetic? And did the lady with arthritis always have arthritis? NO! They did NOT always have these problems. These people LOST CONTROL of their "terrain," summarized as follows:

- Toxicity *beyond* the body's ability to handle it
- Hormonal imbalances as a result of "excesses"
- Intake of food with a *left-spin* energy "footprint"
- Failure to drink biologically friendly water

No one knows from *where* dis-ease comes. No one knows to where dis-ease returns. Live your life in accordance with nature's laws and you don't have to care!

Mind & Body

Never underestimate the power of the mind. Daily, I counsel people who **cannot** be helped because they refuse to control their thoughts.

There are many good books written about the power of the mind. Let's summarize a few points.

1. Negative, unhappy, critical, angry, fearful, depressed thoughts—and words—affect the production of brain chemicals, hormones, depress the immune system, and bring on dis-ease. **Thoughts and words are energy bullets!**

2. The aura diminishes in size when we "think" negative thoughts. **Dis-ease is "thoughts" in the flesh.**

3. A positive outlook promotes healing. A poor emotional/mental attitude hinders healing—no matter how "good" our health habits are. **Guard your thoughts.**

4. Bowel and liver function are affected by our emotions and thoughts. **Good thoughts are better than laxatives.**

5. Positive image visualization brings good results. **What we think we experience What we voice we create.**

6. Beliefs about oneself, life, the future, and others affect us and those around us. **Refuse to harbor bad thoughts.**

7. Exercise is as good for the mind as it is for the body. **Gain control of your thoughts through aerobic exercise.**

8. Incorporate good thoughts, kindness to others, and self-assurance in your life and you will become *Young Again!*

Read *Your Body Believes Every Word You Say*
(see Source Index)

17

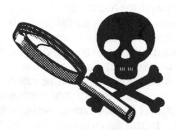

Diagnosis Or Post Mortems?

"The organs of the body can be likened to cities on a road map, each being a unit unto itself, yet, each is connected to the other and ultimately to the composite body."

Dr. Arnold Lorand

The Golden Age of Medicine extended from approximately 1840 to 1930. It was a period that saw an explosion of new knowledge in all fields of science.

The clinical observations of the doctors of this period are of particular interest to us because of their impact on the aging process. Their observations *precede* the advent of modern man's environmental mistakes.

The Golden Age of Medicine was a period of "low tech" medicine. Doctors were forced to rely on astute observation to guide the patient. They also spent more time with patients, often getting to know them better than they knew themselves.

Uncommon good sense was the guiding rule. There was no place to shift the blame if the chosen modality (therapy) failed to cure the patient. The patient was viewed *in camera*—as a unit—rather than as separate parts. The word "syndrome" was not in mode. Cause and effect, diagnosis and prognosis, were anchored in observation, rather than endless tests.

Modern Medicine

Present day medical technology is a mixed blessing. It

excels in the replacement and repair of body parts, and in emergency medicine. Beyond this, it is a never ending process that produces *isolated snap-shots* of the process we call disease—each picture but a *glimpse* of the suffering patient.

"High-tech" medicine only works if the doctor is a good observer. Unfortunately, we are training our doctors to see subclinically sick humans beings in shades of grey, having thrown out our hard won observations of yesterday.

Allopathic medicine has an *unholy* reliance on high tech gadgets and high powered, left-spin chemical drugs. It sees the patient as a flesh and blood machine composed of "parts." Medicine fails to recognize the energy forces at the "invisible" level where vitality is lost before dis-ease is seen in the "visible" realm. Each human being is unique. We do NOT conform to computer generated models. Each of us is an *energy* "dynamic" being of flesh and blood, and we live in a world of dynamic energy forces that interface and **dictate** the body's terrain.

Diagnosis Or Post Mortems?

If it were possible to examine the vital organs of the body, particularly the ductless glands—the pituitary, thyroid, parathyroid, adrenals, thymus, pancreas, and gonads (testes and ovaries)—the effects of our living habits would be plainly evident. But we cannot make such an examination and must therefore learn HOW to assist the *bio-electric* body through a healthy lifestyle and common sense.

Dr. William Albrech, a brilliant professor of soils at the University of Missouri, once commented that we no longer know what healthy animal organs look like because we see only *abnormal* organs. This is the way it is in medicine today.

There was a time when the physician could examine both healthy and *pathogenic* individuals and compare them. By knowing what healthy organs looked like, the doctor could identify dis-ease in its formative stages. In other words, an astute observer could pick up on *subclinical* symptoms before they became SIGNS. The days of humans in peak health are no more. Subclinically sick people are now the norm.

Strange Meanings

To compensate for the universality of a subclinically sick population, the medical schools have rewritten the STANDARDS by which they define health and dis-ease. This is similar to what is occurring in our public schools, where today's "A" is yesterday's "C."

For example, BOGUS holistic medicine, as taught in

"traditional" medical schools, defines **illness** as an abnormal condition where the present level of function has declined compared to a *previous* level. By this definition, *neither* the present level nor the previous level of function meets any defined STANDARD. Traditional definitions have become moot. They no longer define illness as the absence of health, and health the absence of dis-ease. **Today, illness is neutral!**

Today, bogus definitions of health and illness are defined in terms of the individual's *personal perception* of their state of being. In other words, how one *feels* about oneself. Trying to make sense out of all of this reminds me of the Chinese journalist who exclaimed, *"Explain please, strange words and meanings."*

Approximately 85% of the population displays the Rouleau effect in their blood. Rouleau is the harbinger of dis-ease in the formative stage. Personal responsibility for one's own health will drive Rouleau from the blood.

Reversing the aging process requires that we become enlightened as WHY we age. We CANNOT afford to assign responsibility to a medical discipline that ignores the basic root causes of illness, dis-ease, and aging.

The Endocrine System

To further understand the aging process, we must look at the endocrine system of the body. This system is one of two regulatory and communication systems that transmit and coordinate messages to various parts of the body. The other is the nervous system. *(Medical tradition ignores the lymphatic system as a communication system. Nevertheless, the lymphatic system is the primary protein communication system.)*

The *nervous* and *endocrine* systems are *irrevocably* linked to each other, but they function differently. The nervous system transmits electrical impulses (energy) to the tissues via nerve fibers (called *dendrites*) and nerve cells (called *neurons*.) Messages are transmitted in milliseconds (thousandths of a second)—faster than the speed of light.

As we age, the myelin sheath (neurilemma) that covers the nerve fibers deteriorates, precipitating degenerative conditions like Alzheimers dis-ease, multiple sclerosis, myelinoma, neuropathy, and walking legs syndrome.

Aging reversal becomes more challenging if dis-ease is far enough along to warrant a doctor's diagnosis. However, given the opportunity and a "positive" attitude, the body can perform miracles. The body has amazing resiliency. It can rebuild itself, regenerate missing limbs, grow hair on a bald heads, and drive away dis-ease. But to perform these miracles, it needs a functioning endocrine system.

The endocrine system makes its wishes known using chemical **and** hormonal messengers. Chemical messengers are chemical *energy* that causes a *fast* response in the body.

Hormones messengers are *different*. They often take hours to produce a response. Hormone response, however, can last for hours, days, and even weeks. *(Think of the effects experienced in the aftermath of an emergency situation where large amounts of adrenalin were produced to help you cope with the situation. You are wired for hours afterwords!)*

Hormones control our *internal* environment by assuring normal body function and energy balance. Hormone production and balance is absolutely vital to the aging reversal process. The best and safest way to balance your hormones is with the use natural hormone precursors (see source index).

Exocrine & Endocrine Glands

Most exocrine glands secrete into *ducts* which in turn flow into body cavities like the stomach or intestines. Some exocrine glands, however, like the sudoriferous (sweat) and sebaceous (oil) glands, secrete to the skin's surface.

The *ductless* glands of the endocrine system secrete their hormones directly into the extracellular spaces around and between the secreting cells, instead of into ducts. The extracellular spaces—between the cells—are filled with extracellular fluid and house the blood and lymph capillaries.

Some hormones are transported *by the blood* to their tissue destination(s), which may be another gland. Hence, the ductless glands depend on each other and act in *concert*. When one gland becomes stressed, the effect is compounded **throughout** the system. Women with thyroid problems often have underlying problems (subclinical dis-ease) in the ovaries and hormonal imbalances.

Some endocrine tissues are both duct and ductless glands. Examples are the pancreas, ovaries, testes, kidneys, stomach, small intestine, skin, heart and placenta.

Hormones maintain health by changing the *rate of activity* in the body. The amount of hormones released into circulation is based on need, the gland's ability to produce them, and the body's ability to utilize them. **Hormonal excesses manifest themselves as deficiency conditions.**

Some hormones are carried in "free" form in the blood. Others require blood plasma *carrier proteins* to bind and transport them—for example, insulin. Blood plasma carrier proteins are made by the liver.

When the receptors on the target cells have responded

to the hormone, a message is relayed back to the gland that produced the hormones to STOP production. Excess hormones are degraded and disposed of by either the target cells themselves or by the liver and are removed from circulation by the liver and/or kidneys. Aging is the result of general SLOW-DOWN in metabolic function, especially in the liver and kidneys. **The liver, however, is central to all dis-ease.**

Old Age Symptoms In The Young

Some of the SIGNS of early senescence (aging) seen in young adults are obesity, gray or missing hair, wrinkles, weak joints, loss of vitality, and low sexual drive. Symptoms not seen include amenorrhea (irregular menstruation) and impotence [inability to get an erection (penis in men, clitoris in women]).

Other symptoms that serve as excellent *markers* of poor health are accelerated pulse, cold in the extremities, a tendency to constipation, edema, fading memory, mental depression, albumin and casts in the urine.

Albumin is a blood protein that has escaped through the capillaries of the kidney's glomeruli (filters). Albumin in the urine is a SERIOUS indication of loss of kidney function. Since the kidneys are one of the PRIMARY waste organs of the body, the presence of albumin spells trouble.

Casts are composed of salt, hyaline, protein, and chemical and mineral wastes. These wastes take the shape of the kidney's tubules. They indicate *catabolic* activity and degeneration. Weak kidneys are a *prerequisite* to cancer and viral infections. Weak kidneys allow the establishment of clandestine outposts throughout the body and cold war maneuvers by viruses and bacteria fueled by left-spin energy.

Cold in the extremities indicates thyroid disfunction stressed ovaries, and hormonal excesses. All of these are linked to a stressed liver—the body's furnace. An accelerated pulse indicates a systemic condition where the body is overworking to make up for shortfalls or excesses in the system.

Constipation is a systemic condition that influences ALL body functions. The so-called acid stomach is a symptomatic condition experienced after a meal. It is NOT an acid condition at all, but alkaline—the exact *opposite* of what is popularly believed! A little raw apple cider vinegar or Yucca extract can do wonders for this condition.

Detoxification of the body brings rejuvenation and normal hydrochloric acid secretion by the stomach glands. (Be sure to read Patricia Bragg's *Apple Cider Vinegar* book (see Source Index).

Edema (water retention is the tissues) is linked to

excess plasma proteins in the lymph fluids and excess sodium in the cells. Older people should recognize edema—especially in the legs and feet—for what it is: **serious toxicity!**

The legs—including the hair and nails—are responsible for releasing massive amounts of toxic waste energy from the body. As people age, body hair is lost and the nails become thick, yellow, and troublesome. Drugs and protein wastes settle in the legs of older people, further compounding swelling. Edema is a SIGN of trouble. See it as an effect, NOT a cause.

Sodium invasion of the cells alters glandular function and accelerates aging. Tests to determine cellular sodium, drug accumulation in extracellular and/or lymphatic fluids, and plasma protein levels are nonexistent or useless. These conditions can, however, be managed through rebounding, lymphatic massage, walking bare footed in sand or on the green grass, soaking the feet in "pulverized" baby Kombucha mushrooms, using *enhanced* PAC's, and drinking plenty of BEV water with ionic minerals.

Oxidation

As early as 1903, it was demonstrated that the **ductless** glands control ALL the processes of oxidation, and that the diseases of metabolism like diabetes, obesity, gout, arthritis, heart dis-ease, etc. are the direct consequence of *alterations* in the function of these important glands. In other words, the hormones are an important key to rejuvenation of the bio-electric body, especially when combined with PAC's, colon therapy, detoxification, and the flushing of stones from the liver.

The thyroid, like the liver, is central to all metabolic processes. Overwork of this organ or its twin, the adrenals, results in physical breakdown. *Myxedema* (swelling) of the thyroid gland results in a goiter. It also involves the invasion of connective tissue and diminished ability to manufacture and secrete the powerful thyroid hormones T_3 and T_4. *(Women who are dependent upon thyroid medications often return to normal with the use of natural hormone precursors, detoxification, and select supplementation.)*

Stroma & Parenchyma Cells

When the functional cells (parenchyma cells) of an organ or gland die, they are replaced by dysfunctional (stroma) connective tissue, which the medical folks sometimes call scar tissue. In the case of the liver, the parenchyma or functional cells are called hepatocytes (*hepat*-liver; *cyte*-cell).

Stroma cells cover and protect the liver. As the

hepatocytes die from ingesting organic poisons (pesticides, etc.), food additives, or alcohol—the stroma cells invade the liver and form scar tissue.

The liver is VERY dependent on a functioning thyroid gland. Bad living habits, hormonal imbalances, and toxic excesses lead to stress and burnout of the thyroid gland. The thyroid, like the liver, is a MASTER gland. Both depend on functioning adrenals, pancreas, and gonads.

Alcohol • Cirrhosis • Liver Test

Alcohol is a POISON! It kills the hepatocytes in the liver. That is why a drunk person is said to be in**tox**icated. **Tox**—as in **tox**in—means poison. When you drink alcohol you are **poisoning** yourself. If you want to REVERSE aging, you are going to need a healthy functioning liver. Avoid the use of alcohol if you want to see your wish fulfilled.

For your information, the alcohol industry (like the dairy and ice cream industry) is not required to list the toxic ingredients it adds to its brew—ingredients like sulfites (in wine) and urea (in beer). If you insist on drinking beer and wine, make it yourself!

If you know someone who drinks, perform this liver test. First, have the person lie on their back on the floor and raise their knees to relax their stomach. Then, gently but deeply, push down on the right side, just below the rib cage. You will feel a *hard mass*—the LIVER! Be careful, it may be very tender and massaging it harshly can cause the person to become ill!

People with hepatitis, mononucleosis, or chronic fatigue syndrome will also have a distended, swollen liver. These *conditions* place great stress on this vital organ. The liver should be soft, and somewhat hidden under the ribs.

Here is another test. Have the alcoholic person stand and extend their right arm. Next, gently pull down on the arm while your other hand touches the liver region. People with limited liver (or adrenal, or thyroid, or thymus, or pancreas) function will lose their strength and their arm will fall. Some people become nauseated and have to lie down because of the *surge* of electrical energy into their sick liver.

Atrophy Of Sex Glands & Obesity

Atrophy (deterioration) of the sex glands goes hand in hand with systemic toxicity, obesity, and thyroid and liver problems. Obesity is a SIGN of metabolic slow down and hormonal imbalance. Atrophy of the ovaries (which includes the ova and follicles from which the egg springs) and testicles takes years to manifest. Loss of the ovaries, or male castration causes an immediate slow down in basal metabolic activity. Many doctors think nothing of removing a woman's female organs (uterus and ovaries). **Removal of a woman's ovaries is the equivalent of castration for a man. How many men have you seen standing in line to be castrated lately?**

Women MUST learn HOW to stay healthy if they expect to avoid female problems. Hormone precursors are wonderful aids for woman (and men). Women should NOT wait until there are problems to begin natural hormonal supplementation.

Detoxification of the tissues also goes a long way in keeping a woman young and vibrant. Where the ovaries have been lost, a woman MUST learn to manage her own situation and not become dependent on archaic medical advice. I highly recommend that women and men read the special hormone report available from the publisher (see Source Index).

Menstrual disorders like amenorrhea (skipped menstrual periods) and obesity are NOT normal and are heavily linked to hormonal excesses and excess toxicity. These problems should be addressed early on. PMS problems are tied to thyroid and toxicity conditions. If treated early, women can avoid the loss of their female organs.

Obesity is closely linked to hormonal imbalances. Officially, obesity is defined as being 20% over the standard height and weight. If, for example, your maximum desirable weight is 130 pounds, you would NOT be considered obese until you reached 156 pounds according to conventional wisdom.

In good health, you would probably be near the bottom of your table or 118 pounds. The difference here between obesity and ideal weight is 156 less 118 or 38 pounds overweight. Please notice, thirty eight pounds isn't 20% overweight, but 32% overweight and that is a lot of excess!

Obesity is a SIGN that can be verified on a bathroom scale. It is a "marker" condition that indicates loss of vital organ function and hormonal imbalance. It should be considered a red flag—by both women and men!

Osteoporosis

Osteoporosis or *honeycombing of the bones* involves vascularization (invasion) of the bones by the blood vessels. The blood vessels are the body's front line troops. Their presence precedes bone formation as well as bone *dismantling*. Osteoporosis is a systemic (whole body) aging EFFECT. It is not the cause of loss of bone mass. Once again, osteoporosis is related to hormonal imbalances and **excess** toxicity. Osteoporosis is common in older people—and especially in post menopausal women who have lost their ovaries.

Osteoporosis is easily prevented and treated. Osteoporosis has EVERYTHING to do with toxicity, and **NOTH-ING** to do with the need for increased dietary intake of elemental calcium compounds (more later). To treat or prevent osteoporosis, detoxify your entire body, do a liver flush, and get on hormone precursor supplementation. These simple steps will add many "good" years to your life.

Connective Tissue

Connective tissue is one of the four basic types of tissue in the body. It performs the functions of binding and supporting. It consists of relatively few cells in a great deal of "intercellular substance."

The four basic types of tissue are **Connective** *(elastic, collagenous, reticular),* **epithelial** *(skin),* **muscular** *(muscle) and* **nerve** *tissue.*

Beautiful Skin

The last two words of the definition of connective tissue ("intercellular substance") are of particular importance to aging. **Intercellular substance** is the material between the cells. If we are speaking of the skin we are talking about the dermal and sub-cutaneous layers of the skin. This area is served by the blood and lymph capillary system.

It is here, in the basement membranes of the skin, that the body dumps excess metabolic wastes, mineral salts, and FATS. These wastes are deposited by the blood capillaries, and lodge in the spaces "between" the cells. When the tissues become overloaded with waste and can no longer function normally, the connective tissues of the skin break down and the skin becomes wrinkled.

Metabolic wastes **below** the skin break down the connective tissues that bind the skin layers together, and cause *hardening* and *thickening* of the outer skin with LOSS of *elasticity* and resiliency.

Glycolic acid skin cream (mentioned earlier) *fluffs* and *loosens* the dead outer horny layers of the skin while it softens the collagen membranes. It should be used with racemic clay facial balm, hormone precursor creme, and *enhanced* PAC's if a persons really wants to see their skin come alive! The clay draws out toxicity from deep within the skin. The creme hormonally stimulates rejuvenation of the connective tissues, and the PAC's bond to the free radical wastes, prevent their reabsorption, and shuttle them OUT of system and into the toilet. Yucca extract works especially well with the PAC's. Use these things together for double whammy inside/outside effect that simply can't be beat! Wrinkles are nothing to be ashamed of, but who wants them? **Wrinkled skin speaks of loss of vital organ function and buildup of metabolic waste. Wrinkles confirm the arrival of old age!**

Venereal Disease • Sexual Excess

Sexually infectious dis-eases left unattended can cause massive alteration to the body.

Few people who reach adult age are virgins. Most have had one or more venereal (*venus*-love; *al*-pertaining to) dis-eases. VD involves more than simple exposure to pathogenic bacteria or viruses. A healthy body is immune to the ravages of VD! If this were not true, VD would have totally encompassed the entire population long ago. Venereal infections occur when people lose control of their "terrain" (more later).

Sexual excess alters thyroid function, as noted by the ancient Hebrews. They examined the neck of the newly married bride the morning following the wedding night. If the neck was swollen, this was a sign that the marriage had been consummated and a SIGN of heavy sexual activity. Young adults who sexually abuse their bodies lose their youthful appearance early and grow old faster than usual—especially women.

The inability to get an erection in a men or women (penis in men; clitoris in women) is due to hormonal imbalances and poor blood flow brought on by toxicity, insufficient hydration, low thyroid function, a stressed liver, and *atrophy* of the ovaries and testicles. Soy and canola oils also play a part here.

Too frequent pregnancy, prolonged lactation, and poor diet will precipitate a goiter as frequently seen in women. The female body needs at LEAST two years of rest and nourishment between each child. Metabolic stress on the thyroid and liver brings on menstrual and ovarian disorders and sometimes impotence. Atrophy or dysfunction of the gonads precipitate thyroid conditions. Whenever goiter, coldness in the feet and hands, low energy, or inability to get going in the morning, are a problem) **suspect** thyroid, liver, ovary dysfunction, hormonal imbalances and poor blood sugar management.

Regardless of the exact nature of these problems, systemic detoxification, liver stone flush, and hormone supplementation are in order. These things usually turn people's lives around and give them back the most precious gift of all—good health!

Diabetes

Diabetes and obesity are first cousins and represent slow-down and stress to the vital organs. Adult onset diabetes best describes the circumstances under which most people become a diabetic.

There is no question that buildup of metabolic waste and slow-down in organ function precipitates the development of diabetes. When waste energy levels EXCEED the body's ability to cope, blood sugar levels go ballistic. Waste management is a mandatory prerequisite!

The jury is in, and there is also NO question that polio and DPT vaccines mutate and bring on at least 75% of juvenile diabetes cases. Hearing loss in children and adults is also closely linked to vaccinations (more later).

Rene's tea and Yucca extract are being used in mainland China specifically for the treatment of degenerative conditions. Rene's tea is given by IV drip with great success. This vibrational product that knocks out blood born viruses conditions, be it vaccine induced or otherwise.

Enhanced trivalent chromium also works well in cases of diabetes where the problem is related to glucose intolerance or insulin resistance.

Sugar is a carbon-based molecule. In the case of the diabetic, the body keeps the sugars in the blood to BUFFER toxic energy fields. This is why colon therapy, detoxification, and a good liver flush can do wonders for the diabetic. Get rid of the waste, and diabetes moderates and often disappears.

The goal of diabetes management should not to simply lower sugar levels, but to return the entire body to normalcy—which requires a balanced program of supplementation, stimulation, and detoxification. **There is NO root difference between cancer, diabetes, arthritis, and other degenerative conditions. All of them have the same origin. All of them can be reversed.**

Goiter & Iodine

Goiters develop over a long period of time and results in *precocious* senility in women whose sexual and mammary glands are driven beyond their limits. (*Precocious* means occurring at a premature age.)

Iodine supplementation is the traditional treatment for hypo (low) thyroid conditions, along with synthetic and glandular thyroid products. And although iodine is a vital element, it is also a powerful *stimulant* to the thyroid, often making matters worse, not better. **When iodine is given to a person suffering from multiple dietary deficiencies, it can cause a goiter OR exhaustion of the thyroid gland.** Over stimulation in the face of insufficient dietary support is folly. So is the *chronic* use of natural or synthetic thyroid supplements. Both approaches are *palliative* in nature and fail to return the thyroid to normal function.

It is best to avoid the palliative approach (relief of symptoms without treatment of the underlying cause). Instead, try to deal with root causes by returning to the basics.

Let's Review

The organs become stressed from over activity, waste buildup, and malnutrition. Stress produces *alteration* of the vital organs, accompanied by symptoms of dis-ease, and imbalances in the terrain of the "invisible" *bio-electric* body.

Once the *bio-electric* body shifts to a NEGATIVE energy state, dis-ease proliferates. Reversing this process requires commitment plus offensive and defensive measures.

The healing "crises" most people experience during detoxification (which may take many months), directly reflects the toxicity level of the person. Detoxification of the bio-electric body is not fun, but it does return people to a healthy status.

Healing crises are the price you must pay for your sins. I know of NO other investment that brings a higher return than good health and vitality!

The body is more than a flesh and blood mosaic; more than the sum total of its parts. It is a DYNAMIC living energy field that succumbs to the process we call aging through our own mistakes.

We cannot escape death, but we can avoid the degeneration that precedes it. **Post-mortem examination is a poor way to find out that your "chosen" lifestyle was faulty. Change your lifestyle! Get back to the basics today, and you will become an example for others to follow.**

When you assist your body—instead of sabotaging it— you become *Young Again!*

PREVIEW: *Our next chapter discusses HOW the body "manufactures" what it needs by way of the bacteria, and how mineral energy fuels our life processes.*

Stress is negative energy seeking an outlet. Read *vibrations* and learn how to use a vibration chain so you can safely release stress from your body!

TAKE Your Life Back!

If you suffer from poor health or degenerative disease, here's something that will help you get your life back under your control.

It's called **Enhanced Trivalent Chromium** (ETVC). We have known for years that chromium is central to weight control, glucose metabolism, aging, and degeneration. Now we have *trivalent* chromium in an herbal food base and the results people are experiencing are impressive.

Taken in the morning, ETVC raises **energy** levels all day. **Excess body fat** melts away and is replaced by lean muscle mass. Blood sugar problems—like diabetes and hypoglycemia—ease or disappear. Sexual drive increases. Mental acuity and motivation are enhanced.

ETVC is a *transition* product designed to help people "feel" and "look" better. It forces open the door to closed metabolic pathways, and makes the transition from unhealthy to healthy easier—and faster.

When people have energy, they become motivated! Burn off excess fat and the fat person says, "Yah!!" Raise someone's self image and great things happen. Give subclinically sick people a taste of life and look out! That is what ETVC does for people who use it.

ETVC is a boon for insulin dependent and non-insulin dependent diabetics. **It is useful in treating both glucose intolerance AND insulin resistance.**

As insulin levels rise in the blood, production of the adrenal hormone DHEA falls. As DHEA levels fall, Lean muscle mass is lost which goes hand in hand with **obesity** and aging. ETVC helps reverse these conditions. It is especially effective when combined with *enhanced* PAC's, detoxification, and hormonal balancing.

Excess body fat is the result of hormonal imbalances and systemic toxicity. Toxicity ushers in blood sugar problems and **more fat**. ETVC effectively rebalances body metabolism through blood sugar management

Rouleau (sticky blood), high cholesterol levels, and hypertension (high blood pressure) also respond to ETVC.

ETVC supplementation is helps **obesity** in young and old alike. It gets the body moving—even for the sluggish body that generally refuses to respond.

ETVC is a catalyst that helps people remain young or take back what they have lost. It helps them deal with **underlying** health issues that underwrite LOSS OF CONTROL of one's life (see Source Index).

False Readings

Sometimes positive energy **stirs** the system to the point of illness. These reactions are called "healing crises." They often occur in people who are very toxic.

The body has *innate* intelligence. It **knows** and can **anticipate** the effect a positive energy force will produce. Hence, the bio-electric body may reject therapy, or food, or supplements that it actually needs. It does this because it **knows** that the person whose spirit inhabits the body doesn't truly desire to be healed or is unwilling to suffer the pain and misery that can accompany rejuvenation.

Sometimes the body tricks its owner and produces *false* muscle tests, or issues false pendulum and vibration chain responses. To be truly effective, these techniques require the novice or therapist to develop these skills and learn to **clear** the mind and adjoining airspace.

Muscle testing is NOT accurate where heavy metal contamination exists. Heavy metals impinge on the autonomic nervous system and interfere with test readings.

Too many people go through the **motions** and issue **proclamations** based on false readings—and this includes many practitioners. False responses and incorrect interpretation will lead everyone astray.

If you would like to learn HOW to use a pendulum and vibration chain accurately, *The Pendulum Kit, Vibrations,* and *Map Dowsing* are an excellent trilogy on the subject and a good place to start (see Source Index).

The Pendulum

Learning to **effectively** use a pendulum is a MUST in this day and age. Learning to use a pendulum is easy, but many people need help to get going.

I recommend *The Pendulum Kit* because it has proven to be the best and least expensive way to teach people how to plug into the world of *invisible* energy fields that surrounds us.

The Pendulum Kit comes complete with a nice bronze pendulum and a beautifully illustrated book. Many effective techniques are explained. It is very *visual!*

"Dousing" is a phenomenon and a GOD given gift that's available to anyone who desires to come to grips with life on planet Earth (see the Source Index).

18

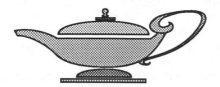

Biological Alchemy

"Since Einstein, Physics has been relegated to Mathematics, the former having lost all contact with reality. Your magnificent discovery of weak energy transmutations should have marked a scientific turning point, (but instead it) encountered a wall of stupidity."

Ren de Puymorin

...speaking of the work of Professor C. Louis Kervran and his discovery that the motion of life derives from the continuous transformation of one mineral into another or—"transmutation."

"**Alchemy!** Impossible! This is a good example of just plain old BAD science!" So ended my official inquiry at the college level—but it did NOT end my inquiry.

What sparked the explosive outburst was the trigger word "transmutation" which means "alchemy." The attacker was a superb college chemistry instructor who did not like the implications of the questions I was raising, questions like...

"*How* do you explain food plants that contain minerals not present in the soil? *How* does the cow produce milk that contains minerals far in excess of her dietary intake? *Where* does the hen get the minerals for her egg shells when they are not in her diet? *Why* does horsetail herb thicken and harden the nails, yet we derive NO such benefit from calcium supplements? *How* can organic manganese produce an increase in the blood serum iron level when it is not iron?" *How* is it that a dried prune has more minerals than a fresh one? How, indeed? The answers to these questions hint of unrecognized genius and ignored or forgotten knowledge.

Asking these type of questions is like proclaiming the invention of a perpetual motion machine. They can get a person in a lot of trouble, especially when put to the wrong person.

In our world of neatly packaged chemicals and defined LAWS of chemistry and physics, these questions have NO answers. However, make no mistake, they DO have answers. These are valid questions—the kind Professor Kervran liked to ask. The problem isn't the questions posed, but the implications they suggest.

Some people of science are intimidated by questions for which they have no answers. Daring to ask them is an assault on DOGMA and enough to get a person branded "science heretic"—and instant burning at the stake!

Mineral Energy

The life work of Professor Kervran (1899-1990) has startling implications for reversing the aging process.

Kervran surmised that the energy *phenomena* we call LIFE is related to the transformation of one mineral into another. He called this process "transmutation." Science calls it alchemy. We will refer to it as *biological alchemy.*

In other words, as the energy forces within an element are changed or rearranged, a new and different element results. In the process, energy is released. Kervran believed this energy fueled metabolic processes and was the energy upon which all life depends. Transmutation, as he described it would require a change in elemental structure at the atomic and subatomic levels and the rearrangement of **an**ions, **cat**ions. In other words, COLD fusion!

Kervran's discoveries came from inside Science's camp. Kervran was a member of both the French and American National Academy of Sciences, the most prestigious watering holes of modern science.

Professor Kervran *dared* to ask the right questions. He *sinned* against Science and dogma when he offered God's answer to his fellow man. He broke the rules because he failed to submit his findings for "peer" review. Great Wizards have NO peers! They see visions of God's handiwork and proclaim the great news!

Like Marco Polo, Kervran's peers *attacked* and *ridiculed* him as they have done to so many other Wizards before him. They ignored him, but they could NOT deny the TRUTH he heralded. When a vessel of TRUTH is opened, it can NEVER be closed again. Truth is a Pandora's Box for those who live in ignorance and who are afraid and intimidated by TRUTH.

Visions

Kervran suspected that minerals held concentrated energy fields within their bonds. His vision of the Creator's handiwork was not unlike that of his contemporary, Dr. Carey Reams. These great men of science never met. Each developed his own vision independently. Each talked about the same phenomena from their own perspective and interpretation of the phenomena they beheld.

Reams called his vision, *The Biological Theory of Ionization.* Kervran called his, *The Theory of Biological Transmutation.* Both spoke of energy forces that grant permission to life. Both spoke of the energy "footprint" of minerals, the same "footprint" described by Vincent and made available in BEV water.

Reams talked of positive energy ions called **an**ions, and negative energy ions called **cat**ions. Kervran spoke of the rearrangement of energy forces and the fusion of these forces at the *sub*atomic level.

Reams spoke of left and right-spin energy and the release of cosmic forces trapped in the bonds "between" minerals (ionic bonds). Kervran, talked of mineral transformation in the gut of animals and in the skin and lymph of the Earth—the soil and water.

The Sun was a central fixture for both men. They saw plants, animals, and microbes as mediators between Sun and Earth. Both men sought the answer to the "Why?" of life that we raised in chapter two—the mystery of life and death, health and illness. God answered both men with living examples of the importance of good, basic food, pure water, and clean, disciplined lifestyles. He answered Reams in English and Kervran in French. Our version will be a combination of both.

Plants • Animals • Microbes

The plant is the link between the Sun and the animal world to which man's body belongs. The plant converts solar energy into carbon sugar molecules with the help of the microbe. Plants bring life and energy INTO the Earth.

The animals—with the help of the microbes—process plant tissue and live off the energy released during the digestion process. Animal waste becomes part of the Earth's bioelectric body and provides the catalyst for new life—both plant and animal.

To Kervran, mineral energy fields in a living system were forever dynamic—shifting and changing one into the other. For example, in multiple stomached animals, calcium compounds, like limestone, can be altered or "transmutated" by the bacteria in order to meet the needs of the host. Humans are not ruminants—we have but one stomach. To be effective, our minerals should be in *ionic, colloidal* form.

Kervran saw "life" energy flowing from a potpourri of mineral elements. To him, health was a manifestation of a microbial *fiesta* in the gut and liver of man and animal!

In order for the *fiesta* to occur, man's body must be electrically balanced so it will attract and maintain a balanced microbial population. The microbe is at the center of the *alchemy* process we call *fusion.* Cold fusion allows life to express and maintain itself. It involves the transmutation of one energy field into another. **Transmutation of mineral energy fields slows aging and brings health.**

The Cow

The cow is a living example of the transmutation process. She eats plants (compounds of carbon, sugars, fats, proteins, and minerals) and converts them into NEW and DIFFERENT energy forms—like muscle and bone.

The cow does this by way of the enzymes and microbes in her liver and GI tract. The bacteria that share her tissues have a *symbiotic* relationship with her. She provides them room and board; they provide her with energy and vitality. Without the microbes and enzymes, the fantastic biochemical reactions Kervran called *transmutations* could not take place. Without the microbes, the cow is unable to nourish herself. Without the microbes, man grows old and dies early.

The microbe is man's passport to a continued presence on the Earth. However, man's disobedience is causing the microbe to turn against him.

Sick cows have much in common with sick people. Both are UNABLE to effectively use the transmutation process. Health and vitality in man is a reflection of the energy process Kervran and Reams called transmutation and ionization. The requirements for healthy organisms are nutritious food, ionic minerals, biologically friendly water, exercise, and a clean, *aerobic* environment.

When the cow drinks water that is chlorinated, the water kills the *friendly* bacteria and creates an energy imbalance that is tailor made for *pathogenic* life forms. One of the side effects of this energy shift is a slow-down in metabolic activity in the gut and liver.

Antibiotics cause a similar effect. They upset the balance of intestinal flora by changing the electrical *terrain* of the body. Once the good bacteria are no longer present to defend their terrain, negative energy microbes move in, set up shop, and live off the negative energy such environments spawn. Without an aerobic environment, aerobes (friendly bacteria) give way to *anaerobic* conditions where anaerobic bacteria colonize the gut unopposed. The end result is a sick cow—or human being.

Fusion & Fission

Life is a tug of war between opposing energy forces. Transmutation and ionization are involved in both positive and negative biological energy shifts which we will call fusion and fission.

"Fusion" involves the joining of atoms to form larger molecules. Under normal biological circumstances, it is a positive energy activity and represents the buildup process we call *anabolism*. Fusion occurs on the surface of the *Sun*, in the *soil*, in plants, and in the gut and liver of man and animal.

An example of *abnormal*, biological fusion would be cancer. Cancer results from toxic waste buildup, hormonal imbalances, the introduction of *radiomimetic* substances that produce or mimic the physiological effects of nuclear radiation (like additives, preservatives, prescription drugs). These things set the stage for uncontrolled oxidation and free radical formation, hence the need for "enhanced" proanthocyanidins. Left unchecked, uncontrolled oxidation leads to "catabolic" fission.

"Fission" breaks down molecules and atoms. Normal fission activity is good. However, once we reach our anabolic peak, the fission process becomes predominantly *catabolic* in nature. Examples of destructive fission reactions are nuclear reactions, irradiation of food, radiation therapy, microwave cooking, etc. Not all fission reactions are anti-life. Fission reactions orchestrated by **friendly** microbes are beneficial. Loss of control of the *terrain* ushers in negative fission reactions, pathogenic microbes, and dis-ease.

Skin • Dirt • Soil

The Earth has skin. Her skin is called soil. Some folks call soil "dirt." Dirt, however, is *dead* unless it is *energized* with microbes, organic matter, and carbon. The microbes *transform* dirt into soil. Soil is biologically *alive*. Soil has *life*.

Water is the essence of life. It is the Earth's lymph, and it is capable of transporting massive amounts of energy. Soil energy and top soil depth is controlled by carbon. Carbon underwrites Mother Earth's aura.

When Earth becomes stressed, her skin forms boils, her lymph becomes toxic, the plants become weak, the animals suffer, and man experiences dis-ease. The condition of Earth's skin and lymph dictates the quality of life AND the life forms that live or die. Life is a microbial affair and it involves transmutation and ionization of mineral energy.

The microbes and the minerals are man's ticket to longevity —if he has the wisdom to recognize their importance and follow nature's rules.

Synchronization

Synchronization can be the end result of a chemical reaction—like mixing vinegar with baking soda—one acid, the other alkaline. When the reaction has run its course, two things have occurred. Energy has been released (heat) and synchronization has occurred between the original reactants. If the reaction stopped because of a shortage of ingredients, *potential* energy remains in synchronized form.

Synchronization of energy in the body is similar. Here, positive energy forces are weak or unable to break the bonds that hold synchronized energy intact. For example, high energy footprint food should provoke a positive response in the body, UNLESS a toxic bowel and sluggish liver stand in the way, in which case, the energy will be lost down the toilet, converted to a toxic form, or become synchronized. Colon therapy can be SHOCK the body out of a state of *modified* synchronization. Yucca extract and enhanced proantocyanidins helps here too.

An anaerobic gut is the perfect terrain for a negative energy takeover—as in cancer.

Synchronized energy is energy that is on hold. It is energy that is NOT available to the body. Synchronized energy fields influence health—for good and bad. People in poor health are in an energy gridlock. They are unable to neutralize *negative* energy fields, yet are too weak to make use of positive energy. Negative energy neutralizes positive energy. Sick bodies produce lots of negative energy. Illness and dis-ease are the end product of a left-spin energy *anaerobic* take over which is a *catabolic* state. **Detoxification can BREAK the deadlock!**

When the bio-electric body suffers *systemic* synchronization, OLD AGE goes into FAST FORWARD and life becomes impossible! As we approach total synchronization, we lose our "radiance." The aura diminishes and dwindles until it ceases to be and the physical body dies. The ghost is gone—yet synchronized energy remains in the form of a cadaver which Earth reclaims. Ashes to ashes! Dust to dust! **Energy is never lost, it merely changes form.**

Energy Takeover

When the chemical bonds holding synchronized energy under lock and key are broken, these energies can go EITHER way. If the bonds are broken in a predominantly *anaerobic* environment, the energy can become a negative force—even if it was originally positive. This is what I meant earlier when I said that right-spin energy entering a left-spin environment can be diverted and used to promote dis-ease. This is how cancer works.

Cancer lives and grows off the negative energy fields produced in a sick, anaerobic body. Learn HOW to manage energy, and you will avoid cancer.
A person suffering with constipation is under metabolic stress—*anaerobic stress*. Constipation SLOWS ionization and transmutation of mineral energy and promotes the development of toxic energy fields. Noxious gas is PROOF.

Positive energy released under anabolic conditions FEEDS conditions like cancer. Cancer proliferates in an anaerobic environment by diverting positive energy to negative purposes—like the growth of a "mass." People with cancer should NEVER be given large amounts of high protein foods—be it meat, fish, fowl, or vegetable before systemic detoxification has taken place. Dietary moderation and low stress foods are best.

Cancer—A Different Set Of Rules

The rules of life are different once a person is under cancer's pall. Cancer is a *catabolic process* and the cancerous person is very fragile.

Cure-yourself health approaches often fail because the person think the rules of the game are the same for the person with cancer. This is where clinical nutrition and many health approaches fall flat on their faces! The rules are NOT the same! Cancer viruses—non-life forms—have the ability to hijack the body's energy fields. Cancer masses are **viral black holes** that draw-in and subvert all available energy and then EXPORT it to outlying colonies. Cancer uses biological alchemy to BREAK **synchronized** energy bonds to produce energy for itself.

There will NEVER be a "magic bullet" cure for cancer. Cancer defies the rules and complies with none of the LAWS of normal health. Cancer has but one purpose: to kill the host and rid the Earth of weak organisms. **Cancer is NOT the enemy, but it is the perfect double agent. First it kills the host. Then it kills itself. SYNCHRONIZATION!**
By controlling your internal body environment, you control the transmutation and ionization processes that Kervran

and Reams described.

Cancer is not inevitable. If you contract cancer, death and misery can be defeated. There is MORE than hope available for people with cancer, but they must understand the rules of the game. The chapter on cancer will outline those rules.

Health and vitality are the EFFECTS of the process we call *biological alchemy*. The process depends on our microbial friends and the internal environment we provide for them.

Kervran and Reams discovered a vital piece of the process we call aging. Their life's work points the way for us to rejuvenation and good health if we understand the rules of the game, and are willing to take personal responsibility for ourselves. When we take responsibility, we become *Young Again!*

PREVIEW: *Our next chapter is about the gut (small intestine) and the E. coli bacteria infections that killed many people and children during 1993. You will also learn what's behind Montezuma's revenge.*

Ozone • Ions

Therapeutic ozone breaks up congestion in the lungs and oxygenates the body while it burns up viruses, molds, and pathogenic bacteria in the air. Odors—from cigarettes to cooking—become a thing of the past.

The newest breed of ozonators double as ion generators for added benefits. Charged ions cause airborne particulates to fall from the air so they can be vacuumed away. They leave NO static dust trails on walls. There are no filters to clean or change or act as breeding grounds for pathogenic organisms. Fleas and dust mites die.

An ozone/ion generator insulates a family from colds, llness and dis-ease. Older folks find them especially beneficial, particularly in the winter.

A single unit can service several rooms at once or an entire house and is totally portable (see Source Index).

Acres USA

The best general interest publication available is *Acres USA*. It has had profound influence in my life. If I could only receive one publication, this is the one. Order a trial subscription and you will see what I mean. Call (800) 355-5313. I will accept your thanks in advance.

Cancer "Craps!"

Conventional cancer therapy has more than a little resemblance to the game of craps.

You have the stakes—your life. You have rules—*house* rules. You have the dealer—a *house* dealer that wears a white robe and who is controlled by the licensing boards and pharmaceutical industry. You have the *house* support team—they wear robes and they have licenses and are trained to do as they have been trained or are told. You have the other players—who appear to be winning enough to justify your joining the game. You have chips—called insurance, life savings, a farm, a house. You have dice—weighted in the *house's* favor. You have liquor—called radiation and chemotherapy. You have the *house* bouncer—his name is Fear. You have the *house* preacher—his name is Hope. You have odds—the 75% the house *dealer* gave you during your "consultations" prior to joining the game.

All games have an end. When you play cancer craps, the game automatically ends when you run out of money, or when you die—whichever comes first.

The *house* always wins when people play *their* game, on *their* turf, and by *their* rules. Is there a solution?

You bet! **Don't play!**

Instead, get into life. Clean up your body. **LAUGH!** Don't cry "poor me!" Don't dwell on hate, anger, and fear. Use the power of your mind to create the body you desire. Never, ever, under any circumstances should you entertain the slightest negative thought. Got it?

What you say your body believes! What you think, you get! It took me fifty years to get this straight, and I am here to tell you that your mind has the ability to create or to destroy! Use it as God intended!

Celebrate! You're **ALIVE** and if you do what you need to do, you will continue to celebrate life and see your great, great grand children grow up and experience the many wonders the future holds for those who love life MORE than those who fear death.

A Life Of Cancer Craps Is A Crappy Life!

V.D. • AIDS • Distemper

Intravenous use of Rene's Tea is producing astounding results on humans in China. US veterinarians use the tea to "cure" dogs and cats of distemper in only 48 hours!

Young Again! Pyramid

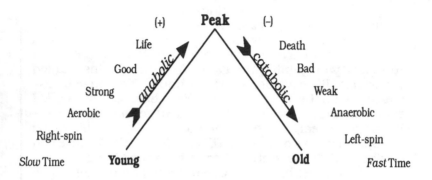

pH Scale

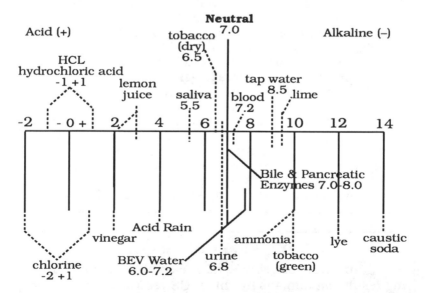

19

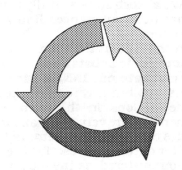

A Tube Within A Tube

Dr. Spot: *"There's always scissors!"*

Earlier we described some of the characteristics of the *integumentary system (skin)* as it relates to health and aging, Now, we will consider our *"inner" skin and see what part it plays in the process we call aging.*

Man's body is a tube within a tube. The skin is our *outer* tube, and the mucous membranes form the *inner* tube. The mucous membranes are the soft tissues that line the mouth, nasal passages, respiratory tract, stomach, gut and colon. They begin in the mouth and end at the anus.

The mucous membranes have tremendous significance to the story of aging and dis-ease. In the mouth, nasal passages, and respiratory system, the mucous membranes are classified as *stratified epithelium* and their primary job is protect underlying tissues AND to transfer energy.

The remainder of the tube is the GI tract. Its membranes are made up of *simple epithelium* whose job is to ABSORB nutrients, protect underlying tissues, and SECRETE mucous and enzymes.

The outer tube, the skin, has a combined surface area of about 30,000 square inches. The pores (openings) of the skin are called *stoma* and there are as many as 3,000 of them per square inch. By comparison to the skin, the mucous membranes have an approximate surface area of 18,000,000 (million) square inches, or 600 times greater. One inch on the outside equals 600 inches on the inside or a ratio of 1:600. THIS IS IMPORTANT!

Eating and drinking gives way to digestion, absorption, and elimination. We absorb so powerfully through the wall of our inner tube that toxic substances find an open doorway through which to enter.

The longer the transit time from the dinner table to the toilet, the more toxic substances we absorb. We must takes steps to rejuvenate our INNER tube.

The mucous membranes are a favorite conduit for drug chemotherapy. Medications in the form of suppositories, sublinguals, and aerosols are very easily absorbed through the mucous membranes that line the rectum, vagina, and respiratory system. A doctor dares not prescribe the same amount of medication to be administered via the mucous membranes as would be given orally, or by subcutaneous or intramuscular injection.

E. coli & The Gut

Most nutrient absorption takes place in the intestinal mucosa. This is the body's most vulnerable and most important terrain. An infection in the gut—Salmonella, typhus, pathogenic E. coli— causes the natural sloughing off action of the mucosa to increase. Normal sloughing occurs at the rate of approximately twenty million cells a day. These cells provide an important source of intestinal enzymes (the enzymes are contained in the sloughed-off cells), and they are also the vehicle of delivery. Pathogenic infection increases sloughing to such an extent that digestion and absorption of nutrients and fluids is NOT possible. Diarrhea and malnutrition result.

The infamous E. coli 0157.H7 bacteria that contaminated hamburger in the USA in early 1993, causes severe sloughing of the intestinal mucosa and "bloody" diarrhea. This is followed by dehydration from loss of fluids, loss of electrolytes, and starvation.

E. coli 0157.H7 produces a toxic waste product called an **exotoxin** *(exo-*to export; *toxin-*poison) that severely stresses the liver, and brings on tissue death and systemic overload of the kidneys. Dead tissue MUST be removed immediately or gangrene will set in (gangrene is petrified necrotic tissue). A dead body left unattended will swell like a balloon due to the gasses produced by gangrene; hence "gas gangrene."

Much of the job of tissue waste removal falls on the kidneys. Hence, the need for kidney dialysis (artificial filtering

of the blood) to assist people suffering with kidney overload and systemic (whole body) toxemia (*tox*-poison; *emia*-blood).
The best protection from dis-ease—bacterial or viral—is a clean colon and a strong immune system.

Old & Young

E. coli infections readily affect older folks because their metabolic functions are limited and their organs and glands are weak. Their energy reserves are low and toxicity levels are high. Their bodies are catabolic and often anaerobic. Lack of resiliency is their Achilles' heel.

Children are at the other end of the continuum. They have high resiliency, but most are malnourished and toxic because they eat the *usual and customary* American diet. Poor bowel habits, bad diet, and insufficient WATER are at the root of toxicity-driven illness. A terrain that is under stress is a **made-to-order** environment for bacterial infections like E. coli 0157.H7. Please do not think that all E. coli are alike, because they are not! Life is IMPOSSIBLE without the strains of friendly E. coli that inhabit the gut. It is only when our *vibrational signature* is off, that pathogenic organism manifest.

Not Everyone Died

Consider that over a million pounds of E. coli contaminated beef found its way into fast food restaurants, yet only a few hundred people became sick and only 6 died. The question is WHY? The answer has to do with the vibrational frequency of these people's "terrain."

Pathogenic organisms "feed" on negative energy fields produced in a TOXIC environment. This explains why, in a family with three children—all of who ate contaminated beef—only one child died. NO mystery is involved here.
The body's energy signature dictates sickness, and death, health and vitality. The aura is a reflection of that signature. It can be measured with pendulum or chain.

Consider the contagious dis-eases that have plagued mankind throughout history: bubonic plague, smallpox, typhoid, typhus, etc. Obviously, everyone did not die. The fact is, most people did NOT die. Those who did die in mass epidemics were those who were weak, who had anaerobic bowels, who were under-hydrated and malnourished. It is that simple!

The panic seen in the recent movie *Outbreak* is understandable in light of the general level of ignorance regarding health and dis-ease. Clean up your act and Ebola plague, Hanta viris, Cryptosporidium bacteria, necrotizing facitis (flesh eating bug), and their likes will bass you by.

A clean body is equivalent to blood on the lintel stone over the doorway. Death passes you by.

Lack Of Understanding

People of science have difficulty understanding discussions like this one because of the way they have been trained. Scientific thought generally embraces the Scientific Method and the Germ Theory of Disease. Our discussion does NOT fit their "model" or their false theories.

Whenever the phone rings and the caller asks, "What are your credentials?!!!" I know I have an "expert" on my hands, or someone who wants to defend something. Credentials are for the ego and the licensing boards. The modest professional who has their ego and prejudices in tow doesn't care about credentials. Credentials are a wonderful thing—IF they don't get in the way. Got it?

Vibrational medicine asks square questions, and it provides square answers. It approaches health related problems from an ENERGY vantage point. It is not hindered by the Germ Theory of Disease and other theoretical artifacts.

Remember, healthy bodies are nourished bodies. Healthy bodies are clean bodies. Healthy bodies are bodies in good physical condition. Healthy bodies are strong bodies. Healthy bodies are vessels of positive energy where negative energy vortexes find no quarter. Healthy bodies have a vibrant aura that *radiates* right-spin ENERGY and repels pathogenic microbes because its terrain is "tuned" for health.

It's The Pits

The small intestine is lined with convoluted folds called the *plicae circularis*. These folds are lined with *villi* (little fingers) and *microvilli* (hair-like structures) that increase the surface area of the intestine to 600 times that of the outer skin. The microvilli contain the cells that absorb and transport food nutrient energy. The area *between* the villi are known as the Crypts of Lieberkuhn. The Crypts are lined with cells that secrete our digestive enzymes and mucous.

As we age, the valleys that make up the intestinal *pits* become shallow. The villi and microvilli shorten. The transit time of food—from mouth to anus—slows. Constipation becomes common. Chronic constipation becomes the rule. As these alterations occur, the pits, villi, and microvilli become smothered in slow moving fecal matter, mucoid substances, and metabolic wastes.

Anaerobic conditions in the colon produce MASSIVE changes in the chemical make up of the fecal matter interfacing the intestinal walls. Fecal matter transforms into a semi-hard, rubber-like, mucoid material that actually *smothers* the intestinal wall. Over a period of years, this *stuff* thickens and narrows the opening (lumen), leaving a narrow tube—like an occluded water pipe—through which the body's wastes pass.

Earlier I mentioned that the colon of a very famous Hollywood cowboy had grown to almost twelve inches in diameter at the time of his death, yet the lumen (opening) for waste movement was only 1 inch. The rest was mucoid waste.

Fully 85% of the population needs colon therapy to get their intestinal house in order. This condition is reflected in the Rouleau effect as is seen in the blood of 85% of the people.

The combined loss of intestinal function, liver function, and a congested integument (skin), cause the average person to **forfeit** 75% of their waste processing capacity! The waste exit portals that remain—the lungs and kidneys—are NOT capable of making up the difference. The result is toxic overload of the entire *bio-electric* body and accelerated aging.

A CLEAN bowel and clean tissues make the difference between youth and vitality old age and death.

Colon therapy may be unAmerican, but it MUST NOT be dismissed. For many others, who have a history of sickness and obesity, colon therapy is the FAST TRACK back to good health. This was the path I took many years ago!

A great book on the subject of colon therapy is *Tissue Cleansing & Bowel Management.* I highly recommend this book because it shows the reader—in forty full color pictures—how to set up and perform colon therapy (see Source Index).

My Story

By 1977 I had reached a plateau in my personal health. I visited a lady who had been trained by Dr. Reams in the Biological Theory of Ionization. Dolly took saliva and urine readings, and read the sclera (whites) of my eyes—which is quite different than reading the iris of the eyes, or Iridology.

The results showed I suffered from congestion in the gut and colon. Subsequent colon therapy confirmed this as I experienced hard, compacted fecal material exit my body. The procedure caused my health to reach NEW heights, as my body immediately **surged backward** to more youthful days.

Without this therapeutic procedure, I would NOT have been able to reverse the aging process, nor could I have written this book today.

These days, colon therapy can be done in the comfort

and privacy of your own home, safely and comfortably.

There is ANOTHER important to equip your home with colonic equipment. In time of severe medical illness (when a doctor or hospital is not an option), or during a period of national emergency or geophysical disaster, a colonic may make the difference between life and death. *(Totally self contained BEV units are also available for emergency situations.)* **Colon therapy rewinds your clock and causes Time to run backwards!**

A *live testimony* from your author, and you can believe it, for I am *Young Again!*

PREVIEW: *Our next chapter is about YOUR aura. Why do people climb rock mountains? HOW could Jesus pass through the wall of the temple?*

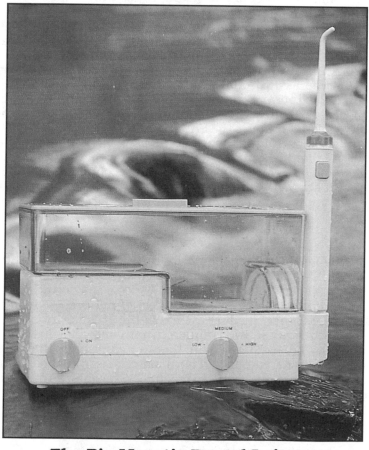

The Bio-Manetic Dental Irrigator

Enhanced PAC'ˢ & Aging Reversal

Enhanced PAC˙ˢ (proanthocyanidins) are **newly** formulated antioxidants and **free radical scavengers.** They are better than any similar substance your author has ever experienced. Their effects are felt within 7 days!

Unlike vitamins A, C, and E, *enhanced* PAC'ˢhave NO side effects. When combined with Yucca extract and Kombucha tea, and a liver stone flush, brown eyes have turned blue or green, and hair now covers bald heads.

Enhanced PAC'ˢ prevent uncontrolled cellular oxidation. Uncontrolled oxidation causes the body to cannibalize itself. Oxidation is another word for aging.

As we age, the tissues oxidize faster and faster. An example of extremely rapid oxidation is a massive heart attack where heart muscle disintegrates almost instantaneously. Doctors sometimes refer to the heart as a "mass of mush" in the aftermath of a massive coronary.

A *free radical scavenger* is a chemical compound that **bonds** to free radicals which are highly reactive chemicals that are missing one or more electrons. PAC'ˢ prevent rapid oxidation and destructive chain reactions.

We ingest massive amounts of free radicals every day. They come from air, water, and food. The body also *manufacture* them from the pollutants we take into the body. Once toxic substances enter the body, they DO change their chemical for and become even more toxic.

Examples would be food additives, fluorides and chlor**amines** in tap water, soy and canola oils, pesticides, microwaved food, and vaccination induced viruses, bacteria, and animal serum proteins that transport them.

Enhanced PAC'ˢ stabilize wastes released into circulation during detoxification and when flushing your liver of stones. They prevent toxic wastes from being reabsorbed as they make their way down 20 feet of intestine on their way to the toilet.

All dis-ease conditions respond favorably to PAC'ˢ. The best formulations include leucoanthocyanins, catechins, bilberry, rosemary, tocotrienols, carotinoids, and CO-enzymes Q6-10. **Per tablet activity should be 135 activity units. Don't settle for less!**

If you want to control aging as your author has done, include *enhanced* proanthocyanidins (PAC'ˢ) in your diet and you will get your wish (see Source Index).

Vitamins A, E, C & zinc don't compare to PAC'ˢ

"Eat your vaccine, dear!"

Did you know that government, the medical establishment, the pharmaceutical companies, and the multinational food giants have hatched a devilish plan that will have disastrous effects on the health of people worldwide and especially in the USA?

The scheme involves using genetically altered fruits and vegetables to transport the likes of hepatitis B, polio, measles, mumps, tetanus, swine flue, and rubella into YOUR body via the food you eat.

Gene splicing of the food supply will produce millions of sick people. It will render "forced" immunization moot while it keeps the hospital rooms full.

If you want to live a healthy, happy, life, you MUST plant a garden, grow some fresh food in containers on your patio, share a community plot, or hire someone to grow "safe" vaccine and chemical-free food for you.

Home grown food—even in small quantities—produces astounding effects on health. The best way to get into gardening is to start today! Don't worry about what you don't know. Just do it and nature will each you the rest.

Normally, it takes many years to build up your soil and neutralize the negative energy fields in the soil. Now, with the use of a product called Bio-Grow, it is possible to completely convert dirt into live soil in less than 30 days.

Bio-Grow creates a positive energy soil environment where microbes and plants prosper. This is a Fourth Dimension product that closely mimics the effects of Biodynamic principles and application.

Bio-Grow is mixed in five gallon buckets and stirred with a wooden stick twice a day in a clockwise direction for 2 days before it is applied to the soil. Application involves sprinkling it onto the soil, or side dressing the plants.

One ten pound box treats 500 square feet. If it is used for foliar application the dilution rate is 20:1. The product must NOT be used in heavier concentrations. We are talking about homeopathic agricultural practices here, so it is important to not overdo.

Bio-Grow tunes the soil and harmonizes Earth frequencies so plants grow and mature in a healthy environment and produce healthy people (see Source Index).

A liver that's full of stones is behind ovary, thyroid, adrenal, and hormone problems. Detoxify and flush your live and life will return to normal.

20

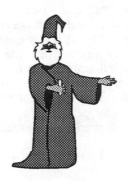

The Aura Effect

*"Man's mind stretched to a new idea never
goes back to its original dimension."*
Oliver Wendel Holmes

The injury had occurred the night before, but Jerry was not aware of any specific damage. As Jerry and I walked into the shop and began browsing, the lady who owned the shop approached Jerry and said,

"OOOH! You must be hurting pretty bad?"

He looked at her blankly and asked what she meant.

"Oh! Your aura! You have a very BIG hole in it in your groin area. Did you injure yourself?"

Jerry was hurting. He had torn a hernia in the connective tissues of his pelvic region the night before.

What was so intriguing about the encounter was that this lady was a total stranger. She knew nothing about Jerry, yet she was able to vividly see his body aura and the hole in it. We had heard of people like this lady, but neither of us had witnessed the phenomena before.

The Glow Of Health

The body has a radiation field surrounding it. This is an established fact. Kirlian photography can capture the aura on a photographic plate—its size, shape, and color in direct relation to the overall vitality of the person.

Jesus was reported to have a glow about Him. Whenever He is pictured, the halo or aura effect is always seen around His head. The halo and aura are right-spin energy. Many people believe the greater your aura, the more advanced human being you are. Perhaps. For certain, each of us has one, and the greater it is, the healthier we are!

When people suffer with dis-ease, the electrical charge of the bio-electric body shifts from one that is right-spin and healthy, to one that is left-spin and pathogenic. When we notice the sickly pallor of another person, we are taking note of a diminished *aura*, though we may not recognize it as such. We also recognize when the person has returned to health—by noting their vibrant *electrical* appearance.

Energy Drain

Some people are exhausting. I am not speaking of the person who runs in *hyper drive*, but the person who drains your energy and leaves you feeling very tired. These folks are energy sinks! They may be nice people, but the *effect* of their presence is less than refreshing. A whole lot less!

Sue owned a massage therapy and iridology clinic for many years. She once commented that certain people drew so much energy from her that she could not work on them. Later, I learned that my wife had severed her friendship with one lady Sue would no longer treat. The reason was that the lady was *exhausting!*

Sue was an interesting person. She had the uncanny ability to *see* and *feel* things about people who came to her for treatments. They call people like Sue, "healer." Sue definitely was a healer. Sue was also a superb organic gardener. Sue had a green thumb and the plants produced abundantly for her. Her plants were "vibrant" and never required any form of poison to control bugs or weeds.

One day I asked her, "Sue, what is your secret?" She just smiled. As I came to know her, I realized that she knew how to accelerate healing—through the laying-on of hands. In her case, it was called massage therapy.

Sue was able to speed up the electron flow in the body of the patient to such an extent that the person walked out of her clinic TOTALLY refreshed and happy.

By accelerating the flow of energy, Sue strengthened the positive energy fields in the body and "draw off" negative energy forces. Sometimes she would shake her hands to dissipate the negative energy. The effects were seen immediately in the patient's *aura* and vibrancy. Sue had mastered the skill of energy manipulation. She understood that **life** is a field of competing energy forces.

Energy & Auras

The world is composed of but one thing: energy! When energy condenses it is called matter. Matter has three states: gas, liquid, and solid—each a variation in the degree of energy density and each vibrating at its own frequency.

Rocks are hard and solid. Touch your skin. It has texture and can be stretched. Rocks and skin are not *really* solids, we just "classify" them as solids. Solids are energy fields joined together in such a way that they take on the shape, feel, and smell of something we learn to identify as rock, skin, or food.

All things living and non-living have an aura. A rock's aura—and the effect it exerts on things near it—can be positive or negative. If the rock's energy state is positive, it will produce a right-spin effect and will be therapeutic, and visa versa.

If we increase the flow of electrons around the nuclei of the atoms in a rock, it will change form. For example, if we heat sulphur, it will change from a solid, to a liquid, to a gas. So will frozen water—ice—although it is not a rock.

Rocks & Mountains

In the Bible, rocks had particular significance in matters of health. Rocks have a sacred place in most religions. Rocks are not *live* in the animal sense, but they do possess *life*. A rock's life is expressed in its energy footprint and signature.

People who climb rock mountains are often asked, "WHY?" The answer usually given is *"Because they are there!"* There is a more accurate reason. People climb rocks because they find it *invigorating*. Climbers absorb fantastic quantities of ENERGY from rock mineral formations. Rocks radiate ENERGY that syncs the climber with Mother Earth frequency.

Man transmutes food energy into fuel energy. Climbing rocks is just another way man taps into nature's energy bank. The same idea applies to swimming in sea water, or walking bare footed in sand or grass. The energy vibrations from these substances is "transferred" to the body and it makes us feel good! People with sore feet, legs, and back respond fast!

Jesus & The Wall

It is recorded that when Jesus was about to be stoned in the Temple, He passed through the wall and disappeared, to the frustration of his enemies. As a child, I accepted this story, but I never believed it because anyone with a lick of sense knows that you cannot walk through a wall.

Today, this story delivers a different message—one that is both factual and explanatory. Christ possessed the knowledge and ability to accelerate the flow of electrons in His body. In so doing, He was able to pass through the wall of the temple. By speeding up His electrons to the point of disintegration (think of ice becoming steam), He squeezed between the atoms of the stone wall and vanished. Neither He nor the wall were solids! Both were condensed ENERGY particles. The Christ did not violate natural law, rather He knew how to manipulate it.

Life is a STATEMENT of positive (+) and negative (–) energy forces. Man give them different names and classifies them in ways that are more easily understood. For example: good and evil, light and dark, right and wrong, left and right, YOUNG and OLD and so on. Regardless, we are referring to the phenomena we call ENERGY!

Reflections

Our body's aura is a reflection of our inner state of health. We can measure our aura with a simple pendulum and it is easy to do. Using a pendulum or vibration chain is simple, but it does require the dowser to focus his/her thoughts. *The Pendulum Kit, Vibrations,* and *Map Dowsing* is a trilogy of books to teach you how to effectively dowse (see Source Index).

A pendulum is nothing but an antenna that sends and receives electrical energy. Our mind receives the information and "interprets" it. You can use a pendulum to measure your aura, and you can use this **reference point** to measure change, or determine the effect a substance is likely to have on the your body systems.

Using a pendulum to determine the electrical energy state of food substances is one of its best uses. A pendulum can identify left-spin or right-spin apples, carrots, etc. Remember, whatever is being measured is like a "radio station" that is sending out ENERGY signals. The pendulum is the receiving antenna. It can also be used to transmit signals.

We send and receive electrical signals when we sense with our intuition, which is a kind of sixth sense. We will discuss these Fourth Dimension concepts in a future chapter.

As you reverse the aging process, your aura expands and physical energy increases. When your aura has returned the level it was at before you began the decent into old age, you have returned to your *anabolic* PEAK. In the precess of getting there, the passage of Time will slow until it finally STOPS altogether. When this occurs, you have achieved agelessness and you are *Young Again!*

PREVIEW: *Our next chapter deals with energy and numbers. Did you know that big can mean small, and weak can mean strong?*

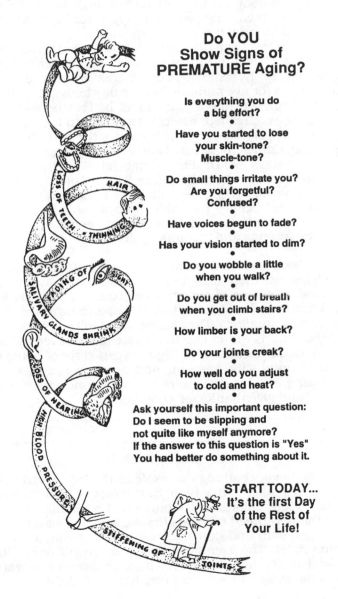

Do YOU
Show Signs of
PREMATURE Aging?

Is everything you do
a big effort?
•
Have you started to lose
your skin-tone?
Muscle-tone?
•
Do small things irritate you?
Are you forgetful?
Confused?
•
Have voices begun to fade?
•
Has your vision started to dim?
•
Do you wobble a little
when you walk?
•
Do you get out of breath
when you climb stairs?
•
How limber is your back?
•
Do your joints creak?
•
How well do you adjust
to cold and heat?
•
Ask yourself this important question:
Do I seem to be slipping and
not quite like myself anymore?
If the answer to this question is "Yes"
You had better do something about it.

START TODAY...
It's the first Day
of the Rest of
Your Life!

Fresh Air • Deep Breathing • Ozone

Fresh air is very important to good health, yet people do not get enough of it. Fresh air is full of energy. It helps the body rid itself of toxic energy fields via the lungs. Deep breathing provides oxygen for both external (lung) and internal (cellular) respiration.

Practice deep breathing regularly. A good method is to close your mind to everything and concentrate on breathing deeply. Listen to yourself breathe in and breathe out. Do this for five minutes twice a day for a great effect.

Fresh air allows you to rest better and wake up feeling more refreshed. Sleep with your windows open—even if it is very cold. Cold air causes the body to build brown fat. Cold increases metabolic activity. Sleep outside under the stars like Dr. Paul Bragg did. Read the Bragg's new book on deep breathing (see Source Index).

An ozone (O_3) generator is the smart way to clean up dirty air (smog, pesticide sprays, etc.). An ozone generator is of tremendous benefit to people who suffer with emphysema and respiratory disorders—especially in the winter time.

People who have suffered for years with respiratory problems, see them disappear in a few short days due to the healing effects of ozonated/ionized air. The medical establishment would doesn't want people to earn of ozone's therapeutic qualities. They know they can't compete with a device that is dirt cheap to operate (see Source Index).

Good health and a high oxygen state of being go hand in hand with fresh air and deep breathing. Open your windows, breathe deeply, ozonate and ionize your home—and give thanks for good health!

Shower & Bath

Make your bathing water safe and biologically friendly with a three stage redox filter that removes toxic organic chemicals like chlor*amine*. Common shower filters don't touch the new breed of toxic chemicals in our water.

The skin and hair respond to biologically friendly bathing water. The liver stays healthier. People feel better and live longer. The skin absorbs massive amounts of water borne chemicals—avoid them (see Source Index)!

21

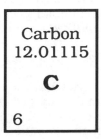

Carbon
12.01115

C

6

Avogadro's Number

*"The health of the people is the foundation
upon which their happiness depends."*
Benjamin Disraeli

It was a hot August day in 1975—the mercury had reached 95° Fahrenheit. Out of nowhere came what looked to be a hippie carrying a clip board. He said, "I'm from the City of Velvet and I'm checking all buildings for proper address numbers and you don't seem to have any!"

"Do too!" I retorted.

"Well, I looked and I didn't see any and I want to know what you are going to do about it?" he rattled as he flashed a copy of the local business ordinance in my face —expecting to cement his authority and intimidate me.

"Do too!" I said again, "And I can prove it!"

As we proceeded to the front of the building, I motioned to Dale to follow my new found acquaintance and me.

There we stood, the three of us, facing a 4x4 "blank" post that formed the door jam, and I said;

"Dale, this fine gentlemen is here from city hall and he says that we are not in compliance with city ordinances regarding having our building properly posted with our street address."

"Right there!" I said. "See! It says, 505 S. Main. What's wrong with that?"

And the man looked at me and said with a strange look on his face,

"There is no address there! It's blank!"

"Hmmm!" I buzzed, as I turned to Dale and said,

"Dale, do you see 505 S. Main St. posted here on this post?" Dale look at me and fired back,

"Sure do! Right there on the post!" With that, the man looked at me, then at Dale, shook his head—unsure WHO was crazy—gave up and just *walked away.*

Things Not What They Seem

Things are not always what they seem. Nothing can be something. Something small may actually be big. Something weak can be strong. We cannot always trust our eyes, and sometimes logic does not make sense of conflicting circumstances or experiences. Sometimes we must follow our instincts or we lose our direction, go insane, or just *walk away.*

The man in our story knew when to *walk away.* Science does not. Instead, science tries to make natural energy phenomena comply with its LAWS, and in the process, it misses nature's lessons.

In homeopathy, something weak is actually strong. Something that should not exist actually does exist. Something that is nothing can be made into something.

These *apparent* "contradictions" cause science and medicine to ridicule instead of open mindedly inquiring. They demand *scientific* proof, backed by a "body" of knowledge, when they should be interested in RESULTS. They get caught up in theory and method, and forget that their studies and discoveries are riddled with contradictions.

Phenomena

Here are a few examples of electrical phenomena. Let's see if they shed light on the aging process.

Biodynamic agricultural practices transmute raw cow manure into a potent, yet *different* substance. It then mixes a "pinch" of the *potentized* substance in twenty gallons of high energy water to *transfer* the energy from the "new" substance to the water through certain stirring procedures. Applied to hundreds of acres of dead soil, the *energized* solution causes an energy *explosion* in the soil and life bursts forth. *Science cannot explain this phenomenon because it does not fit its model.* Science wants "scientific" proof, when it should be interested in results.

Homeopathic medicine uses the principle of *dilution,*

succussion, resonance, and *transference* to create energy substances (called remedies) that effectively treat dis-ease on the Fourth dimension energy level.

If you were to add one drop of black paint to one gallon of white paint, you would have a MIX of both colors. The black paint would, of course, be very diluted and would exert little influence on the white paint. The more white paint added, the less influence the black paint has. However, black paint is still there, albeit in smaller amounts each time more white paint is added. This is a "physical" dilution, and our example deals with the **physical** influence of the black paint on the white paint.

Homeopathic medicine is concerned with the influence of energy fields upon each other, rather than the physical influence in our paint example above.

Potentiation

Remedies work on the basis of "similars." Homeopathy starts with a substance that has a *similar* vibrational frequency as the dis-ease energy field. The substance is then **diluted.** At each dilution, the remedy is pounded (succussion) so that it will absorb various frequencies (10x, 20x, 50x, 100x, 200x, etc.). This process is referred to as "potentiation," and the remedy as a "potentized" solution.

The idea is to create multiple dilutions of different frequencies that, when taken into the body, will "cancel" disease target frequencies. A "potentized" remedy treats the patient in the Fourth Dimension realm. In homeopathy, dilution and succussion add power, where in our paint example, the black paint became less influential each time we added more white paint.

Homeopathic dilutions are different than physical dilutions. They are electrical phenomena instead. Remedies are CONCENTRATED "energy fields" that are derived from the vibrational frequencies of "physical" substances. The more the remedy is *diluted,* and the more it is "succussed," the more energy the remedy contains and the more effective it becomes against dis-ease. Logic says a "remedy" should NOT exert any influence because the original substance is weaker—maybe even nonexistent—and energy transference through *succussion* pushes the "scientific" mind too far. Logic, however, is faulty here because it is usually based on Third Dimension physics instead of Fourth Dimension understanding of energy phenomena. Homeopathy **manipulates** and **transfers** the electrical *signature* (frequency) of one substance to that of another, hence *resonance* and *transferance.* In homeopathy, something that should not exist DOES exist. *Science cannot explain this* *phenomenon because it does not fit its model, so they ridicule and expresses contempt!*

MORA technology is a spin off from homeopathy, just like the word processor is a spin off from the typewriter. MORA duplicates electrical *signatures* and *transfers* them to the patient INSTEAD of using the actual *remedy* itself.

The *remedy* is placed into an scanning "well" where its frequency is *duplicated* (think of a computer scanner that reads a typed page and converts it to codes and signals so the computer can use it). The duplicated frequency is then *transferred* into the sick person's body and the desired *cure* takes place. The process can be repeated over and over without consuming the remedy itself. In homeopathy, something that doesn't appear to exist actually does exist.

Whether or not a healing modality "fits" accepted medical theory, models, dogma, or the "LAWS" of science doesn't matter. The only thing that really counts is results!

It's In The Numbers

Amedeo Avogadro (1776-1856) was an Italian chemist who saw big numbers in small things. He developed a method to estimate the number of atoms that exist in a substance by comparing it to a known reference substance whose number of atoms were known, at least in theory. This reference number is called Avogadro's number, or [N], in his honor. Like Reams, Pauling, Caisse, Semmelweis, Carson, and Gerson, Avogadro was ridiculed by his "peers" for his vision, and the TRUTH to which he bore witness. *(Wizards don't have peers. Wizards are surrounded by copy cats who want to put their name on someone else's discovery.)*

Avogadro's reference substance was 12 grams of carbon-12. The carbon atom is extremely small. The number of atoms in 12 grams of carbon-12 is *extremely* large! It is estimated to be approximately 602, 000, 000, 000, 000, 000, 000, 000 atoms!

In homeopathy, the most powerful remedy is one where a substance has been **diluted** and **potentized** to a point that NONE of the original substance remains. Physically, a substance no longer exists once it goes *beyond* Avogadro's number or *twenty-two places.* Logic says that when the original substance ceases to exist—you have reached NOTHING! Yet, a homeopathic remedy has an enormous energy "footprint" for something that supposedly doesn't exist.

Each time a substance is diluted and potentized, its energy footprint increases exponentially. Hence, a 200X remedy may actually be a MILLION times more "potent" than the energy frequency of the original substance.

Aging & Avogadro's Number

Avogadro's number is VERY important to the aging process. If the positive energy contained in a homeopathic remedy can cause MASSIVE change for the "good," then the negative energy transference of a poor lifestyle, bad food, and polluted water should be DISASTROUS to health and longevity. The some reasoning holds true for **negative *actions* and thoughts** that produce effects millions of times greater than the actual event—similar to the ripples that are created when a rock is tossed into a pond—each negative thought and action creating a compound and reverse negative effect on health.

Dr. Samuel Hahnemann

Samuel Hahnemann (1755-1843) is the father of homeopathic medicine. He was a brilliant German physician. The electrical phenomenon he discovered is known as the medicine of **"similars"** or homeopathy.

Let's compare homeopathic medicine to allopathic medicine and see if a contrast of the concepts involved can help us to understand the aging process.

Allopathic medicine (conventional medicine) attempts to treat dis-ease with chemicals that are *antagonistic* to dis-ease. It treats dis-ease by inducing a **pathologic** reaction that is antagonistic to the dis-ease being treated—an **"opposite cures opposite"** approach. A pathologic reaction is one where pathology (dis-ease) is "created!" Drugs are prescribed based on the benefit : risk factor we discussed earlier. Pharmacology recognizes that all drugs carry risk and all drugs damage the vital organs. Allopathic medicine thinks short term by attempting to *overpower* dis-ease with drugs that SHOCK the body into a condition of *subclinical* illness. Allopathic medicine uses powerful, *left-spin* energy fields (drugs) and shoots these negative energy bullets—"magic bullets"—into the vital organs, tissues, and glands. Allopathy is the medicine of "opposites."

Homeopathy is the exact opposite of allopathy. It is the medicine of "similars." It is "legitimate" holistic medicine. It uses energy fields with "similar" vibrational frequencies to CANCEL offending disease energy frequencies. Homeopathy relies on a **"like cures like"** reactions.

How Homeopathy Was Discovered

Hahnemann, was extremely disillusioned with conventional medicine. While treating patients with yellow fever, he discovered that if he gave a "healthy" person—who did NOT have Yellow Fever—a tea of cinchona bark (which was known to be effective against the fever), intermittent fevers would spontaneously develop as if the person actually had the condition. Thus, a "similar" effect!

Hahnemann discovered that a "diluted" substance is more powerful than a large amount of the substance. He refined his new method of treatment and eventually included the physical, emotional and mental disturbances of the patient. Remedies were developed by *trial and error* based on their ability to *produce* a response similar to the sick person. If a trial remedy produced a **similar** reaction, it was further tested on a sick person to see if it would bring about a cure. *(Present day homeopathic remedies do NOT bring on actual illness or dis-ease in a healthy person. They can **only** cancel offending energy fields if they **exist** in the patient. They are NO side effects.)*

Hahnemann experienced much success applying his "similars," but noticed that the effectiveness of his remedies increased in direct proportion to the dilution and potentiation factor. In other words, the MORE he diluted and "pounded or succussed" the remedy, the more effective it was on the patient! His findings were in serious "conflict" with the orthodox medical dogma of his day. The conflict continues to this day!

Dosage-related effects—as practiced in modern pharmacokinetics (the study of the dynamics of chemical drugs in the body) looks at the action of drugs on body metabolism with emphasis on the time required for absorption, duration of action, distribution in the system, and method of excretion from the body. These things determine the **activity level**—*the saturation level of the drug in the blood and tissues.*

Allopathic medicine is acutely aware of the problems brought on by drug usage. It walks a tight rope between short term benefits and short term damage to the vital organs. Long term damage is NOT an issue because it cannot be proven. Long term effects are instead given "new" dis-ease names.

Hahnemann got wonderful results using remedies that *exceeded* Avogadro's number. This conflicts with Newtonian physics which states, "where there is an action, there is an equal and opposite reaction." Newtonian LAWS are the basis of modern drug chemotherapy mentality. Pharmacology and medicine as we know them, rely on HUGE quantities of drugs to produce an **activity level** that can be MEASURED. Medical science uses a sledge hammer approach that is based on "opposites," where homeopathy uses *gentle* remedies that are based on "similars."

Allopathic medicine loads you up with drugs to a

point BEYOND the ability of the kidneys, liver, lungs and skin to excrete them. The cells and tissues are forced to accept drugs by default, and life force is diminished! Damage to the glands and organs mirrors the *type* and *quantity* of drugs used and the *duration* of time they remain in the system.

Homeopathy is the modality of **preference** for patients and physicians who are interested in "healing." Remedies *interface* the subtle energy level where dis-ease has its roots.

Homeopathy & Agriculture

Modern agriculture uses new SUPER *potentized* poisons to try and stop insects and weeds. Until recently, large amounts of poison was called for. Now, VERY small amounts of poison is mixed with huge amounts of water. The idea is the same as biodynamics, but the effect is the exact opposite.

Agricultural and pharmaceutical companies have cloned Hahnemann's principles of *dilution, potentiation,* and *transference* and have turned them to **EVIL** purposes. The *experts* are using God given knowledge against Earth and her inhabitants.

This is why I encourage the reader to plant a garden and grow some food. Home grown food can cover a plethora of poor choices and mistakes in personal lifestyle. Real food is a gift from God. It will cause your cells to resonate "healthy!"

Think Small

Americans like to think big—big cars, big houses, big meals, big surgeries, big bottles of pills! In fact, the "big" syndrome is so prevalent that people complain and feel cheated when they pay a lot of money for a small bottle of pills!

In health related matters, we must LEARN to think *small* as in terms of the HUGE side effects created by negative energy substances. We must understand that the bio-electric body interfaces both positive and negative energy forces, and that even "tiny" amounts of a toxic substances can exert massive long term effects on health.

When we consume potent negative energy substances, we misapply the principles of homeopathic medicine.

If you want to experience and maintain PEAK health, you must think in terms of Avogadro's number—or you will not become *Young Again!*

PREVIEW: *Our next chapter looks at our multi-dimensional body. It looks at the "terrain" of the bio-electric body and reconsiders Pasteur's obsession with "bugs" and the Germ Theory of Dis-ease.*

SUPER Ionized Mikrowater

Mikrowater is a special type of *therapeutic* water being used in Japan to treat everything from diabetes and cancer to gout and connective tissues disorders.

In Japan, Mikrowater is made using special equipment and common tap water. In the USA, water contaminant levels require **extensive clean up** of contaminants to create non-toxic ionized Mikrowater.

Medical grade ionized Mikrowater is made using BEV water plus ionic sea minerals. Medical grade Mikrowater enjoys many advantages over plain Mikrowater.

The advantages of **medical grade** SUPER ionized Mikrowater derive from the ability to create highly *reduced* alkaline water or highly *oxidized* acid water with pH ranges that are far BEYOND plain ionized Mikrowater.

Mikrowater ionizers create extremely **fine** water molecules that powerfully interact with body tissues at the *subtle energy level* where dis-ease and illness have their roots. Ionizers concentrate acid and alkaline mineral ions **along with** *contaminants* found in tap water *and* drinking water made with conventional purifiers and distillers found in most homes. (Purity is critically important!)

Mikrowater ionizers create two types of water: acid ionized Mikrowater and alkaline ionized Mikrowater. Each has its own special uses in healing the body. **Acid** ionized Mikrowater is used externally to heal infections and promote beautiful skin, while **alkaline** ionized Mikrowater is taken orally or used as colon irrigation water.

For example, alkaline Mikrowater is **saturated** with charged electrons that are loaded with available energy. The body uses this energy to **heal** a sick body. Sick bodies are acidic bodies. Alkaline ionized Mikrowater neutralizes body acids similar to way *Far Infrared* products work. Super Mikrowater a **quantum leap** over *plain* Mikrowater.

With the advent of BEV water and its marriage to ionized water, we have created **medical grade** SUPER Mikrowater with pH ranges from 2 to 11.5, with unsurpassed purity and contaminant protection. The **healing potential** that comes with purity and additional pH range is astounding.

SUPER **medical grade** Mikrowater is the single biggest health advance in medical history. Existing BEV and Mikrowater units are easily retrofitted.

(See pages 17-110 and Source Index)

22

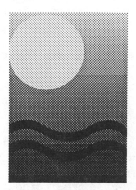

Change The Terrain

"No tree has branches foolish enough to fight among themselves."
"Watashi Wa" Lampert

The great French bacteriologist, Pasteur, said, *"Le microbe c'est tout!* The microbe is everything!" A contemporary, Claude Bernard retorted, *"Le microbe c'est rien. Le terrain c'est tout!* The microbe, that's nothing! It is the terrain that's everything!"

When we look *beyond* the bacteria, we see that they are only participants in a grand scheme. Bacteria take their cues from the *signature* of the bio-electric body—the "terrain."

The bacteria cannot prosper unless the *terrain* is conducive to their growth. Therefore, it is the *terrain* that must concern us. The terrain is the doorway through which dis-ease enters and old age expresses itself. The electrical terrain of the bio-electric is *beyond* the physical body and the Third Dimension world in which we live.

Multi-Dimensional Body

The human being is a *multi-dimension* creature. We act out our lives on three levels—mental , physical and spiritual — but life goes beyond these. We learn early to perceive and interpret our world in physical terms and geometric concepts we call length, width and height—the First, Second, and Third Dimensions.

We experience other levels of existence—higher levels—such as the abilities we exhibit and or experience from time to time like intuition, telepathy, dowsing, and maybe even the ability to see holes in another person's aura. These things belong to higher levels, like the 4th and 5th, dimensions.

Aging & The Fourth Dimension

These higher dimensions are *invisible* dimension for all but a few. Aging occurs in higher realms before it is experienced in our Third Dimension world and seen in the mirror.

Vitality and health are controlled by the electrical energy forces of the Fourth Dimension. Anything that impacts the Fourth Dimension electric body affects the Third Dimension physical body and visa-versa.

Health and dis-ease are expressions of the "energy" tug-of-war constantly going on in the invisible world of the Fourth Dimension.

When we die, the tug-of-war is over. The negative energy forces won! Simultaneous with death, vital force (spirit) leaves the body. We *"give up the ghost!"* The "ghost" returns from whence it came. It returns to a *higher* energy level, perhaps the Fourth Dimension. Maybe higher. No one knows for sure. Call it heaven, hell, hereafter. Suit yourself.

The Fourth Dimension body goes by different names like—**subtle energy** body, **soul, astral** body, **spirit, invisible** body, **bio-electric** body, and **etheric** body, **Chi, Qi, Prana**. They all refer to the same thing, depending on your view.

Our Fourth Dimension existence is generally invisible, but it is there none the less. We can deny its existence, but doing so will NOT change the reality of its existence, or its influence on our earthly journey.

When we attempt to heal the physical body, but ignore the spirit body, healing is incomplete. If we allow the electric body to become old, the physical body follows suit. If we experience death in the physical realm, but maintain our hold on our spirit, we are NOT really dead, and we return to our physical world with tales of after death experiences. If death occurs in the Fourth Dimension realm—where our spirit body resides—we experience physical death and life on Earth ceases.

Vantage Point

The electric body should be viewed as an *extension* of the physical body, and the physical body as the *expres-*

sion **of the electric body. The Fourth Dimension interfaces dis-ease and health, life and death.**

It is important that we become comfortable with these concepts. They will help us to understand our earthly dilemma. Long before dis-ease manifests itself in the physical realm, the electric body is undergoing *vibrational* changes that set the course for the physical recognition of illness. This is what Bernard meant when he said, *"The terrain is everything!"*

Before we can learn how to *manipulate* the energy forces that interface the physical AND electric body terrains, we must adopt a *vibrational* view of health and dis-ease.

In order to understand the forces of aging, one must understand the idea of an "invisible" world of *antagonistic* energy fields. We only feel the influence of these spiritual forces when they BURST into our physical, *visible* world in the form of SIGNS confirmed by the doctor's diagnosis.

The *invisible* world is poorly understood. Yet, this is the arena where the war for health and dis-ease is fought. We are concerned with the terrain of BOTH worlds—the *visible* and the *invisible*—and the energy forces fields that influence and govern them. Examples of these energy fields are bio-junk food, polluted water, negative thoughts and words, drugs, and bad living habits in general. Humans are a reflection of the universe as are all other life forms.

Food Plants & Insects

We have much in common with plants and insects. They can help us to better understand our *dual* existence because they too have a *dual* existence.

Plants have many functions. Two functions are the production of food nutrient energy, and the infusion of solar energy into the soil. In the process of synthesizing food molecules, the plant brings CARBON from the atmosphere into Mother Earth's dermal *skin* layer—the soil.

The plant is the mediator of solar energy. Plants capture it and use it to form complex organic food molecules. Organic food molecules contain carbon, oxygen, nitrogen, hydrogen, sulphur, and "ionic" minerals. These molecules are biologically active. They participate in anabolic activities we call *growth and repair*. Healthy soils equate to healthy plants and right-spin molecules, unless the plants have been genetically engineered like soy and canola (rape), which are good examples of plants that feed on left-spin energy fields and produce toxic oils and proteins that charade as food.

Mediators

As mediators of energy, plants receive solar and cosmic energy forces and convert them into new and different energy forms—like food and wood. **Energy is never lost, it merely changes form!**

Plants are ANTENNAS. They are *living* pendulums. They receive energy constantly—by day from the Sun and by night from the cosmos. By day, plants convert solar energy into hydrocarbon sugars (*hydro*-water. *carbon*-atomic element #12.) with the help of mineral ions and enzymes supplied by the soil bacteria. By night, plants use sugar molecules and earth minerals for growth, the "dew point" being the **"peak"** of their feeding period (that point at which sufficient heat is given off to cause the formation of condensation or "dew."

In Paul Hermann's fascinating book, *Conquest By Man*, he mentioned reports of early Viking adventurers who landed in the New England and sipped the "sweet dew" from the blades of grass.

Plants CANNOT create by themselves. They need the trillions of unpaid workers in the soil—the bacteria to complete the miracle we crudely refer to as photosynthesis. All (so called) higher life forms—plant, animal, and man—require microbial assistance in order to express their existence.

The bacteria live on cosmic energy as well. They eat the carbon sugars plants manufacture. They eat the energy released in the breaking of covalent bonds when carbon based cellulose (carbonaceous matter, like leaves, stems, manure, etc.) is dismantled.

It is the microbes that are responsible for breaking the bonds that hold earth minerals and rocks together and releasing bonded energy. They live off that energy—as do humans.

Plant submit their order for nutrient energy at the *root level*. The bacteria receive and fill the order IF the soil is a POSITIVE energy soil environment. Unfulfilled orders create **"stress"** that weakens the plant and causes an energy shift to the left. Stress related changes in the plant's "terrain" lower its vibrational state and causes it to transmit negative energy signals to nature's garbage crew—the insects and viruses.

The health minded person must learn to MANAGE "stress" if he or she expects to enjoy good health and endless vitality. Techniques like yoga, deep breathing, prayer, Qi Gong, Tai Chi, walking barefooted in sand or on grass, sleeping under the stars, exercise, laughing, meditation, positive thoughts, etc. buffer stress.

NEVER forget, *stress* seeks an outlet, just as electricity seeks ground. Be alert and PROVIDE a safe outlet for it to dissipate. Energy is never lost, it merely changes form! Spinal and knee problems are two good examples of stress disorders.

The Carbon Connection

A healthy body is built around carbon. Organic molecules and compounds have carbon in their structure. Carbon is number 12 on the chart of atomic elements.

Carbon is UNIQUE because it can *bond* with so many different elements and *participate* in millions of different reactions—all of them *unique* unto themselves. It is this characteristic that allows toxic **organic** poisons to *hitch* a ride on the carbon atom. The R-group (stands for reactive group) and its location on a carbon molecule determines whether something is DDT, malathion, or dioxin—all being organic poisons!

Toxic organic chemicals are POTENT left-spin substances. When used on plants, the health of the plant suffers greatly. Animals and humans that eat poisoned food suffer too. Sometimes the doctor provides the sufferer with a label.

In only a few decades, man-made organic poisons have spoiled life on Earth. Yet, poisons rate high on science's benefit to risk scale which says "cheap food at politically popular prices is desirable." **There is an implied threat in the cheap food argument which says, "cheap food is better than no food." These ideas are dangerous, immoral and wrong.**

Plants are more than green things. They are living miracles. The *experts* tell us plants only need NPK (nitrogen, phosphorous, potassium) to produce food that will sustain life. This is NOT true! It is an covert effort to mislead and confuse.

A gut full of poisoned, empty calories does not produce a healthy human being or a happy nation. When we eat left-spin food, the results eventually manifest in the physical body and in violent crime statistics. First, we become toxic. Next, we suffer hormonal imbalances and partial shutdown of the vital organs. Later, much later, the changes are confirmed upon post mortem examination. **Too soon old, too late smart is a sorry excuse for a life that ended on a sour note.** People must understand that agricultural practices control nations.

Explosions

Carey Reams did most of his life's work in the agricultural arena. He believed that plants and animals live on the energy released during the breaking of mineral bonds. He referred to these reactions as "explosions!"

Explosions occur when WATER reacts with soil—especially rain water! Rain greatly accelerates plant growth! The grass leaps; the corn jumps. Rain water is biologically active water—as is BEV water. It reacts with the soil minerals and acids and releases energy so plants can grow.

The reader will recall that water functions as a solvent. Water dissolves things and forms solutions that makes things come alive by feeding still more reactions.

The roots of a plant secrete carbonic acid (carbon + hydrogen) which dissolves and frees mineral ions from rock. The bacteria absorb the water and dissolved mineral ions into their bodies, digest them, and either hold them or secrete them as a kind of glue-like substance. It is this sugary secretion that gives organic soil its crumbly texture, and causes it to flocculate and hold together.

Carbon-rich soil is **young** soil. It is **active** soil. It is **anabolic** soil. It is soil that is *alive* because it is high in what Leonard Ridzon calls "biogenic carbon" in his book *the Carbon Connection.* Soil rich in biogenic carbon will NOT leach. It holds minerals and nutrients in **colloidal** form [charged (+) (–) ions] for the plants and earthworms. Colloidal mineral ions are held in this form until the plant places an order for them. If the plant orders ions that are *different* than what is on hand, the bacteria use the *alchemy/transmutation* process we described earlier to produce the mineral ion the plant needs. This process takes place at both the *atomic* and the *sub-atomic* levels and can be best described as "cold" fusion.

Carbon acts as a bridge in cold fusion reactions—be it in the soil, or in the gut and liver of man or animal. Carbon controls health and aging. It is the basis of life.

Transmitters & Receivers

Plants grown as nature intended have a healthy aura which radiate 'healthy' energy signals. Plants grown with commercial fertilizers and poison sprays radiate signals in the "*I'm sick, Come and eat me!*" band.

Dr. Phil Callahan discovered how insects use their antenna to pick up these distress signals and navigate by them—like an enemy war plane homing in on the target plants.

Insects only attack *sick* plants. Insects are NOT the enemy, and the arena is not a war. Insects comply with nature's order to destroy weak organisms—in this case, plants!

In the human arena, toxic waste buildup puts stress on the bio-electric body by weakening the vital organs. Microbes detect stress in humans. They operate like insects by *tuning* into our "I'm sick, come and do away with me!" signals. They follow nature's decree and attack, but they are NOT the enemy.

Insects have antenna on their heads, and cilia (tiny hair

like projections) on their body. Both structures are tuned to vibrate in the "sick" band—where stressed crops broadcast their signals.

Insects know exactly which plants represent a meal and which ones do not. Different insects are tuned to different frequencies. You won't find Colorado Potato Beetles eating sweet corn. Nature tunes each insect's antenna to its own "I'm sick, come and eat me!" frequency. Signals are transmitted in spectrum outside the range of white light. The near and **far infrared** are neither audible nor visible to man.

White light contains all visible color frequencies and is part of our Third dimension experience and world. Light is electrical in nature, and anything electrical in nature is related to light. Color therapy, cold laser therapy, and ultrasound are applications and variations of **therapeutic** light vibrating at frequencies that stimulate healing. Microwaves and radar are light, but they are anti-life energy frequencies. **Dis-ease belongs to the world of invisible energy frequencies.**

When a plant is sick and stressed, you will see the insects gorging themselves. When farmers have to spray insecticides to produce a crop, you can bet the food crop is a "compound" negative and you can measure it with a pendulum or vibration chain, or the *soon to be available* **Biotester.**

Any crop that requires poisons to keep the insects at bay is sick. Eat it, and you will absorb those freak energy frequencies and will become sick too.

Organic Poisons

Organic poisons are potent negative energy fields. They are the equivalent of a homeopathic remedy working in REVERSE. Their "combined" negative effect on the body of man or animal is beyond comprehension. Dis-ease and old age has its roots in the negative energy arena of poisoned, sick food and biologically unfriendly water.

Organic poisons are a band-aid approach to food production. Their use is NO different than medical science's insistence on mass immunization of the population.

Sprays and immunizations mask health problems in plants and people, and create new ones. Both are "potentized" energy fields that perpetuate sickness and destroy lives.

The Refractometer & The Terrain

If sick plants attract predatory insects, viruses, and molds, can we assume that healthy plants repel them? The answer is a big YES! The same rules apply to the bio-electric body and aging. A positive energy terrain does not support disease, it repels it! Negative energy attracts more negative UNLESS a concerted effort is make to break the cycle.

Dr. Carey Reams discovered a unique way to determine the health and nourishment level of food plants. **He discovered that healthy plants have a high level of dissolved mineral solids in their juices.** This is determined by way of a refractometer, which is a simple, hand held device that refracts light and measures the *brix* level of natural sucrose sugars in plant juice.

The higher the "brix" level (brix is the unit of measure—like a foot or a pound, same idea), the higher the mineral content of the juices. The higher the level of sugar and minerals, the healthier the plant and the more nourishing the food. *(Do you remember the story earlier in chapter nine about satiety and Reams' dinner party for his neighbors?)*

When sugar levels are high, plants do NOT radiate negative energy in the *"I'm sick, come and get me!"* band. Moreover, if an occasional insect stops by to have a bite, it promptly dies because high sugar levels—which the insect is not equipped to handle—quickly turn to alcohol in the bug's system and it dies! **Instant and total intoxication!**

Alcohol is a toxin (POISON) to living systems. Yet, when sick, it can be beneficial to take a hot Epsom salt, hydrogen peroxide and fresh ginger bath followed by a shot of whiskey before going to bed. The alcohol kills invading organisms and SHOCKS the system. The alcohol serves as a drug and the effect is palliative, but it often brings relief. A better solution is colon therapy, followed by the bath water mix and a shot of Harmonic silver water. The results can be spectacular!

Plants grown in highly mineralized soil that is high in carbon and loaded with microbes will have high brix readings, which is a "marker" of the dissolved minerals in the plant's juices. The higher the brix readings, the MORE nutritious the plant, and the greater is its "life force."

The refractometer scale is from 0-32 brix, "0" being the bottom and 32 the top of the scale. **The lower the numbers, the more insect infestation and plant dis-ease that will be seen.** In the case of sweet corn, nature's garbage crew will back-off at 18 brix and will cease to be a problem above 24 brix. The insects will not be seen at all at maximum brix levels. High brix means NO dis-ease and food that is extremely nourishing for man and animal. Crops raised by conventional wisdom of the "experts" will be low brix and insect infested.

Ninety-nine percent (99%) of the food grown in the USA is low brix, low vitality food. Low vitality food spoils easily. It breeds violence in children and adults. It is the **perfect** food for perpetuating a militaristic society that will do as it is told by the forces of influence behind the scene. There is a STRONG correlation between sick food, weak minds, violence, and our obsession with sports. Rome experienced these same phenomena. They always appear as a civilization is winding down.

"In a nation whose legions once commanded the known world, the people cry but for two things; bread and more games."   Pliny

Civilizations wind down because nature's dietary laws are ignored with reckless abandon. Poor nutrition manifests itself in a plethora of ways. Populations under nutritional and biological stress are weak. Sick food and water produces social EXCESSES, not the other way around. Birth defects are part of the "terrain" story. We have *known* for a very long time that birth defects are linked to food and the creation of free radicals and uncontrolled oxidation in the tissues. Offset these negative things by using PAC's. They are harmless to pregnant women.

Eat Your Vaccinations, Dear!

Inferior food is what is behind the drive to *irradiate* America's food supply. Ditto for the genetic manipulation of plants, especially since mad scientists have begun gene splicing Hepatitis B and dozens of other dis-ease organisms into fruit and vegetable DNA.

If historical myth has any substance, I would remind the reader that Atlantis and its people were destroyed for genetic cruelties and cross breeding of life forms. Genesis speaks of kind begetting kind in the order of things.

I predict that people who eat genetically manipulated food will become sick sooner, suffer miserably, and die early. Furthermore, their offspring will experience gross pathologies with no hope of cure. Darwin's "survival of the fittest" will become a horrible reality.

We are breaking the rules when we cross specie lines. Like with like. Kind begets kind. Cross breeding of species produces offspring whose vibrational *signatures* can only be described as "freak!" The effects will be beyond comprehension.

We are making another horrible mistake by classifying animal fats and liquid oils together just because they have similar characteristics. The difference between them is more than just a matter of liquid, solid, saturated, unsaturated, short chain, long chain fatty acids, omega this and that, etc.

Vegetarians and meat eaters alike MUST to strive for balance in their diets or they will suffer and die young. The answer is to be found in fresh, homegrown fruits and vegetables. Real food covers a lot of dietary mistakes. **For those** who can't grow their own food, I highly recommend the use of juice capsules and tablets. They belong in every kitchen and <u>travel bag</u>! We use them, and we live out of our garden!

Parenteral Nutrition

Glucose is our blood sugar and our primary fuel. When stored in our liver and muscles, it is called glycogen. We cannot live without glucose, and we cannot live on it alone.

It is now standard medical procedure to add various minerals and vitamins to glucose solutions if a person will be on any form of parenteral nutrition in the hospital for more than a few days. Parenteral nutrition is any form of nutrition administered other than by way of the mouth and stomach. For example, intravenous feeding or the use of a feed tube directly into the small intestine.

Parenteral nutrition is a band-aid measure. It is the best medicine has for people who are on the edge. It is also a glimpse of life to come for those who think they can eat bio-junk food, drink toxic water, and IGNORE nature's dietary laws!

The Terrain Of Weeds

Weeds are a yardstick of soil fertility. They tell a story AND they hold meaning for those who desire to reverse the aging process. For certain, weeds do not have to be a curse to the farmer or gardener, if we understand them and their part in the scheme of things.

The popular definition of a weed is "something growing out of place." This definition is based on ignorance. Weeds grow where they choose because they have a job to do. Their job is to *absorb* negative energy from both the soil and the atmosphere for the benefit of all life. Their job is to *rejuvenate* soil energy. **Weeds—like bacteria and viruses—only grow where the "TERRAIN" is to their liking!**

We bought a home with a 1/4 acre garden space that was infested with quack grass. The neighbors laughed when we told them we would be rid of the quack grass and have a nice garden the following year. They stopped laughing when we gave them beautiful vegetables. All we did was change the energy TERRAIN—and no more quack grass!

Quack grass only grows where the soil is low in organic matter, low in calcium, high in pH, has an unbalanced decay system, and is high in aluminum. The solution was simple. We "hand" dug, shook, and piled the quack grass. We built four or five compost piles around the garden site using organic matter of all types —including quack grass, leaves, fresh manure, grass clippings— plus bacteria starter, granite dust, gypsum, soft rock phosphate, and red wigglers (worms). We turned the piles weekly. After two months, we spread the finished compost and dug it into the top four inches of soil.

After this process, we could NOT get quack grass to grow. The reason? We changed the "TERRAIN" of the soil. We helped Mother Earth energize her skin.

Every weed has a place and a time. If you change the environment, that weed will cease to be a problem because you have altered the terrain. Some weeds grow where food plants cannot grow. Some weeds also grow along side food crops. Their job is to maintain energy balance.

I remember a story an acquaintance of mine told me about how the pioneers abused the soil as they came west. They found virgin soils high in life giving energy and nutrients. They would move on as soon as the soil had "burned itself out." Later, after the deserted farm had sat for eight or ten years, Tex's father would come along and pick the farm up for next to nothing and presto, the soil produced! Tex's father understood that weeds play a very important part in life on this planet. Weeds ONLY proliferate when the "TERRAIN" dictates their presence. **Weeds, insects, bacteria, and viruses are our friends. Understand them and life makes more sense.**

The food supply is sick because the soil is sick. We should not be surprised that man, who eats sick food and drinks sick water, is also sick!

Hybrid Food

The advent of the hybrid seed has particular significance for the health minded person. The hybrid was heralded as a wonderful thing. Bigger crops, sweeter corn, better germination, and more control at harvest. Some of these things are true, but there are serious trade-offs—like unbalanced enzymes and vitamins, freak proteins, and poor mineral uptake.

Hybrid crops CAN, however, withstand the hard salt fertilizers used to force food crops to produce when they are grown on sick soil. These same crops can withstand the poisons used to keep nature's garbage crew at bay.

Hybrid seeds came into "fashion" because the seed companies wanted to *patent* them. The farmer—ever dependent on bank loans—was *persuaded and often strong armed*, to use these new seeds. **The "experts" in the ag schools and government extension offices said, *"Hybrids are the wave of the future!"* (Whose future?)**

In the words of one farmer, *"We traded open-pollinated seed left over from the past harvest—which was a FREE gift from*

God—for these damnable hybrids that we have to buy every year!" Powerful interests took control of people's food supply. We exchanged high vitality food, produced on healthy soils, for empty calories and poisoned crops grown on sick soils. **The Earth and her inhabitants are paying the price.**

Native Wisdom

We live in a world beset with conflict. The four corners of the square are at odds with each other. Philosophy, science, law, and religion have lost their moorings. The people gyrate from pole to pole—confused, mad, frustrated, depressed, violent—at odds with their world and themselves. They need wisdom and guidance.

David Lampert comes from the Lakota nation of American indians. His native name is *Watashi Wa,* which translates *"I am here!"* I am glad he is.

Dave offered some Lakota wisdom that every health-minded person needs to understand and incorporate into their lives. ***"No tree has branches that fight among themselves."***

We cannot enjoy good health and longevity when we are at odds with the world and ourselves. We cannot fulfill our destinies when we eat food and drink water that is *anti-life.*

Hybrid Inferiority

When we eat food grown from hybrid seeds we are eating food that is genetically weak. Hybrids do not reproduce true to their own kind. They *defy* the ultimate test of viability for any living thing: viable offspring.

Hybrid seeds are the freak offspring of controlled breeding techniques. They are *inbred* and they are inferior. Their energy spin is LEFT! Home gardeners get by with them because they generally have healthier soil. **Hybrid food is INFERIOR and should be avoided!**

Food crops grown from hybrid seed play into the hands of those who CONTROL the commodity prices and markets—and the food supply of the entire world.

Remember these points when the *experts* in the "media" hype the wonders of genetically engineered crops and irradiated food. Behind the rhetoric, you will find sick food, less competition, higher profits, and GROSS human suffering in third world countries—AND in the United States.

Food is a gift from God. It was NOT meant to be a plaything. Eat good food and drink friendly water. Do these things, and you will enjoy health and vitality as you become *Young Again!*

PREVIEW: *Our next chapter is about "OBESITY." Learn the "real" reason for obesity. Whether you are thin or not, the chapter contains VALUABLE information that you will need to understand the remainder of this book.*

Magnets Heal

Next time you mash a finger, sprain your ankle, work in front of a computer terminal, strain an arthritic joint, suffer a serious injury, feel stress in your neck, pull a muscle, have a headache, suffer with PMS, want to stimulate your immune system, suffer from prostate pain, etc., use a Super Magnet and watch what happens.

When a Super Magnet is placed over an injury, first north pole, then south pole in alternate fashion, healing is accentuated when worn over the thymus gland, a Super Magnet enhances the immune system.

People often ask, "What side of the magnet works best?" The answer is north, south, both. Effectiveness is enhanced by alternating magnetic polarity.

How do you determine what side of the magnet is best for you? How often should you use a magnet? How long should you use it? The answers are easy to discover.

Determine your magnet's polarity by going outside and dangling your magnet by its cord. Whichever side of the magnet faces north is the south side or south pole.

Next, have someone hold each side of the magnet to the skin approximately 3 inches below the collar bone in line with the right breast nipple while you extend your right arm even with the shoulder. Have the person test you for strength using both sides of the magnet while gently pulling down on your arm. The strong side should face the body. Use a vibration chain to determine how long to wear the magnet, and how often it should be worn. *The pendulum Kit* and *Vibrations* will teach you how to check your results.

Off and on usage generally works best. For immune enhancement, wear the magnet over the thymus (two inches below base of neck) for one hour, then five minutes, and finally 30 seconds through the day. For a bruised finger, injured joint, etc. alternate the magnet's poles every few minutes and the pain will lessen or disappear and you will suffer little discoloration from bruising.

Life is a scrapbook of lessons—never mistakes!

Colon Therapy

Colon therapy speeds the removal of waste and accelerates detoxification of the tissues and fluids. Toxins include fecal matter, mucoid material, metabolic wastes, drugs, and poisons circulating in the blood and lymph.

A *coffee* colonic stimulates the liver to dump bile. Bile secretion is the liver's equivalent of a bowel movement! Kombucha tea is another great colon solution. It cleans the colon and restores microbial balance and pH.

One half of a fresh lemon squeezed into a cup of warm water taken on an empty stomach heals the liver and breaks up mucous congestion. Lemon is especially effective during therapeutic fasts, providing enemas or colon therapy are used to move waste out of the system.

The proper "colonic" begins with colon equipment and 3-5 gallons of percolated coffee (never use instant coffee!), kombucha, or BEV water. NEVER use tap water! If you do not have a BEV system, use spring bottled spring water—not distilled water. Use a tepid solution. Alternate with a cold solution to stimulate peristaltic activity in the gut. Yucca extract and PAC's taken daily cause the colon lining to break loose easier and go down the toilet.

Start by infusing about 1/2 gallon of solution into the colon while on your back in birthing position. Massage deeply along the descending colon (left side of the abdomen), along the transverse colon (below rib cage from left to right), and along the ascending colon (right side of the abdomen) from the ribs down to the appendix.

After the water is held for a few minutes, release your bowel and begin again. Repeat the process until you have used 3-5 gallons of fluid or more. The final infusion should be held for fifteen minutes, if possible. The process takes between 1-2 hours. Do a colonic weekly if you are toxic. You will NOT harm yourself. Once you get your health back, once a month will be sufficient.

Wait 2 hours after eating before doing a colonic. Allow 15 minutes on the commode to empty your colon after the final infusion, shower, and go to bed if possible.

After one month of Yucca extract and PAC's, **flush your liver of stones.** This is very important!

Read The Tissue Cleansing Book !

23

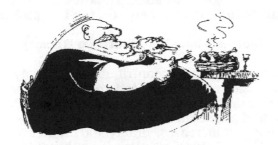

Fat Falstaff

Shakespeare's Prince Hall to grossly overweight Falstaff:

"Leave gormandizing; Know the grave doth gape?
For thee thrice wider than four other men!"
Shakespeare

Obesity is the curse of the industrialized world! We eat the wrong things instead of the right things. We live to eat, when we should eat to live. We eat much when we could eat little. We dig our grave with our teeth.

Obesity is an EFFECT. It has little to do with inheritance and everything to do with incorrect living habits. We are concerned with the causes of obesity and its influence on the aging process.

Obesity is dis-ease. It is a forerunner of multiple secondary conditions! Lifestyles that precipitate obesity involve *under activity* and *over activity* of the vital organs (pancreas, thyroid, parathyroid, thymus, pituitary, testicles, ovaries, liver and adrenals). Over-activity stresses the vital organs, causing them to exhaust themselves, while lack of exercise stresses the entire system and produces toxicity.

Obesity plays by its own rules—like cancer. Fat bodies respond *differently* than they did prior to becoming obese. The dietary approach to obesity has merit, but other modalities like hormone balancing, detoxification, exercise, and water.

Obesity is confirmation of metabolic "slow down" and loss of vitality in all of the organs and glands. Obesity is the most obvious SIGN of aging. It is **not** something that just happens to people—it is a self-imposed condition brought on by ignorance, lack of self love, and poor choices. **Obesity is maintained through ignorance, reliance on conventional beliefs, and "experts" who perpetuates the problem.**

Factors That Contribute To Obesity

Excess food intake contributes to obesity, but hormonal imbalance and bio-junk food are much worse. Bio-junk food is the equivalent of "sabotage." Hormonal imbalance slows the system and accelerates waste buildup.

As body fat increases, vitality and organ function slow. Fat does not *cause* the body to slow down, but it is a confirmation that slowdown is in progress. Obesity gives way to diabetes, hypertension, gout, poor self-image, frustration, and a wardrobe full of unusable clothes.

As waste levels increase, radiance of the aura dims, mirroring the condition of the electric body. The aura can be compared to the defense shields on the Star Ship *Enterprise*. If our defense is strong, negative energy forces cannot penetrate it. If it is weak, dis-ease becomes reality.

A fat body has LIMITED electrical capacity which is reflected in low energy and drive. As body fat increases, the fat person's body slows down even more. Hence, the fat person gets fatter and the path to a youthful existence becomes ever more difficult.

Obesity is a vicious cycle. Sluggish blood and lymph flow impinges on cellular respiration, mitochondrial oxidation, and SLOWS movement of waste to the liver where bile wastes can get to the intestines and eventually the toilet.

The obese person often fails to understand that because they are obese, they will have to go the extra mile to get their health back. Colon therapy is mandatory.

Detoxification of the fat person's body produces **many** healing crises. Healing crises occur when toxic waste energy fields are released into the **blood, lymph**, and **intestines**. These wastes must be quickly flushed from the system or headaches, gas, cold sweats, dizziness, etc. often result. Therapeutic fasting combined with colon therapy works wonders for the obese person. **As waste begins to leave the system, body response accelerates.**

The liver dumps bile wastes just 3 inches below the outlet from the stomach—or twenty feet UP from the anus. If waste mucoid and fecal matter impedes the flow of bile wastes, healing crises occur as a result of the wastes being "reabsorbed" because they cannot get OUT of the system.

As toxic waste exits the fat person's body, the organs and glands must be supplemented to avoid hormonal shorfalls. Obese people burn fat ONLY under specific conditions. We must come to understand those conditions.

We see and feel FAT on the physical level. We must learn to understand FAT on the invisible energy level.

Eat Less • Live Longer

Little food is required to maintain good health, if the food is biologically friendly to the body. Examples of high vitality foods are Harmonic pollen, Klamath algae, and predigested, organic liver. It's important that people learn to measure food vitality with a pendulum, and vibration chain (the electronic Biotester should be available in 1996). Avoid over cooking of food. Eat one third of your food RAW! Foods like kale, collards, beets, apples, carrots, and fruit are excellent choices.

It has been demonstrated over and over again that animals live longer when their food intake is reduced to approximately 75% of their optimum intake level. In order to be able to reduce food intake and not feel like you are starving, the body's nutritional needs must be met. Otherwise, a hungry body will CRY for more food!

There is risk involved in lowering food intake unless the dietary base is carefully constructed. Eating less food is NOT a viable approach to weight control. Eating "quality" food, however, IS a viable approach. Smart eating includes things like fresh fruits and vegetables (home grown if possible), clean, non-toxic meat, fish, and fowl, and raw milk. Good food makes people thin and full of energy. *Enhanced* trivalent chromium greatly assists energy production, fat metabolism, and blood sugar related problems.

When we are healthy, we can eat as we please. But when glandular reserves become exhausted, bio-junk foods cause us to become obese.

FAT should be understood in terms of positive and negative energy management, as well as in terms of *what* we eat, *when* we eat, and how *much* we eat. If we eat highly nutritious food, drink biologically friendly water, balance our hormones, and rid the body of EXCESSES, weight control comes automatically and vitality returns.

Sabotage & Body Instinct

Bio-junk food and unfriendly water stand in the way of

a healthy lifestyle. They short circuit our fat burning enzymes and shut-down our fat burning pathways. They block mito-chondrial production of cellular energy. Once momentum is lost, the body has difficulty getting going again. A fat body *resists* movement—the very thing it needs most!

Body fat contains lots of toxic waste. But before the body will burn fat, it MUST be assured that the waste left behind will be flushed from the system.

The body has *innate intelligence*. It is intuitively smart. It knows what to do to keep us alive—like getting the toxic wastes out and away from the vital organs to minimize damage.

Turning on the body's metabolic pathways requires that we meet all of our basic needs from dietary intake and exercise, to detoxification and hormone supplementation.

Even the most nutritious food can become a *liability* when put into an anaerobic, left-spin environment Here it is quickly *converted* to left-spin energy and fat. A fat body is a sick body. Sick bodies REJECT the very nutrients they need. They often REBEL and become sicker in the presence of nourishing food unless colon therapy, and PAC's are used to stabilize the system during detox. Rejection and rebellion are **symptoms.**

It's not that the "fat" body has forgotten how to handle nourishing food. It's that it instinctively "knows" that doing so—in the face of accumulated waste—can cause suffering and intermittent misery. The body's inability to process and me-tabolize right-spin nutrient energy is linked to a EXCESSES in the system plus hormonal imbalances.

Obesity and constipation go hand in hand. Obese people usually have to resort to colon therapy and PAC's to clean up their body and speed the rejuvenatory process.

Kindling Wood & Fat

Once detoxification are under way, the body will accept balanced meals of quality proteins, **complex** carbohydrates, and "fresh" green leafy vegetables. Complex carbohydrates are "long burning" food molecules—like those contained in multi grain cereals, home made, whole grain breads made with *blackstrap* molasses, fresh greens, and organic potatoes.

Complex carbohydrates can sustain a person for four to six hours. Greens are extremely nourishing and provide the very best type of bulk for a healthy bowel. They are loaded with cholorophyl, which is the plant's "blood!" Everyone should grow comfrey. Comfrey leaves are very delicious when lightly steamed and dressed with a little olive oil and apple cider vinegar. Kale and collards greens are also excellent choices. Greens purchased in the store are not as good.

People confuse complex carbohydrates (CC)with the worthless processed starches and sugars in processed foods. Complex carbohydrates do not make people fat. However, the body needs them to "burn" fat. **CC's are to fat burning what kindling wood is to a wood fire.**

In other words, fat won't burn unless you have something to get it burning and keep it going. Body fat is the **LAST** energy source the body will use to fuel in its energy needs. The body will draw on muscle tissue protein BEFORE it will draw on body fat reserves. Again, the body is reluctant to release fat bound toxicity unless it knows that the waste can be gotten out of the system. Quality food and water is the fat person's ticket to greater health and longevity. When quality food is combined with aerobic exercise, enzyme activity accelerates.

Oxidation Of Fat

Aerobic exercise activates fat-burning enzymes. Exercise should demand 60—80% of the maximum heart rate (MHR) for a minimum of twelve minutes. This causes the **liver** to produce and release enzymes to oxidize (burn) small amounts of fat during exercise AND large amounts of fat throughout the *entire* 24 hour day.

Exercise stimulates metabolic activity—which includes oxidation of waste and fat—and stimulate circulation of body fluids (blood and lymph).

Obesity is experienced when mitochondrial activity is low. But, the more exercise you do, the more fat you will burn, not because exercise burns fat (it burns little), but because it increases enzyme and metabolic activity.

Exercise should NEVER be used to offset poor choices in food, water, and lifestyle. Obesity ceases to be a problem when people adhere to a healthy lifestyle, which for the fat person should include all of the things discussed so far.

Basal Metabolism

Basal metabolism refers to the *minimum* energy requirements necessary to keep us alive. Basal metabolic rate is usually measured at wake up, twelve hours after eating, before pulse and temperature rise, or the emotions become stirred. Nutritional needs—as reflected in charts and graphs dealing with height, weight, and "activity" are based on this rate.

For example, I am 5' 11" and weigh 158 pounds. According to the nutrition folks, my body needs approximately 2200 Kcalories (a Kcalorie is 1000 calories) a day to meet my minimum requirements based on my *activity* level. This is my total daily energy requirement. Kcalorie energy units should derive from ALL food sources (carbohydrates, proteins, fats; vegetables, fruits, meat).

Of the 2200 Kcalories I need, over 80% are used to meet my **minimum** physiologic energy needs—heart beat, body heat, breathing, peristalsis, mental processes, etc. If I add twenty minutes of hard aerobic exercise to my daily routine, I raise my energy needs by **only** 300 Kcalories—very little. If I do NOT add those Kcalories to my dietary intake, my body will **withdraw** them from fat reserves **providing** that my diet supplies enough high quality protein and toxicity problems are not a threat to my system. This is very important!

One of the reasons fat people stay fat is that their body has not been "programmed" to lose weight. This is where mental preparation, meditation, and DETOXIFICATION come into play. The body *anticipates.* It has a *sixth* sense. It has *innate* intelligence. Detoxification should precede fat reduction. Reduction by any other means may get rid of fat, but it always returns. Program you body and the fat won't return. **The fat person MUST pay attention to the basics!**

Exercise—not to burn fat—but to form fat burning enzymes, circulate blood and lymph, and become aerobic. As you become aerobic, the appetite diminishes because the body's energy requirements are satisfied, AND because body EXCESSES are moved out of the system. DO NOT FORGET IT!

Thermogenic Supplements

Thermogenic supplements (*thermo*-heat; *gen*-production of; *ic*-pertaining to) cause the body to burn its fat. Certain herbs like MaHuang (Ephedra), Guarana, and Capsicum accelerate *thermogenic* activity. When these are "complexed" with a full array of other herbs plus trivalent chromium, they do not WHIP the body. Poorly complexed or isolated thermogenics hype the system and are no better than synthesized drugs.

Thermogenic supplements work best when used with hormone precursors. The idea is to balance the hormones (estrogen, progesterone, insulin, testosterone, thyroxine, etc.) while burning of excess fat. Newgestrone creme that is compatible with DHEA precursors helps reduce fat while meeting female needs.

PAC's greatly assist thermogenic supplementation. So does Kombucha tea and Yucca extract. The flushing of stones from the liver and gall bladder brings about the most dramatic change in thermogenic activity. Water intake is central to fat reduction by whatever means. Men should try to drink 1 gal/day; women 3/4 gal/day. Include 5 drops of liquid sea minerals per glass. Raw, peeled beets, small amounts of fresh beet juice, and fresh lemon juice in water between meals is dynamite.

Oxygen • Exercise • Salt

Fat will NOT burn unless oxygen is present. No oxygen, equates to no oxidation. BEV pure water, aerobic exercise, and ozone generators help supply oxygen to the mitochondria in the cells so they can burn body fat.

If you are obese, exercise may be difficult for you. Obese people find it difficult to get their body *moving*—especially aerobically. Use aerobic exercise equipment that does not jar the joints. Start slow. Each day increase your time a few minutes. Push yourself to reach twenty minutes duration as your metabolic rate increases and fat comes off.

Next, get OFF the salt. Get OFF all prepared foods. Stop eating restaurant food. Avoid seasonings that contain MSG (monosodium glutamate). Get your mineral electrolytes from liquid ionic minerals and nutritious food. **If you insist on using granular salt, use Keltic salt.**

Common table salt and sea salt from the health food store contain 98% sodium chloride. Keltic salt contains 35% sodium. It's best to use neither. Both upset body chemistry, however, Keltic salt contains far more trace minerals than regular sea salt. Liquid ionic sea minerals are 99.5% trace minerals with less than 1/2% sodium. **The obese person needs these mineral ions to clear the Rouleau effect from the blood and feed and cleanse the cells.**

Obesity and toxicity go together. Whenever waste proteins accumulate in the extracellular fluids, sodium will invade the cells, and water follows. Obese people are **endematous** (water retention in the tissues). Detoxification moves wastes to the blood for transport to the liver and disposal via bile secretions into the small intestine. Cleansing the cells of sodium occurs naturally PROVIDING plenty of *organic potassium* is available. Fresh green leafy vegetables and juices are excellent sources. Juice capsules and tablets are a lifesaver. They are very convenient to take and most folks like them.

As sodium is exchanged for potassium, cellular mitochondria multiply and produce more energy. The liver hepatocytes use enzymes to convert body fat into a usable energy that can be used to make adenosine triphosphate (ATP). The mitochondria don't burn fat, but the ATP energy molecule. **The bio-electric body needs energy to POWER the transformation from old to young, and the mitochondria produce it.**

Obesity ceases to be a problem when the liver is detoxified, the liver stones are flushed, the lymphatic system is on the move, and sodium levels are reduced. Physical activity is a mandatory prerequisite, not for the sake of exercise, but for waste movement and enzyme production.

Fats • Proteins • Allergies

Fats and fatty acids are extremely important to normal body metabolism. They should make up 20% of the diet. Do not be afraid of naturally saturated fats like coconut oil, and animal fats. They will not hurt you. Butter, olive oil, flax, sesame, sunflower, and nut oils are excellent choices.

NEVER use margarine, soy, or canola oils. Medical science and the media claim they are good for us, but they are wrong. Always do the *opposite* of whatever the "experts" tell you.

NEVER eliminate all oils and fats from the diet—the body needs them! In John Noble's wonderful classic *I was A Slave In Russia*, Noble told how, when he was in the Soviet gulag prison system (1945-1954), the human slaves were given a thimble full of sunflower oil each day. Without it, the prisoners would die! **Up to 40% of the body's NORMAL energy needs come from the metabolism of dietary fats.**

Proteins should be carefully scrutinized as to quality, quantity, and source. Go easy on animal protein. Don't overdo! Avoid cheeses altogether. Eat only real proteins, not artificial bio-junk like TVP (textured vegetable protein) and the like. When you get to the hereafter and you look in God's recipe book for healthy living, you are NOT going to find any recipes calling for TVP. The quality and spin of manipulated proteins CANNOT sustain life. Lentils, beans and legumes (except soy), Klamath algae, biogenic liver tablets, and Harmonic pollen are superb protein sources. Food reactions follow in the tracks of obesity.

So called food allergies are protein related. People with allergies are **TOXIC**—believe it! When checking for body response, always cross reference your testing techniques (muscle testing, pendulum, vibration chain, etc.) to determine how your body may respond to different foods or supplements.

Bias has NO place in vibrational testing! Too many people (professional and lay alike) go out the window in this area. They don't use good sense. They plant their feet in cement just because something tests negative or because of something they read. Patients LOOK for excuses not to become well. They allow their mind to control body response. Always test things in the hand, out of the hand, for present and future reactions. Seek answers to questions regarding long term effect DESPITE initial negative reactions. Good questions from a properly "cleared" mind produce valuable insight. Poor technique is worse than none at all. Learn to use the speedometer test. It is one of the best! Hopefully, the new electronic Biotester will be available in 1996. *In the meantime, every person should learn how to "effectively" use a pendulum, vibration chain, dowsing rods, and aurameter.*

Klamath Algae & Harmonic Pollen

Klamath algae is a superb FOOD product that greatly enhances the rejuvenation process. It is one of most powerful, naturally occurring, right-spin food substances known. Harmonic pollen is another. They are possibly the two best foods on the planet. I use them both.

Klamath algae is indigenous to Upper Klamath Lake, Oregon. Harmonic pollen comes from the wilds of northern British Columbia. Both foods are pure, raw, and wild. They are "low stress" foods because they require very little digestion.

The vitamin B-12 content in Klamath algae is easily assimilated. This is an important issue for vegetarians. The hormones and enzymes in harmonic pollen are nothing short of impressive. A couple of alga tablets, a spoonful of pollen, and an apple makes a very good **low** stress, **high** energy, **no** letdown lunch. Both foods are very complete proteins!

The electrical *signature* of Klamath algae corresponds energetically with, and has an affinity for, the lymph more than for the blood, which explains its role in detoxification. When used together, Klamath algae and harmonic pollen enhance the immune system and play a KEY role in fat metabolism.

Klamath algae serves the function of janitor and free radical scavenger while fine tuning and regulating the entire metabolism. It is particularly effective in balancing the obese person's metabolism and putting an END to hunger. People who eat Klamath algae and harmonic pollen STOP craving food.

Klamath algae and Harmonic pollen are NOT hybrid foods, nor have they been genetically *manipulated.* They contain massive amounts of chlorophyll. They fuel cold fusion reactions in the liver and gut of humans and pets alike.

The bio-electric body takes on the vibratory *signature* and energy *footprint* of the food and water it is given. Quality food enhances a person's life (see Source Index).

Raw Milk • Real Food • Obesity

Raw milk is a wonderful food and a good source of nutrients and enzymes. Few people raise milk cows or milk goats, but they can buy raw milk from someone who has these animals. Older people especially benefit from drinking raw milk. It is a very good food. (Raw milk is neither pasteurized nor homogenized. Both processes are destroy good food.

Do not be frightened by the **scare tactics** of government health officials who are doing their best to end public access to raw milk. I find it most convenient that outbreaks of E. coli and Cryptosporidium have occurred just when they were needed to scare the public into accepting the "wisdom" of *experts!*

Bureaucrats mean well, but they usually *regurgitate* the lines they memorized and believe in. You can bet they are not privy to what is going on behind the scenes in regard to the manipulation of America's food supply. I *strongly* suggest every reader see the futuristic movie *Outbreak* to understand what I am referring to.

Obesity and good food do not go together. Neither does **hunger and violence in a well fed society. Instead, people take control of their families, lives, and country.**

Making BEV Water

BEV water is important to the obesity scenario. The best source of BEV water is from your own tap. All that is required is BEV processing equipment.

At my home, we use a counter top unit. It is portable, and that is important to me. If I am on the road, I can take it with me and hook it up at the motel. If we move or go on a vacation, we have biologically friendly water immediately.

Under the counter models are also available. Whole house systems produce superb conditioned water throughout the house, but only provide BEV grade water at the kitchen sink. (BEV water cannot be moved in metal or plastic pipes.)

People who are survival oriented, who use alternative power sources, who visit the wilderness, or who travel or live in Third World Countries use the "alternative" self-contained BEV model that runs on 12, 110, or 220 volt power OR on a self-contained solar power panel that powers the pump, which creates the pressure needed to run the unit. The multivoltage pump draws only 5 watts! Other models do NOT require electricity and there is NOTHING to clean!

BEV units work flawlessly on standard household water pressure. They do NOT use electricity. There are no boiler elements to clean (as in distillers). Filters are not expensive. A small, hand held scientific instrument called a "conductivity meter" is used to monitor water quality and determine when it's time to change the filters.

BEV units are made in the USA and the technology behind them is **"proprietary."** They are shipped to the end user ONLY after each unit is **individually** bench tested to insure it exceeds BEV standards.

BEV equipment is NOT available door to door, through multi-level companies, or in stores. Extremely strict quality control insures customer satisfaction. Water is made for as little as 5-10 cents per gallon.

BEV water is strange stuff. It must be stored in glass or in its own tank—away from atmospheric contaminants—so the water will NOT draw pollutants and negative energy from the air. Glass and polycarbonate are the only substances that do not react with this water. Polycarbonate bottles come in pint, 1/2, 1, 3, and 5 gallon sizes.

BEV water affects obesity at the most fundamental level. It stands to reason that you can't detoxify the body if you can't move the waste out of the system. Distilled water won't do it. Its structure and energy charge is distorted and ruined.

Magnetic Sponge

BEV water is like a magnetic sponge in liquid form. When it comes into contact with body toxins, it bonds to them and carries them OUT of the body. In the process of flushing negative energy substances out of the system, it creates positive energy vortexes that EXCITE cell chemistry and stimulate metabolism. Toxic mineral deposits in the tissues (basement membranes of the skin and arteries) are carried out of the body. Atherosclerotic plaques diminish. Capillaries in the posterior eye, ears and scalp respond well. Lastly, BEV water *feels* different in your mouth and throat.

BEV is a ***proprietary*** water processing system. While purity is very important, the magnetic *signature* and biological activity of BEV water that makes it ***unique.*** There are many traditional water filtration systems on the market. Unfortunately, they don't go far enough in toxic waste removal, nor do the stand up to BEV proprietary process. (BEV manuscripts that discuss BEV theory are available (see Source Index). **We may not be able to dictate the quality of the air we breathe, but we can control the nature and type of water we drink.**

NOTE: Avoid distilled water. It has been boiled and the water molecules are contorted. The water biologically dead. Toxic substances like fluorine, chlorine, chloramine, and trihalomethanes are actually *concentrated* in distilled water, It tastes flat and it is a breeding ground for viruses and bacteria.

Chain Reactions

The body functions through a continuous series of biochemical reactions. These reactions stall out if the body is missing the raw materials it needs. Unanswered needs are *limiting* factors that slow metabolism. When metabolism slows, we become wrinkled, degenerative, old and **FAT**. When the body is forced to process bio-junk food and water, it has but three choices: dismantle the molecules and dump them via the kidneys and bowel; burn (oxidize) them; or store them in NEW body fat produced specifically for this purpose.

Bio-junk food and water contain "radiomimetic" chemicals that "mimic" hormones. They are so potent that the body has to isolate and store them in FAT to protect itself. The liver cannot process these freak molecules for lack of needed catalysts, enzymes, and energy. Most people's livers are so loaded with **stones** that bile flow is limited. Parasites in the liver (flukes) live on these toxic energy fields, reproduce and spread throughout the body. The kidneys cannot process these toxins because they are too "hot." Hence, body fat increases and aging accelerates. **We "become" what we eat.**

Blood & Lymph Circulation

As body fat increases, blood and lymph circulation slows. The life insurance companies use height and weight as the basis for their rates. They *know* that obesity is an excellent *indicator* of trouble in the making. It is no accident that thin people are thin. They are thin because they metabolize and burn excess energy. **The fat person is up against the same problem as the person fighting cancer. Metabolism is slow, toxicity is high, excess rule, and hormones are unbalanced.**

Feel Worse First!

During the early stages of detoxification, expect to feel worse BEFORE you will feel better. A response indicates things are happening! A enema provides quick relief in severe cases by sending toxins down the toilet. You feel better fast!

It's best to do serious detoxification on weekends and rest during the work week. Fasting is recommended in conjunction with detox procedures (see *Miracle of Fasting* in Source Index). Eliminate ALL food while fasting. Fruit and vegetables should be eaten the day before a fast begins. Get plenty of fresh air, mild exercise, and rest! Colon therapy before and after a fast is HIGHLY recommended. **Use of *enhanced* PAC'ᵉ is highly recommended. They speed progress.**

Diuretics

NEVER use diuretics (water pills) to reduce weight!

Diuretics cause a loss of vital body fluids—and with them — your **reserve** of potassium. Potassium pills do NOT adequately replenish lost potassium. Potassium loss promotes sodium invasion of the cells, shut down of the mitochondria, and loss of energy. Loss of energy means poor fat metabolism.

    Sodium chloride (table salt) sets you up for a good case of cancer by creating energy EXCESSES in the body. **Organic potassium drives OUT sodium!** As sodium exits the cells, the mitochondria come alive and burn more fat. The obese person needs ENERGY to become thin! Shedding of fat and release of excess fluid proteins comes with detoxification and blood sugar management. Enhanced trivalent chromium helps the obese person to become thin. When the obese person becomes thin, no one needs to tell him or her that they **ARE** *Young Again!*

PREVIEW: *Our next chapter deals with the relationship between lightning, energy, vitality, and BROWN FAT!*

Breast Implants: Silicone or Soy?

    Thousands of women are suffering from the toxic side effects of silicone breast implants because they trusted the *"experts"* who told them they were safe.

    A pendulum and vibration chain would have saved these women from the experts had they know how to use them. These devices indicate that silicone implants are left-spinning energy fields and dangerous to the body.

    Now, the experts are promoting soybean oil breast implants—because they are "safe!"

    I hope no one believes them. Soy oil is an industrial oil. Avoid it in your food and don't be foolish enough to implant it in your breasts. **Never listen to the *experts!***

People Getting Fatter Worldwide

    People weigh an average of 10 pounds more than they did 7 years ago. Lack of exercise is blamed, but the problem goes deeper. Obesity MUST be addressed at the *subtle energy level* of our existence.

    Enhanced trivalent chromium takes off the fat, puts on muscle, and levels blood sugars (see Source Index).

Gerivital GH₃ Plus

We get a **NEW** body ever 7 years. But as we age, the process slows down. Sub-clinically sick people take up to 12 years to get their "new" body . and when they get it, it isn't as good as the one they traded in.

If you would like your new body to be *younger, stronger,* and *better* than the one you are in the process of trading in, I recommend you implement the ideas in this book and try some Gerivital GH₃ Plus (GGH₃ Plus).

Gerivital is a cell rebuilder. It has been used in Europe for over 25 years with startling results. Over 25 MILLION hours of research make it the most studied compound ever developed.

GGH₃ Plus rejuvenates the tissues over a period of several years with NO side effects of any kind. The jaw line regains a youthful appearance (as people age their jaw changes). Liver spots disappear from the skin.

The skin takes on a youthful appearance. Sagging tissues tighten up due to rejuvenation of the elastic, reticular, and collagenous fibers that compose the connective tissues 'beneath' the skin.

GGH₃ Plus is known for returning white and gray hair to its youthful, natural color. *(I use GH₃ Plus along with Kombucha tea and "enhanced" PAC's with great results.)*

The FDA has blocked the importation of Gerivital into the USA for over fifteen years on the flimsy excuse that it is a "drug" because it contains **procaine** (novocaine). Procaine is totally harmless. It decomposes into two natural B vitamins PABA and DEAE. *This is the same stuff my holistic dentist used to erase the scar memories from my skin (earlier in this book).*

American made GGH₃ Plus uses two **natural** B vitamin instead of procaine which removes it from FDA control. If you would like to enjoy a *youthful* appearance as seen on the faces and bodies of the movie stars, use GGH₃ Plus. The stars have used it for years. Its effects are enhanced with Kombucha tea and PAC's (see Source Index).

A youthful appearance is PRICELESS! It translates into a good job, respect, and self esteem.

"The difference between an old man and an old gentlemen is the way he dresses and looks."

The Vaccination Dilemma

Vaccinations are part of life in the Western World. In fact, they are so *pervasive* that health-minded people need to "tune in" to their Jeckyl and Hyde nature if they hope to enjoy a long, healthy life.

Vaccines encourage the body to build immunity and antibodies against future exposure to contagious diseases. The process involves the introduction of **pathogenic** life forms into the body in a serum of **foreign** proteins.

While immunity—and the antibodies that go with it—is desirable, the side effects of vaccinations are not. The immune response (reaction of body to foreign proteins) is an act of *self-preservation.* Antibodies in the blood are evidence of past microbial warfare on a systemic level.

Natural immunity is *different* than vaccination-*induced* attempts to *force* antibody formation and immunity. Vaccinations establish "resident" enemy troops in outposts throughout the body. Later, when we are weak or old, these foreign troops bring about insurrection from *within!*

Vaccines create electrical "static" because their magnetic *signature* is *foreign* to the body. Their vibrational frequency interferes with health and longevity by creating "disharmony" at the *subtle energy* level of our being.

Once antibodies are formed and immunity is conferred, it is VERY important to eliminate vaccination induced proteins from the body. If these substances are not **driven** from the body, they will participate in the development of crippling degenerative dis-eases.

The best way to deal with vaccination-induced energy proteins is to **"erase"** their *signatures* from the body. This is accomplished with the use of *biogenic,* full spectrum, homeopathic remedies in mixed, multiple potencies of 9x, 20x, 30x, 100x, and 200x. **The process does NOT affect immunities and antibodies already existent.**

The goals of immunization are admirable, but the side effects can be heart breaking—especially in young children whose immune systems are undeveloped. Always **buffer** vaccinations to avoid the risk of hearing loss or inducing Type 1 diabetes in your child.

Adults MUST be concerned about the insidious, **long term** effects of immunizations on their body. The solution requires that you clear *your* body of the "baggage" that came with those *innocent* vaccinations. If you do, you will **enjoy** a longer and healthy life (see Source Index).

Homeopathy

"Homeopathy is wholly capable of satisfying the therapeutic demands of this age better than any other system or school of medicine."
                                        Charles F. Menninger, M.D.

Homeopathic detoxification is a *crucial* step in the treatment of dis-ease and chronic health conditions.

Homeopathy teaches that *symptoms* of a "disease" are a *natural* part of the healing process, and their expression should be **encouraged** rather than be suppressed.

Recent advances in homeopathic formulation have led to the enhancement of *traditional* remedies with *biogenic* and nutritional support (Homeovitic+Bio+Nutritional). Enhanced support intensifies the *innate* healing energy of the body through *vitalization*.

Vitalization enhances the energy *footprint* of a substance by a stepwise series of dilutions + succussions designed to increase **resonance** (vibrational frequency) so energy can be transferred from the "vitalized" substance to a less active one.

Transfer of resonance to toxins occurs when the vitalized substance (vitic) is similar (homeo) to the less active one. Thus, all vitalized substances obey the law of similars (homeovitic), which says *"like is cured by like."*

"The cause is the cure" is even more specific. For instance, the use of mercury in its *vitalized* form removes mercury residues from the body through "resonance" and "transference."

"Transference" of energy from the *vitalized* substance to offending toxin(s) speeds healing and eases stress on the body's vital energy reserves.

Enhanced homeopathic remedies in *combined* strengths of 9x, 20x, 30x, 100x, 200x provide *biogenic* support, promote cellular rejuvenation, and deal with underlying health problems at the **subtle energy level.**

These remedies are now available and are very effective in dealing with conditions that involve:

Alcohol	Allergies	Tobacco	Bacteria
Viruses	Chemicals	Dentals	Yeast
Fungi	Metals	Parasites	Radiation
Stress	Spider Bites	Food additives	Free Radicals

"Enhanced" Homeopathic Remedies Work!

24

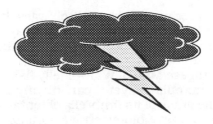

Brown Fat

"Where I am, death is not. Where death is, I am not."
Epicurus

In 1976, Peking, China (now Beijing), suffered a massive man-made earthquake that killed 650,000 people. The events prior to its occurrence were exactly in line with the predictions of the electrical wizard, Nicola Tesla (1865-1942). Tesla said earthquakes could be *created* by manipulating massive amounts of electrical ENERGY!

Tesla predicted a highly charged ionic atmosphere would be exhibited. Buildings and objects may have an iridescent blue green glow about them. Multi-colored lightning—red, blue, and gold—may be seen in the early morning sky around the epicenter for hours before the event. The earthquake would be the EFFECT of a massive electrical energy shift, NOT the cause.

The lightning we see in the sky and the electrical phenomenon of the *bio-electric* body have much in common. BOTH are *expressions* of electrical energy. Both are electrical phenomena.

The *physical* body is *condensed* energy that we can see and touch. It belongs to our Third Dimension world. The *electric* body, however, belongs to the world of the Fourth Dimension—an electrical world that is *invisible*, but there nonetheless.

Our aura also belongs to the Fourth Dimension world. It is a "generated" electrical field that radiates from the physical body. Energy that is *generated* must have a source—something that is producing it. We are interested in the body's source of energy because it DEFINES the aging process in terms of *rate* as well as our *ability* or *inability* to reverse aging. Bio-electric energy is the body's version of *lightning!*

Bio-electric Lightning!

Animals produce electrical discharges that mimic lightning. For example, electric eels and electric rays— creatures of the ocean—release enough electricity to light the dark at night or even kill a man.

The Portugese Man o' War—a jelly fish—is but a mass of transparent protoplasm, yet it can kill any living thing that comes within the grasp of its umbrella of tentacles. It kills with a MASSIVE discharge of bio-electric *lightning.*

Consider the electrical spectacular that occurs when the human sperm enters the ovum at fertilization. At that instant, over 480,000 volts of electricity (Yes! 480,000 volts) are released!

The discharge of electricity coagulates the outer surface of the ovum and prevents penetration by other sperm. The event is the beginning of a new organism. It is an *electrical* event of massive proportions that *generates* a new life! Death is a similar—but opposite—electrical event where "spirit" energy returns from whence it came and metabolism synchronizes.

While we are on this earth, it would behoove us to understand the SOURCE of *lightning* that keeps us alive. Understanding it is the key to becoming *Young Again!*

The Body Electric

The body is a flesh and blood electrical storage battery, and power generation system in one. Peak health depends on the bio-electric body's ability to generate and store electrical ENERGY! We are dependent on a source of *fuel*, a storage system, a *transmission system* to distribute the energy, and a method to *control* the ebb and flow of that energy. Energy is our BRIDGE between youth and old age—life and death.

We draw on our electrical energy reserves as needed and we replenish them through rest, detoxification, and nourishment. When we fail to restore electrical balance, we lapse into partial or total energy synchronization. A corpse is a good example of total energy synchronization. Aging is partial synchronization. It is the crock-pot version. Aging is the effect of a LOSS of electrical vitality. It is *slow* death. **As vital organ function slows, we LOSE the ability to generate and store energy, which speeds the passing of Time!**

The Mitochondria

The mitochondria are bacteria that inhabit the cells of all animals. They were first observed through the microscope around the year 1800. However, they were not officially identified as "living" organisms—capable of independent existence—and given a name until approximately 1935.

The *mitochondria* derive their name from the Greek *mitos*—a thread, and *chondros*—a grain. These root words describe their shape, NOT their function. Originally, the mitochondria were thought to be artifacts (waste), or organelles (tiny bodies) found within most cells. Eventually it was discovered that they are our SOURCE of *bio-electric lightning!*

Life is impossible without the mitochondria. They process our glucose sugars and produce and burn the energy-carrying molecule adenosine triphosphate (ATP), which is our energy carrying molecule. Glucose is our sugar fuel. It is stored in the liver and muscles as glycogen. When energy is needed, the cells convert glycogen back to glucose and the mitochondria oxidize the glucose and produce our energy.

Conversion of body fat to energy takes place in the liver. Aerobic exercise helps the liver's functional cells (the hepatocytes) to produce enzymes that CONVERT body fat into usable glucose fuel that the mitochondria can burn.

The mitochondria CONTROL aerobic respiration which is also referred to as internal respiration because it occurs in the cells as opposed to external respiration, which occurs in the lungs.

Mitochondria Control Aging

The mitochondria are BOTH power generators and storage batteries. They convert food energy into metabolic electricity. They are referred to as the **power house** of the cell.

The mitochondria replicate (reproduce) on their own. This is important! They are not dependent on the host even though they reside in our cells and are influenced by the body environment. They have their own DNA code. (Think of DNA as cellular programming *software*, genetic instructions, and a road map all in one.)

Mitochondrial activity is what *drives* anabolism— the process of build-up and repair of body tissue. Anabolism is a youthful condition and the opposite of catabolism.

As we age, anabolism gives way to catabolism. When we reach our *anabolic peak,* growth and repair of body tissue slows. Energy production slows. Hormone production slows. Health and vitality diminishes and old age becomes reality.

Mitochondrial energy is right-spin, positive energy. It keeps us alive. When mitochondrial function becomes limited, the effects are seen in the mirror. When energy production falls short of our minimum requirements, life ceases.

Growth Plates

Medical science's *dividing line* between youth and old age is based on long bone extension. When the growth plates between the diaphysis (shank of the long bones) and the epiphysis (end of the long bones) "close," science says we cross the threshold into that *twilight zone* between youth and old age. Whatever growth or lack thereof that has occurred is a done deal. We have officially *stopped* growing. This event usually occurs between ages 18 and 22. Science's definition of aging focuses on the extension of long bones. It is incomplete.

Our definition of aging focuses on the body's *shift* from anabolism to catabolism, which can be accelerated or reversed at will. Our focus is on *perpetual* growth and repair of body tissues, instead of long bone extension. We are NOT concerned with closure of the epiphyseal plates.

When the mitochondria cannot produce enough electrical energy to meet the body's needs for growth and repair, we age by default. Aging and the passing of bio-electric TIME are one and the same. Our friends, the mitochondria, control TIME.
We must learn HOW to assist the mitochondria if we want to reverse aging and stop the passing of Time.

The Sweat Zones

The sweat zones of the body are areas of heat production and waste energy release. Concentrations of mitochondria in the sweat zones confirm the relationship between mitochondrial function and waste ENERGY release. These zones experience heavy lymphatic fluid movement (lymph is our non-blood body fluid. Good lymph flow is crucial to good health.

The lymphatic system is cancer's electrical highway. The lymph nodes are the power stations along the way. They are located in the sweat zones of the body.

The lymphatic system's job is multiple in nature. It includes toxic waste management. It recirculates extracellular fluids back into the blood supply. It is the body's primary *protein* communication system.

The lymph nodes **hold** toxic energy fields and release them only when the body can handle them. This is why body hair is found in areas of high toxicity—like the groin, arm pits, scalp, face, and legs. Hair siphons off and releases left-spin energy wastes. (Hair analysis is a measure of EXCESSES.)

Hair Analysis

Hair analysis speaks of EXCESSES. It should not be used to measure *deficiencies*. We do not suffer from deficiencies, only excesses. Hair analysis provides "clues." It is a tool and a window into the body, but in a PAST TENSE time frame.

Hair is analyzed and found to contain mercury. The heavy metal may be coming from the amalgam fillings in the teeth or some other source. Whatever the source, the person IS excreting mercury—via the hair. That's good! We know that the body is releasing the mercury.

But what if this same individual showed no mercury in the hair? Is mercury free? No! This is the dilemma that all health practitioners face—conventional and alternative alike. **They diagnose and treat on the basis of deficiencies when there is NO such thing!** Practitioners and patients have been schooled in "deficiency" thinking. It should be thrown out.

So the person who is dumping mercury (or whatever) via the hair, suffers from a condition of excess, where the mercury is MOBILE rather than stagnant, which is desirable. And the person whose tissues retain mercury residues, but it does not show up in the hair? That person is mercury toxic AND stagnant and hair analysis CANNOT be relied upon to guide treatment. (Anyone who has mercury amalgam fillings should assume they ARE toxic and have them removed by a "competent" holistic dentist. Enhanced homeopathic remedies plus Yucca extract and PAC's can remove and ERASE mercury signatures from the tissues where amalgam removal is not possible for whatever reason (see Source Index).

Hair is a storehouse of toxic waste energy OUTSIDE of the body. Body fat is just the opposite. And if we expect to reverse aging and experience boundless energy, we must provide a body-friendly environment where the mitochondria can produce the energy needed to drive waste disposal—which includes excretion via the integument (skin, hair, and nails), the lungs, the urine, and the bowel. The exit portals rely on a FUNCTIONING lymphatic system, which, in turn, relies upon adequate exercise, lymphatic self-massage, colon therapy, dietary discretion, body-friendly water, and ionic sea minerals.

Insects • Birds • Sperm

Insects and birds have heavy concentrations of mitochondria in the muscles that are responsible for flight. The mitochondria furnish that energy.

The human sperm makes the long trip into the woman's fallopian tubes to fertilize the ovum, with *power* generated by the mitochondria. The base of the sperm's tail is saturated with mitochondria. When the sperm fertilizes the egg, the electrical discharge of 480,000 volts of electricity comes from both the sperm and the ovum. Both are energy bodies—one is huge, the other is tiny.

The discharge of the ovum is only .19 volts. The electrical discharge by the sperm is 25,263,157 times GREATER than that of the ovum—a huge difference!

There is a massive difference in physical size between the sperm and ovum. The volume of the ovum is $1,760,000^2$ microns. The volume of the sperm is only 21^2 microns. When we divide the size of the ovum by the size of the sperm we find that the egg is 83,809 times greater! These MASSIVE differences in physical size and electrical potential results in the release of the 480,000 volts of electricity we call *bio-electric lightning!*

At Birth

When we are born, the number of mitochondria in our cells is very high, as is the level of BROWN FAT, which we will discuss shortly. This explains why children and young people are warm blooded and **prematurely** aged people (especially pre, post, and menopausal women & andropausal men) suffer from internal coldness. The mitochondria produce huge amounts of energy needed for us to grow to adulthood in a few short years, and maintain internal warmth. Hormonal imbalances (excesses) are **very much** a part of the *coldness* people experience.

As we grow, we experience the ebb and flow of energy called health and sickness. By the time we reach adulthood, the growth plates in the long bones have closed and we achieve our maximum height. When we cross the threshold of our anabolic peak, we experience a shift from right to left-spin energy dominance and we begin our descent into old age—UNLESS we are willing to **take control of our life** and **responsibility for our condition** and **begin the rejuvenatory process.**

As the *bio-electric* body comes under the dominance of negative energy fields, mitochondrial activity slows and so does their rate of replication (multiplication). In other words, we lose our energy and drive due to conditions of EXCESS. As health and vitality wanes, dis-ease manifests itself and the doctor provides the label in the form of a diagnosis.

So aging is really nothing but condition(s) of excess, which produce hormonal imbalances, which impact the vital organs, which brings on a scenario of suffering and eventually death. **It does NOT have to be this way!**

Rest • Detoxification • Illness

Rest is a part of the rejuvenation process. Rest allows the *bio-electric* body to heal. It *frees* and *redirects* mitochondrial energy so critical metabolic processes can rebound.

Illnesses ARE healing crises. When someone suffers with the flu, hepatitis, cancer, etc.— there is NOT enough available energy to both heal the body and carry on normal activities at the same time. We go to bed by default!

When we force the body to work under conditions of high metabolic stress, be it *diagnosed* OR *sub*clinical illness, we "squander" mitochondrial energy that should be used for detoxification and healing.

To get the system back on stream, the mitochondria NEED our assistance. They will automatically increase their numbers and activity if we will flush the system of EXCESS metabolic waste. This is best accomplished via colon therapy, Yucca extract, and PAC's, and **the flushing of stones from the liver and gall bladder** (a painless procedure).

Mitochondrial replication involves the doubling of DNA and genetic material —so two bacteria are created out of one. This process is called *mitosis*. As the mitochondria increase their numbers, power generation comes back on-line.

When the mitochondria FAIL to return to former activity levels, we break through a Time "barrier" and experience aging. All of us have seen our parents and friends jerk and slip their way *down* the catabolic side of the pyramid. Metabolic slow down produces *plateaus* in the aging process. **Aging accelerates in direct relationship to slowing of cellular respiration and oxidation, loss of mitochondrial function, and blockage of bile flow due to stones in the liver.**

Sodium & Waste

Aging, toxicity, and catabolism are peas in a pod, and where you find one, you will find the others. Toxic waste comes in many colors and sizes. Sodium chloride is one of them.

Sodium chloride (table salt) is of particular importance to our discussion of the mitochondria. Sodium is a *poison*. Sodium is a *preservative*. Sodium is an electrolyte. Sodium conducts electricity in a solution—as in the **intra** and **inter**cellular fluids in the tissues (between and in the cells respectively)—as well as in the blood. Intercellular or interstitial fluid is between the cells. Blood is in the vessels. Neither fluid is sterile as commonly taught in medical schools. They are dynamic, live, *organism-bearing* body fluids. Their energy profiles are *easily* altered by diet and circumstance. The elimination of the Rouleau effect (see page 136) from the blood is PROOF of the effect liquid ionic sea minerals have on toxic blood. Soft drinks dramatically alter blood and body pH and should be considered as toxic as alcohol.

In our society, it is impossible to get too little sodium. Many people, however, do suffer with symptoms associated with low electrolytes. Conventional medical *protocol* calls for increased sodium intake. This approach is wrong because it fails to address the issue of EXCESS toxicity in the tissues. Excesses always manifest as deficiencies. A safer and better approach calls for serious detoxification therapy and the use of liquid ionic sea minerals.

Under **normal** conditions sodium remains OUTSIDE the cell membranes—out in the **extra**cellular fluid—**between** the cells. Potassium is sodium's twin. It is found on the INSIDE of the cell membrane—in the cytoplasm (*cyt*-cell. *plasm*-fluid.).

A healthy body maintains a balance (ratio) of sodium to potassium. Because our foods are devitalized and over pro-cessed, we ingest EXCESS sodium and insufficient potassium to maintain a proper ratio. The more sodium we consume, the greater will be the on loss of potassium from the cells. Salt brings on death. *The word* **death** *is mostly "eat."*

STOP The Salt

Under normal conditions, few sodium ions (Na^+) are allowed inside the cells. Excess sodium (Na^+) ions gain entrance to the cells as potassium ions (K^+) are given up by the cells for use elsewhere in the body. This is a one for one trade and occurs in the face of a sodium **excess.** As each K^+ ion leaves the cell, it is replaced by one Na^+ ion. An unbalanced diet will FORCE the body will *steal* potassium from the cells to sustain itself.

The body depends on the process we call biological alchemy to meet its dietary needs. It can make what it needs **if** all systems are functional, but he alchemy process fails under conditions of excess. Hormonal and toxicity excesses bring on PMS, thyroid conditions, and obesity. Supplementation should be used only as a "bridge." Using supplementation to "cover" their bad living habits is foolish. I am here to tell you that this approach does NOT work. **Peak health and longevity re-quires change in one's daily habits and mental thoughts.**

Sodium and potassium ions BOTH carry a (+) charge and are close in size. This allows them to swap positions. Ion swapping occurs whenever the sodium to potassium ratio is upset. Hence, EXCESS sodium drives out potassium.

When Na⁺ ions invade the cells, the cells become dysfunctional—along with the mitochondria therein. Sick cells fail to contribute to overall health and vitality and additional excesses occur, creating a vicious circle. Excess waste and dietary shortfalls of potassium eventually result in auto digestion or "self-cannibalism."

Older people and people suffering with degenerative conditions, build up **MASSIVE** amounts of toxic wastes in their tissues. Under conditions of EXCESS, edema appears and turgor is lost (turgor is resistance of the skin to deformation). This *waterlogged* condition is common in the extremities (hands, legs, ankles and feet).

Edema is **more** than water retention. It is a SIGN of excess waste proteins in the tissues, diminished heart function, and kidney slowdown. NEVER use diuretics! Instead, detoxify immediately and regain the loss of vital organ function.

Allopathic medicine relies on diuretics (water pills) to drive EXCESS fluids from the tissues. In the process, more potassium is lost, and the body cannibalizes muscle proteins and body fat as fuel sources. When it runs out of reserves, the person's weight **collapses** overnight—leaving skin and bones.

As waste and toxicity increase, body hair decreases. Again, this is very common among older folks who go "bald" all over their body, especially the legs. Same for fungus under the toc nails, fcct problems, toe nail irregularities. **When body hair is lost, the system is on its way down. Hair is crucial to detoxification of the skin. Clean up your body, and your will restore hair with "color" from your head to your feet.**

STOP or reduce the use sodium chloride (table salt) at the dinner table and in food preparation. Instead, try lightly misting your food with liquid sea minerals. Home grown food doesn't need salt. It is loaded with mineral ions.

Salt's effects are insidious. Cancer loves high sodium environments. Cancer tumors and masses are surround themselves in a field of sodium saturated tissue. Sodium and cancer go together. Sodium does not cause cancer, but it is ALWAYS a player. The elimination of table salt is an important step in reversing the aging process.

Cancers are strong, sodium saturated energy fields. Cancer <u>tumors</u> "import" and "condense" negative energy. <u>Masses</u> export negative energy (see page 307).

The invasion of sodium into the cells is the equivalent of shutting off the power in Jurassic Park. When the power goes off, nature's dinosaurs—the cancer viruses—follow the lead and take control of the DNA and RNA software in our cells and they multiply. Their proliferation rate is exponential (2, 4, 8, 16,

32, 64,128, 256, etc.). Their job is to eliminate weak organisms.
Viruses ONLY gain entrance to our cells when our electrical defenses have been sabotaged. We are our own saboteur when we include table salt in our diet!

BEV water and liquid ionic sea minerals are critically important to sodium detoxification. BEV water is the PERFECT *carrier* solvent due to its high energy *footprint*. It transports sodium OUT of the cells and OUT of the body, but it can only do this with the help of ionically balanced sea minerals. Either eat a diet high in natural organic potassium, or get it from sea water derived ionic minerals. **Sodium must be DRIVEN OUT of the cells. It will NOT leave on its own.** Fresh juices are rich in organic potassium. So are juice capsules and tablets.

As the sodium in the cells is replaced with potassium, the mitochondria come alive and multiply—producing the cellular equivalent of lighting! The electricity is turned on. The shields are raised, and the viruses revert to their dormant state because the *terrain* that catered to them has changed; conditions are no longer opportunistic. Health and vitality return.

Pricking the finger is a good way to gauge the overall health of the bio-electric body. If you prick your finger and the blood fails to stand-up with a very distinct "pearl," but instead produces a low profile ball, or flows or oozes onto the skin, you have NO time to waste! Detoxification is mandatory.

Blood should be BRILLIANT red, never dark red. Blood that has a low *crown* and dark color is in a *pre-cancer* state, and the Rouleau effect will be present.

Brown Fat & Mitochondria

Brown fat has a great deal to do with vitality and rejuvenation. Understanding it sheds light on WHY some people are fat and other people are thin.

Officially, brown fat is called *brown adipose tissue* (BAT). BAT was only recently discovered. BAT is brown because of the extremely heavy *concentrations* of mitochondria in it, which makes it is very active biologically speaking. Except for the word fat, BAT has NO resemblance in appearance or function to its shirt-tale relative, *white adipose tissue* (WAT)—which is the normal body fat commonly thought of.

Officially, BAT is responsible for **"non-shivering thermogenesis"**—the generation of heat in the absence of shivering. Shivering is a normal body function that is part of heat production under cold OR high stress conditions (people shiver during and after a serious emergency). BAT is heavily vascularized (lots of blood vessels) compared to WAT.

Babies have much higher concentrations of BAT than

do adults. People who live and work in cold climates have more BAT than people in warm climates. Japanese women skin divers have very high concentrations of BAT and are able to bear frigid ocean waters for hours at a time. They can do this because of the high concentrations of BAT in their tissues, and because of a right-spin energy diet. BAT produces massive amounts of cellular lightning.

Healthy people have more BAT than do sick people. Thin people have more BAT than fat people. The more BAT you have, the thinner you will be and the more energy you will have!

To understand BAT, let's review the physiological process called *thermogenic hyperphagia.* Dissected it looks like this: *thermo*-heat. *genic*-pertaining to the production of. *hyper*-above normal. *phagia*-that which eats.

People who are subclinically sick, or who suffer with degenerative dis-ease have low concentrations of BAT!

Obese people do not have enough BAT. Instead, they have too much WAT (white adipose tissue). As WAT increases in a person's body, BAT decreases. As we discussed earlier, obesity is the most obvious SIGN that a person's body is aging in the internal organs, and that EXCESSES and hormonal imbalances exist. **BAT diminishes when we lose control of our body terrain. BAT and good health go together.**

When we reach our anabolic peak, loss of BAT accelerates, obesity becomes a problem, vitality diminishes, and aging accelerates. This downward spiral normally begins in the middle twenties to early thirties.

In industrial societies like the USA, BAT loss among women (and men) is *epidemic!* Premenopausal symptoms are now appearing 10 years AHEAD of the onset of menopause and andropause. Symptoms that used to manifest in the late forties and early fifties, are now **rampant** among people in their late twenties and early thirties. Signs and symptoms of aging develop in direct relationship to loss of BAT, development of hormonal imbalances, and toxic excesses in the body.

Hormone precursors encourage BAT formation and help reverse menopausal and andropausal symptoms in BOTH sexes with NO negative side effects. Detoxification is basic. Aerobic exercise, rebounding, and lymphatic self-massage are important. Subjecting the body to cold is VERY beneficial. Swim regularly in a cold pool, ocean, or lake. Do ease your way into the water. Never plunge in as it can cause temporarily paralysis and death due to the "gasp reflex." Perform yard and garden work and take walks during the cold months dressed in only a light, short sleeved shirt to encourages BAT formation and build immunity. Finish your shower with an ICE COLD shower. It's VERY stimulating!

My favorite cold therapy is to do my aerobic exercise OUTSIDE in nothing but boxer shorts—year around! "Cold" workouts stimulate the body and train the mind to focus beyond the immediate present.

Enhanced trivalent chromium is also very effective in encouraging BAT formation and it has no negative side effects.

Increase BAT and you will BACK your way "up" the aging pyramid to your former anabolic peak. When you reach that peak, you have become *Young Again!*

PREVIEW: *Our next chapter is going to SHOCK you! You are going to learn WHY men and women are going bald—and what they can do about it! You are also going to discover the relationship between certain cooking oils and the HIV/AIDS virus.*

Look at all the sick and dying people!

Medical Studies

People rely on the advice of their practitioner. Practitioners, in turn, rely on the *credibility* of medical studies to guide them.

Unfortunately, too many medical studies are flawed. For the patient, *bogus* medical studies can mean the difference between life and death at worst, and pain and suffering at best.

In front of me is a news article captioned, *"Fraud Mars Breast Cancer Research."* Investigators uncovered more than a *decade* of fraudulent breast cancer research. And another report condemning mammograms for damaging women's breast tissues.

These reports are frightening, but the **message is clear**. We cannot afford to lose our health, NOR can we afford to rely on science, studies, and experts to save us. Instead, we must personal responsibility for our health.

And please, do NOT fall into the trap of conjuring reasons why tried and proven alternative modalities will not work for you. If you want your life back, be willing to do what needs to be done. Sick people cannot afford excuses.

Follow the steps outlined in this book and you can look forward to a dis-ease free life. Health and longevity is a gift we experience in the wake of *personal* responsibility and action. Start today!

25

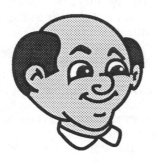

Bald Heads & Oils

"Hair on my legs, hair on my chest, but no hair on my head?"
Uncle Ross

Balding is a SIGN of premature aging. So is thin hair. Balding is *loathed* by men, yet it is accepted as inevitable if it "runs" in the family. The *experts* tell us balding is a genetic trait. They are **wrong!** Balding is neither inevitable nor genetic, nor does it have to be permanent. Balding is related to oxygen deficiencies in the scalp tissues, reduced mitochondrial activity, waste EXCESSES in the scalp, and hormonal imbalances in the system. **Hair follicles die or go dormant in a toxic environment!**

Scalp toxicity and congestion are linked to the consumption of certain dietary oils. If you eat the oils the *experts* tell you to eat, you will likely go bald or develop thin hair. And you will succumb to degenerative conditions like arthritis, gout, coronary degeneration, and cancer.

Almost *everything* the public has been taught about dietary oils and fats is false. We have been manipulated and lied to. It's time to wake up.

A Short History Of Oils

Beginning in the 1930's, cotton seed oil became the primary "liquid" dietary oil substitute for fats like butter and lard. During WW ll, cotton seed oil was hydrogenated to create a butter substitute that was SOLID at room temperature. They called it **oleo**margarine, margarine, or oleo for short. War mentality caused the public to accept oleo, and by the 50's—when I was growing up—margarine was considered an *acceptable* butter substitute. By the early 1960's, Americans experienced ANOTHER fundamental shift in the TYPE of dietary oils and fats they were eating. This time it was away from solid fats like butter, lard, and margarine to liquid oils. (Today we have *soft* margarines to bridge the gap).

While the media and the *experts* vilified butter and lard, the Cholesterol THEORY of Cardiovascular Dis-ease became the new scientific "buzz phrase" within the halls of academia. **The cholesterol theory was hatched to *stampede* the public into giving up butter and eggs.**

Later, more buzz words were added to the American vocabulary. Words like *unsaturated* and *poly-unsaturated.* Corn and safflower oils appeared on the scene. These replaced cotton seed oil for those with finer tastes and fatter wallets. Margarine was in its hey-day. Fewer people were eating butter. Lard was only for the poor.

By the late 1960's, SOY BEAN oil began to appear on supermarket shelves and in thousands of *processed* foods. Cotton seed, corn and safflower oils were still in wide use, but there was a new focus—health! Soy bean oil became synonymous with **health and the health food movement.**

The shift away from natural fats—like butter—to liquid and *hydrogenated* seed oils, coupled with chlorination and fluoridation of public water supplies, caused Americans to experience a dramatic increase in degenerative heart dis-ease.

The *experts* blamed naturally occurring *saturated* fats and *cholesterol* for the rise in cardiovascular problems, while they ignored the horrendous increase in degenerative dis-ease conditions. They ignored balding because it was considered to be a "genetic" problem, NOT a dietary one.

The experts like to razzle dazzle us with oily words like omega 3's and 6,'s phrases like long vs. short chain fatty acids, and concepts like monounstaurated and polyunsaturated. These terms are meaningless to the average person. What does hold meaning are the effects of premature old age. For instance, LOOK at the huge increase in young men with balding heads! And young women with thinning hair! Ignore the fancy talk. It is designed to keep you confused.

With the advent of the new "healthy" oils, the occurrence of balding and *thinning* hair increased in both sexes, both young and old. The only person who noticed that something was going on was Dr. Carey Reams. Reams however, worked in the agricultural arena. He was a voice crying in the wilderness.

For your benefit, we will define some commonly used medical terms that will help you to understand the dilemma people face in regard to oils, fats, and dis-ease.

Arteriosclerosis—Hardening of the walls of the arterioles (small arteries) due mainly to fibrous thickening of the connective tissues in their walls, hyalinization, and infiltration of lipids (fats) into the intima (innermost wall) of the arteriole.

Atherosclerosis—a form of simple intimal arteriosclerosis with atheromatous deposits within and beneath the intima of the arteries.

Atheromatous deposits—the fatty *degeneration* of the artery walls with infiltration of those walls by lipids(fats)—as in arteriosclerosis. Cellular debris, toxic waste, and calcium deposits are usually involved.

Intima—the innermost layer of the three layers that compose the artery wall.

Hyalin-a clear substance that has undergone amyloid degeneration; material deposited in the glomeruli filters of the kidneys.

Amyloid-the abnormal deposition of hyaline in the tissues during pathological state (dis-ease).

Hyalinization—normal infusion of hyaline; seen normally in the matrix of cartilage and abnormally elsewhere; any alteration within the cells or extracellular spaces which involves the deposition of hyalin.

Plaque—-a cholesterol containing mass in the intima or tunica of the arteries; means *patch.*

The Soy Connection

Dr. Carey Reams often commented on the rise in balding, but it was my friend, Tom Mahoney, who provided the clue that solved the puzzle. It was an *agricultural* clue.

Tom talked of a strange family of plants known as the **Fabales**. He noted that if cows are allowed to graze on soy they will *die*. And if sheep graze on soy, their hair "falls out."

Tom's observations were the trigger I needed to solve Dr. Carey Reams' thirty year old question. Reams was sure there was a link between the soybean, balding, and deterioration in the blood.

Soy Oil & PHG

Soybean oil and soy bean curd (tofu), contain a toxic biochemical called **"phyto-hema-glutinin"** or PHG for short. Dissected, the word looks like this: *phyt(e)*-that which comes from plants). *hem(e)*-blood. *glutinin*-a vegetable protein "glue." **PHG is a large protein molecule that has proven to be specific in its ability to *agglutinate* human blood.**

Agglutination means to "glue," to cause to "adhere," to combine into a "mass!" The Rouleau effect we have been referring to is a good example of agglutination. Soy oil—and soy based products that contain the oil—are especially rich in PHG.

PHG causes blood circulation to slow. It causes blood to clot. It combines with impurities in the blood and forms plaques in the walls of the arterioles, and closes off the fine capillaries in the posterior eye, ears, and SCALP. It magnifies the Rouleau "sticky blood" problem now affecting 85% of Americans. PHG numbs the immune system's T cells, and it negatively influences the central and peripheral nervous systems. It alters hormonal activity, and it influences endocrine and exocrine activity while it slows vital organ function.

PHG kills rats DEAD! It is poisonous to *all* living things. As with any systemic poison, the *quantity* consumed, *length* of exposure, and *individual* predisposition are KEY factors that explain why the body *seems* to be able to tolerate soy oil and tofu. **The effects of PHG are "cumulative," and the reader must forever remember the insidious nature of this word.**

Soy & Digestion

Soy oil interferes with *normal* digestion. Soy beans produce gas and upset body chemistry in *sensitive* people. Peanuts are a *famous* member of the Fabale family of plants, and many people cannot digest peanut butter. Peanuts contain little PHG in comparison to soy. More examples of the Fabale family of foods are garbanzo beans (chic peas), fava beans, lentils, mung beans. These contain *almost* no PHG.

Two Fabale legumes that cause serious problems for *grazing* animals are clover and alfalfa. In the field, they can be deadly toxic and cause bloating in ruminants. Cows, horses, and sheep thrive on grasses which contain growth energy proteins. Grasses have a different "spin" on their protein molecules than do legumes like alfalfa, clover, and soy.

Soy oil (PHG) reacts with circulating minerals and dissolved gases in the blood like chlorine, chloramine, and fluorine. It forms substances that resemble bath tub scum—like that which comes from Grandma's lye soap.

Municipalities use chemicals like sodium hypo-chloride (sodium hydroxide + chlorine) to treat public water supplies. Sodium hydroxide (lye) is what Grandma used to make her lye soap. It is extremely alkaline (pH 12). Chlorine is extremely acidic (-2 and +2 pH) and is used to kill bacteria. The hydroxide is used to drive up the pH so that the acidic water will not kill you. Halogenated (chlorinated and fluoridated) tap water reacts with dietary oils and other circulating wastes and produces left-spinning energy fields that feed pathogenic microbial life forms.

Oils and fats are absorbed by the lymphatic capillaries called lacteals. They are NOT absorbed directly into the blood capillaries as are proteins and carbohydrates. Lacteals give way to larger ducts that transport and deposit dietary oils and fats into the blood. The junction of the lymphatic system and blood system is at the subclavian veins that feed the superior vena cava vein which empties into the right side of the heart. The heart then pumps the blood to the lungs for oxygenation AND left spin energy *detoxification* before it is returned to the left side of the heart for distribution to the body.

Forty percent (40%) of the blood leaving the heart goes up the neck and into the head. In the process, soy oil REACTS with blood toxins and chemicals and settles OUT of the blood. These precipitates are electrically "charged" energy fields that cling to the walls of the coronary arteries that **service** the heart. They slow or close off blood flow to the heart muscle. These precipitates are called *plaque!*

Plaque formation causes the lining (intima) of the arteries to deteriorate and form clots. When a clot or plaque deposit breaks lose, it can migrate up the neck and into the brain and produces a stroke. If on the other hand, the oxygen supply to the heart becomes severely limited due to plaque formation, a heart attack will result.

As blood enters the neck, waste settle out, narrowing the carotid arteries that feed the head and brain. Waste finds its way into the VERY FINE capillaries that feed the cells of the posterior eyes, ears, and scalp and closes them off. Lymph capillaries become sluggish and deteriorate in the form of eye problems, poor hearing, and balding accelerates.

Balding and gray hair are SIGNS of premature aging. Balding means your body is in trouble. Reversing the process involves helping the body remove the waste deposits from the cells, tissues, lymph, and blood, so dormant hair follicles will awaken or new ones will form. Detoxification requires the application of ALL of the health principles in this book: diet, water, colon therapy, exercise, and a few select supplements.

Ingestion of soy oil—and canola oil—accelerates mental deterioration in the young and old alike. Recall of information becomes difficult. Further deterioration leads to things like Alzheimers and the horror that comes with it.

Alfalfa Sprouts

Alfalfa sprouts are a popular food delight for many health-oriented people. However, the effect of sprouts on the bio-electric body is questionable at best.

Alfalfa **sprouts** contain powerful *phyto* chemicals that are detrimental to people with weak immune systems. In dry leaf form, as used in food supplements—alfalfa has a different make up and vibrational spin and does not pose a problem.

Cancer patients should NEVER, EVER eat alfalfa sprouts. Sprouts depress the immune system. They create a condition of EXCESS and must not be eaten by anyone with—or recovering from—cancer. Sprouts cause cancer to attack with a vengeance! (Mung bean sprouts do NOT pose a problem.)

People with immune conditions or liver problems (hepatitis, mononucleosis, chronic fatigue, cirrhosis etc.) should avoid alfalfa sprouts. Alfalfa sprouts create excesses, and it is the liver's job to moderate energy imbalances, manage excesses, and detox the body via the flow of bile.

Occasional sickness is good. It means that your immune system is functioning and that your body KNOWS when things are out of balance.

Eyes • Ears • Scalp

Bio-junk food diets accelerate aging. Balding, glaucoma, retinitis, and macro degeneration are directly linked to poor blood and lymph flow and waste accumulation. Translated, this means *insufficient* oxygen and nutrients reach the cells, and cellular waste removal is hindered. These conditions produce an energy EXCESS beyond the ability of the hair to manage. *(Hair loss from chemotherapy is a confirmation of this observation).*

The primary purpose of body hair is to transport toxic energies from the "skin" and connective tissues.

Hair follicles are heavy nutrient energy feeders. They require good blood and lymph circulation. Slow growing hair—and nails—is a SIGN of toxic stress. Loss of body hair is worse—especially leg hair. Buildup of waste means shut down of the vital organs and sore feet. Walking legs syndrome, corns, bunions, and deformed toes indicate nerve and connective tissue disorders. Thin hair is but an early version of balding. Gray hair paints a similar story of poor assimilation, hormonal imbalances, and toxic waste buildup in the system.

Supplementary Information On Soybeans

Soy beans are *unlike* other beans. Soy is a *toxic* weed! It is one of two toxic oil producing weed plants grown for human and animal consumption. Insects will NOT eat soy bean plants because they are poisonous.

Soy bean plants—and canola too—thrive on left-spin energy. They *prosper* on the most toxic soils and air. They convert and store toxic energies in their "oil" which is contained in the beans. **Humans do likewise by entombing toxic waste energy fields in their fat—or tumors!**

Soy is a the second strongest left-spin energy food plant grown! Few people know that soy beans were genetically altered in the middle 1950's with that "harmless" process called "*irradiation.*" This was done to INCREASE the soy beans "oil" content. Powerful interests made sure government funded the research. These are the same interests that promote the Cholesterol Theory. They wanted an oil crop that would grow and prosper on negative energy soils—like those where hard salt fertilizers and poisonous sprays have destroyed healthy soils. They are not concerned about the long term effects of soy on people.) **Soy oil is an "industrial" oil, NOT a food oil!**

Sticky Oils • Sick People

The toxic nature of soy has been known for a long time. yet soy oil is added to THOUSANDS of processed and prepared foods (read the food labels and see). Soy products are even substituted for dairy products—like milk and butter.

Heat olive oil, butter, or lard by themselves in a skillet and you will observe that they become "thinner." Soy and canola oils become thicker, sticky, gummy, especially after they cool. Put soy and canola oils into a 98.6° human body and thousands of unpredictable reactions will occur. They oxidize fast! **Industrial oils do not belong in the human body.**

Peanut oil is an interesting oil. It makes a nice massage oil for the skin. But put it in the body, and all hell breaks loose. It is toxic inside, but not outside. Edgar Cayce told of this scenario over fifty years ago.

The best oil available is OLIVE OIL! Olive oil is the product of a **fruit**—the olive! If olive oil was good enough for Jesus, it ought to be good enough for you and me!Nut oils are nice oils. So are sesame, sunflower, and flax. Avoid corn, safflower, and cotton seed oils.

Tofu is a very popular food among vegetarians. Tofu is the curd of the soy bean. It is rich in PHG because of its high oil content (up to 52%), and therefore toxic. If you make Tofu a regular part of your diet, your health will suffer and you will grow OLD. Tofu should NEVER be eaten by recovering cancer patients! NOTE: 99% of vitamin E capsules use soy oil as the carrier. Wheat germ oil is a safer choice. PAC's are a **far better** source of antioxidants than vitamin E, C, or A.

Many people ask, "What about soy protein?" My answer is avoid it if you can. It isn't toxic like the oil which contains the PHG. However, it is the wrong "kind" of protein, meaning it is a *maintenance* protein, as opposed to a *growth* protein. Humans and animals can handle some "whole" soy proteins, but more than a little will result in metabolic degeneration.

Scientists tell us that protein is protein, but they are wrong. All substances have an energy "footprint" or "signature"—including proteins. The problems associated with soy protein occur when it is used in its "raw" form! Avoid soy proteins where possible.

Food products that contain the "free" amino acids that comprised soy proteins are okay because the negative *signature* of the native soy protein is neutralized. Bragg Liquid Aminos is a good example of a "safe" soy derived amino acid food product with a positive energy *footprint.*

Debating The Issues!

I am fully aware that the contents of these pages are totally contrary to what the press and "experts" are saying about the wonders of soy (and canola) oil.

A week doesn't pass that some new "study" lands on my desk with a note asking me to debate the issues regarding soy. Sorry! There is nothing to debate.

Believe whomever you like. The choice is yours. Go ahead. Believe the experts. Ignore common sense and logic. In the end, I can assure you that I will be vindicated and the scoffers will be "dead" right!

Rotenone • Fish • Insects

Rotenone is used by organic gardeners as a "natural" organic pesticide. It is also used for poisoning unwanted fish species in lakes throughout North America.

Rotenone comes from the *soy bean. Roten* is Japanese for *derris.* It means to destroy, to tear apart. Derris is the specie name for the soybean within the family Fabale.

Home gardeners have been told by the *experts* that rotenone is great stuff. However, if you read the label you will be warned against breathing the dust.

When inhaled, rotenone is absorbed through the mucous membranes of the respiratory system. The mucous membranes are a direct conduit into the blood and lymph. These membranes provide easy access to the body's IMMUNE system. A breath of rotenone dust is a direct shot at the central and peripheral nervous systems. It is the **glycosides** in the rotenone that brings on paralysis of the muscles.

We can LEARN from watching an insect that has been dusted with rotenone (PHG). Insects react to rotenone in a matter of seconds with TOTAL paralysis! This harmless stuff from SOY BEANS shuts down the insect's nervous system and muscles. Soybean oil does the same thing to people by destroying their nervous and immune systems, but it does it a day at a time over a period of years!

When used to poison lakes, rotenone causes a complex *series* of changes within a fish's body. The net result is that it prevents the fish from extracting ENERGY from nutrients!

Rotenone kills ALL the fish in a lake with an application as minute as 1 part per million (ppm).

One-half pound of rotenone is equivalent to 60,000 ppm. One-half pound equals 8 ounces or 7,500 ppm per ounce. The *experts* tell us that it would take **1 ounce** of rotenone to kill a 150 pound man. If 1 ppm can kill all the fish in a lake, do you think it would require a concentration that is 7,499 times greater to kill a human being?

It would appear that the *experts* calculations as to what is a "safe" amount of this **poison** that the human body can handle is less than accurate. The truth of the matter is that the *experts* do NOT know how much is a safe amount. These number games remind me of the "experts" Rachel Carson struggled against in her effort to warn mankind of the inherent danger of pesticides. Read *Silent Spring* (see Source Index).

When you eat soy oil, you are eating PHG—which gums your blood and puts your IMMUNE and NERVOUS systems under severe stress. Avoid it!

Sweet Proteins

Glycine is an amino acid. It is one of approximately twenty-three amino acids that form larger molecules called proteins. Sow peas (soybeans) are very rich in glycerine containing proteins because they have been *irradiated* and *genetically engineered* to produce proteins that are high in glycine. Industry, in turn, concentrates glycine through a process called hydrolysis. The result is a glycine-max (glycocide) concentrate (*glyc*-means sweet, as in glycogen which is glucose in storage form in our muscles; *cide*-death by prevention of glycolosis). Glycolysis is the process by which we produce ATP energy molecules for mitochondrial production of energy (*glyc*-sweet; *lysis*-to cleave, breakdown, burn).

Concentrated glycine is produced using *saponification* (the same process Grandma used to make her lye soap). A liquid glycer**ol** is produced that is extremely sweet and syrupy. These molecules have an *alcohol* molecule attached.

An -**ol** on the end of a chemical name means it is an alcohol. Alcohols are excellent *non-polar* solvents, that is, they dissolve fatty substances like those that comprise our cellular membranes. Alcohols destroy our cells and attack the myelin sheath that protects our nerve dendrites (fibers).

The chemical industry likes *glycine-max* glycer**ol**. It is widely used as a *solvent* and as a **plasticizer** in the manufacture of hundreds of plastics, including PVC water pipe.

BEV water cannot be transported in common plastics of any kind, or processed through a carbon block filter because it reacts with the plasticizers and glues and dissolves them. Bottled water—especially distilled water—is loaded with plastic isolates leached from the plastic bottles. That is one of the reasons distilled water tastes so bad. Concentration of poisonous volitiles is another.

When the soy molecule is subjected to heat in the presence of organic compounds like those in our blood, thermoplastic synthetic resins are formed.

The result is **sticky blood** that clumps and closes off the capillaries. Keep in mind, this is a "subtle process." It occurs SLOWLY over a period of years! The body cannot tolerate these resins, so it stores them in the soft tissues (blood is liquid *tissue,* muscle is soft tissue), organs, and fat. Blood vessel degeneration and plaque formation are part of this scenario.

Glycosides • Opium • Morphine • Atropine

Glycosides (rotennone) from soybeans causes physiologic reactions in humans and animals. *Morphine* and atropine are examples of drugs that contain high concentrations of glycosides. Morphine comes from opium and attacks the **central nervous system**. It affects muscle control, pupil dilation, and is extremely reactive in the body. *Atropine* comes from the belladonna family of plants. It alters response to electrical signals and causes paralysis of our **parasympathetic nervous system,** the part of our nervous system over which we have NO direct control, like the heart muscle, breathing muscles, and other involuntary body functions. Digitalis a glycoside that comes from Foxglove. **Morphine, atropine,** and **digitalis** are controlled substances that have been *isolated* and *concentrated.* Substitution of **synthetic** glycosides is common and one reason behind the negative reactions associated with their use in the medical arena.

Soy & Dog Food

In front of me is a label from a can of a well known brand of dog food. You will find it on your supermarket shelves. It says "Soy FREE • Highly Digestible."

The implications of the words on the label and those on TV ads (January 6, 1994) indicate that there is a serious problem with whole soy protein in dog food. Some dog food people tout *digestibility* because they have removed the soy. They are very closed mouthed about the **long term** *degenerative* effects of soy on dogs. They are afraid of retaliation!

The dog food and grazing animal connection confirms the problem of soy in animal metabolism. Soy causes serious degenerative problems in humans, but it is NOT being taken out of our food. Instead, it is being **promoted** by one expert after another as the "perfect" food. Someone is wrong!

If food that contains soy is toxic to dogs **(carnivores)**, and grazing animals **(herbivores)**, what do you think it will do to human beings **(omnivores)** who are a little of both?

Maybe "people" should decide what dog pedigree they would like to be so they can qualify for *soy free, highly digestible food—arf, arf!* Avoid foods that contain soy oil, soy protein solids, and tofu.

Bragg Liquid Aminos

Bragg Liquid Aminos is derived from soybeans, but it is not toxic because it contains NO oil and the proteins have been reduced to their individual amino acids. It is an acceptable substitute for soy and tamari sauce, which are highly toxic, not because of their PHG content (they contain none), but because they are LOADED with sodium.

Liquid Aminos was developed by Paul Bragg, in whose memory I dedicated this book. It is a "pure" amino acid product in balanced form. If you like soy sauce, you will love Bragg Liquid Aminos. It can be purchased at health food stores or directly from the company by calling 1-800-446-1990.

Amino acids (also known as aminos) are composed of carbon, nitrogen, oxygen and hydrogen. Liquid Aminos is made to exacting specifications. **None** of the soy -elated problems we have discussed apply to this product. It takes someone like the Braggs to so it right!

Note: Private interests, via the "government," have recently strong armed the largest hamburger chain in the world (guess who) from going back to using animal fats for their french fries. It appears that soy bean interests in the commodity market control government. Deep frying is bad enough, but using soy oil is much worse than lard. Everyone is getting in on the act. Even the movie theaters push soy/canola oil popcorn!

Conclusion

We know the cumulative effects of soy bean oil, canola oil, tofu, and alfalfa sprouts on humans and animals. We know their effects on the blood, the central and peripheral nervous systems, the immune system, and the environment. **The evidence is obvious for those with eyes to see.**

Please **do not** call the publisher and demand to know the sources of the research that went into this and the following chapter. No one funds this kind of research. There are NO formal studies. The pieces are there if you want to do your own research, on your own time, and at your own expense. In the meantime, I suggest you take my advice and do whatever you have to do to avoid soy oil, soy products (with a few notable exceptions), and canola oil!

Take the time to learn how to effectively use a pendulum and vibration chain and you will be able to confirm the negative effects of soy—and a thousand other things—on your own body. Hopefully the new electronic *Biotester* will be available in 1996. It will be a wonderful tool to help everyone become *Young Again!*

PREVIEW: *In our next chapter, you will learn about the connection between blindness, glaucoma, and canola oil!*

Gulf War Syndrome

Gulf War veterans were <u>ordered</u> to take a drug called Pyridostigmine Bromide (PB) every day. This drug interferes with *acetylcholinesterase*—an enzyme that is critical to nerve synapse function (nerve signal transmission). **The side effects were known & predictable!**

PB produces the symptoms being experienced by Gulf War veterans. The question is WHO ordered its use, and WHY? The answer is "the experts!" They know best! The same experts that tell us to eat soy and canola oil, and promote the use of *(harmless)* poisons like malathion.

Yucca extract, *enhanced* PAC's, and a liver flush to rid the liver of stones will turn these people's lives around!

War In The Marketplace

It takes twenty years to create a market for a product. Early on, consumers fight back IF an enemy can be identified. In time, fight gives way to resistance. After twenty years, fatigue sets in, memory fades, and the metamorphosis is complete.

The rules for *creating* a bogus market are the same as for waging war. I refer the reader to Sun Tzu's 6th century B.C. book *The Art Of War*, summarized as follows.

Outline an agenda, disseminate disinformation and misinformation, create confusion and dissension, raise an army of experts, use subversion, quote statistics, and finally create fear. Fear leads to panic, and panic to victory.

Perhaps now you can see how *they* developed antipathy towards butter, coconut oil, and lard while creating a high demand, consumer-friendly market for **industrial** oils like soy and canola.

Sun Tzu was correct! The game is called **divide and conquer!** It's simple. It works. His book was the official training manual in the rise of the Soviet empire.

Hear what the experts preach. *See* which way the masses are moving. *Tune-in* to what the media is pushing. **Now! Go the other way as you spread the word!**

The "250" Club

The "250" Club is for anyone who would like to live to the age of 250 vibrant, healthy, years *young!*

Please do not dismiss such a goal as impossible or ridiculous. It's within the reach of anyone who truly desires to make it become a reality in their life.

Society needs goals and role models. Think of the good things that would spin-off from a core of people who have healthfully lived five generations?

Instead of each generation starting over every fifty years because wisdom and experience are lost, the "250" Club would act as a *transition* team to help other humans worldwide to connect with Earth and learn to live in harmony with Nature and each other.

Think of the suffering and strife that could be eliminated through the transfer of correct living to our g...r...e...a...t grand children. Life on Earth would become a joy—and a new paradigm. "Power" would lose its grip.

The "250" Club is an exciting and worthy goal.

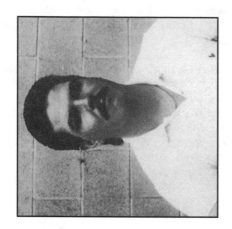

Before

After

Glen Roundtree is living proof of the effectiveness of Harmonized Silver Water on severe burns. His face healed "scar free," but his hands and arms are scarred where he was treated by allopathic doctors using conventional therapy.

Harmonized Silver Water is "tuned" to hertz frequencies that complement the bio-electric body. It goes beyond common colloidal silvers that are based on PPM (parts per million). This Fourth Dimension product uses the homeopathic principles of *resonance* and *transference* to promote healing. Everyone should have a bottle on hand. Great for colds and flu and dozens of other uses.

26

Blindness & Oils

"Since the days of revelation, the same four corrupting errors have been made over and over again: submission to faulty and unworthy authority; submission to what it was customary to believe; submission to prejudices of the mob; and worst of all, concealment of ignorance by a false show of unheld knowledge, for no other reason than pride."
Roger Bacon

Millions of people have suffered the loss of their vision from glaucoma, a dis-ease involving *atrophy* (deterioration) of the optic nerve. For years, the *experts* have been telling people that glaucoma results from fluid pressure buildup in the eye which causes the optic nerve to deteriorate. This THEORY was based on an incorrect medical model. They were wrong!

The *experts* have now admitted that these things are NOT true and have given birth to a new theory. Their new theory says that glaucoma is caused by a deficiency of oxygen and blood flow. Finally, they are on the right trail. In the end, they will discover that glaucoma is the result of insufficient blood flow due to agglutination of the red blood cells (sticky blood) and waste buildup in the cells and **inter**cellular fluids.

Agglutinated blood corpuscles CANNOT squeeze through the extremely tiny capillaries of the posterior eye and therefore cannot deliver oxygen to the mitochondria. This is what the problem has been all along. If people continue to eat soy and canola oils, a lot more people are going to experience vision irregularities—like retinitis and macula degeneration.

Death of the mitochondria in the cells of the *posterior* eye is due to oxygen starvation, sodium toxicity, and waste accumulation. When they die, the cells die and the tissues of the posterior eye *atrophy.* Glaucoma has much in common with hair loss, Alzheimers, multiple sclerosis, cerebral palsy, and hearing problems.

There are several things a person can do to reverse these debilitating conditions. Biologically friendly water is basic to all rejuvenation, as is fresh, viable food. Detoxification of the tissues and body fluids is accomplished with Yucca extract, Kombucha tea, PAC's, and colon therapy.

Rape or Canola?

The name **Canola** is a "coined" word. It is not listed in anything but the most recent reference sources. It is a word that appeared out of *nowhere.*

The flip side of the canola coin reads: RAPE! You must admit that canola sounds better than "Rape." The name *canola* secreted the introduction of **rape oil** to America.

Canola oil comes from the rape seed, which is part of the Mustard family of plants. Rape is the **MOST** toxic of all food oil plants. Like soy, rape is a toxic weed. Insects will not eat rape. It is deadly poisonous. **The oil from the rape seed is a hundred times more toxic than soy oil!**

Canola oil is a *semi-drying* oil that is used as a lubricant, fuel, soap and synthetic rubber base, and as an illuminant for the slick color pages you see in magazines. Canola is an **industrial** oil. It does NOT belong in the body!

Canola oil has some very interesting characteristics *and* effects on living systems. For example, it forms latex-like substances that cause *agglutination* of the red blood corpuscles, as does soy only MUCH more pronounced. Loss of vision is a **known characteristic** side effect of rape oil. Rape oil *antagonizes* the central and peripheral nervous systems—like soy oil, only worse. Deterioration, however, takes years.

Rape (Canola) oil causes pulmonary emphysema, respiratory distress, anemia, constipation, irritability and blindness in the bodies of ANIMALS—and humans.

Rape oil was in widespread use in animal feeds in England and Europe between 1986 and 1991 when it was thrown out. Do you remember reading about the cows, pigs, and sheep that went **blind,** lost their minds, and attacked people? They had to be shot!

Not long after the first edition of this book appeared, a woman called me from Chicago to tell me that she was in England at the time the Mad Cow Disease was at its peak.

She told me that she personally witnessed a news report on television that told people not to panic if they had been using rape oil in their diet and were over 65 years of age. The "experts" added that the effects of rape oil ingestion takes **at least** ten years to manifest, and in all likelihood, most of these people would be dead by then anyway. Interesting!

In the reports I read, the "experts" *blamed* the erratic behavior on a viral dis-ease called *scrapie*. However, when rape oil was removed from animal feed, "scrapie" disappeared. Now we are growing rape seed and using rape (canola) oil in the USA.

Canola oil is now *our* problem. It is widely used in thousands of processed foods in the USA—with the blessings of government watchdog agencies, of course.

Officially, canola oil is known as "LEAR" oil. The acronym stands for *low erucic acid* **rape.** The *experts* in the industry love to tell the story of how canola was developed in Canada and that it is safe to use. They admit it was developed from the rape seed, but that through *genetic engineering* i.e. irradiation, it is no longer rape seed, but instead "canola!"

The experts love to talk about canola's "qualities"—like its unsaturated structure, omega 3's, 6's, and 12's, its wonderful digestibility, and its fatty acid makeup. They turn us against naturally saturated oils and fats, while they come to the rescue with Canola oil. They even tell us how Asia has warmly embraced Canola due to its distinctive flavor. *Isn't it wonderful how internationalist brokers "help" third world peoples? Doesn't their tune remind you of the introduction of microwave ovens?*

In the old west, there was an **earthy** expression that sums up the industry flim flam that accompanied the introduction and promotion of rape oil into the diets of unsuspecting people world wide. It was, ***"Horse Shit & Gun Smoke!"***

The term *canola* provided the perfect cover for commercial interests who wanted to make billions in the USA. The name "canola" is still very much in use, but it is no longer needed. I suggest you go to the grocery store and look at the peanut butter ingredient labels. The peanut oil has been removed and replaced with **rape** oil.

Chemical Warfare

Rape oil is used to produce the chemical warfare agent, "MUSTARD GAS." This is the chemical agent that was responsible for blistering the lungs and skin of hundreds of thousands of solders and civilians during WW I. Recent reports from the French indicate mustard gas was used during the Gulf War.

Between 1950 and 1953, white mustard seed (rape seed) was **irradiated** in Sweden to increase seed production and oil content. *Irradiation* is the process the *experts* want to use to make our food "safe" to eat. Genetically engineered fruits and vegetables—which will soon have innocent things like hepatitis-B spliced into their DNA—are another example of man's misuse of technology and abuse of public trust by powerful interests and "head in the sand" watchdog agencies.

Canola oil contains large amounts of **"iso-thio-cyan-ates"** which are **cyanide** containing compounds. Cyanide INHIBITS mitochondrial production of ATP. ATP is the chemical acronym for adenosine triphosphate, which is the energy molecule that fuels the mitochondria. ATP energy powers the body and keeps us healthy and *YOUNG!*

Canola Oil & Body Metabolism

Many substances can *bind* metabolic enzymes and block their activity in the body. In biochemistry, these substances are called *inhibitors*. We have spent a great deal of time talking about inhibitors, only we used terms like bio-junk food, toxic waste, negative energy, drugs, left-spin, etc.

Toxic substances in canola and soy oils encourage the formation of covalent bonds. Covalent bonds are normally *irreversible* and usually CANNOT be broken by the body once these molecules have synthesized (formed).

For example, consider the pesticide **malathion.** It binds to the active site of the enzyme *acetylcholinesterase* and stops this enzyme from doing what it is supposed to do, which is to divide acetylcholine into choline and acetate.

Malathion is the "harmless" pesticide spray used to kill the Med Fly and blanket every living thing in California a few years ago and again in February and March of 1994, and in Texas in April of 1995. Malathion is an **organophosphate**.

Nerve Function & Organophosphates

Acetycholine is critical to NERVE impulse transmission. When inhibited, nerve fibers do not function normally and the muscles do not respond.

For example, think of your garage door opener. If no signal is sent, the door does not open. In the case of the body, your hand or leg does not respond. Perhaps you have noticed the tremendous increase in disorders like systemic lupus, multiple sclerosis, cerebral palsy, myelinoma, pulmonary hypertension, and neuropathy in recent years. Soy and canola oils are players in the development of these dis-ease conditions. So are the **organophosphate** insecticides used in food production in the name of efficiency.

Acetylcholinesterase inhibitors cause paralysis of the striated (skeletal) muscles and spasms of the respiratory system.

That is why malathion is the pesticide of choice by the *experts*. It kills insects by causing **muscle paralysis**—just like *rotenone* from soy beans! It inhibits the insect's *enzymes*. It inhibits the enzymes of humans too!

Agents *orange* and *blue* that were used in Vietnam to defoliate jungle cover are organophosphorous compounds. The Vietnam Vets and the Vietnamese people know first-hand about them. Government *experts* who okayed their use and chemical companies that manufactured them have finally owned up to their toxic effects on PEOPLE and the environment. Nevertheless, present day experts in academia and government continue to "abba dabba" the public with stories of "safe" science and cheap food through the use of poisons.

Canola oil is rich in glycosides. Glycosides cause serious problems in the human body by blocking enzyme function and depriving us of our life force, Chi, Qi, Prana, call it what you like.

Glycosides interfere with the biochemistry of humans and animals. Consider the effect of a rattlesnake bite. It is the glycosides in the venom that **inhibit** muscle enzymes and cause instant immobilization in the target host.

Canola Oil • HIV & AIDS

Soy and canola oil glycosides depress the immune system. They cause the **white blood cell defense system**—the T-cells—to go into a stupor and fall asleep on the job. These oils alter the bio-electric "terrain" and promote dis-ease.

The alcohols and glycosides in canola and soy oils shut down our protective grid—the immune system. Fluoride, immunizations, antibiotics, and bio-junk food play a similar role in immune system collapse.

An *alcohol* is a chemistry term for the "reactive" chemical group on an organic molecule. "R" groups are what make organic compounds work—for good and bad! Canola alcohols and glycosides are very reactive. They are as toxic as fermented alcohols, but their effects manifest differently. **The damage takes years to show up.** *(You may wish to review our discussion of sweet proteins in the soy chapter.)*

When the medical experts check your blood for the presence of the HIV virus, they are looking at your white blood cell "count." If the numbers are normal, they will tell you that you do NOT have HIV. What they don't see is that the T-cells are in a toxic *stupor*. This *opportunistic* condition causes life forms in the blood and lymph to metamorphose and manifest as hepatitis, pneumonia, and **HIV,** and to *bypass* the body's immune system defenses (the T-cells) and get a foothold. As Claude Barnard said, *"The terrain is everything!"*

Once inside the cells, HIV⁺ takes over the RNA and DNA. They uses the mitochondria to produce energy for their own use. Quietly, they multiply (replicate) and one day—BANG!—you wake up and you are dying of AIDS.

Aids & Green Monkeys

In his earth shaking book, *AIDS The End of Civilization,* Dr. William Camball Douglass asked, "Do you really think some Green Monkey all of a sudden bit some guy in the ass and presto, AIDS all over the world?"

Dr. Douglass was examining the hype that the Centers for Disease Control in Atlanta has been *peddling* to the public about the AIDS virus—HIV. Douglass' book tells the "whole" story of the development of HIV at the Ft. Detrick, Maryland) military installation. His story is a well documented, and confirms the theme of the futuristic movie *Outbreak.*

Lorenzo's Oil

Another movie *Lorenzo's Oil,* offers another good example of how far off course medical science has strayed, and how muddled is the scientific mind. Early on in the movie, the *experts* said the problem with the dying child was not in the math i.e. pH. They were wrong.

Had the experts determined the pH of the saliva, urine and blood they would have *instantly* known what they were up against. That dying boy had a chronically low total body pH! So low that his body fluids were *dissolving* the myelin sheath that protects the nerve fibers. This was causing his nervous system to disintegrate. *Does this description smack of the dozens of degenerative nerve related disorders plaguing people today?*

The boy was given Lorenzo's oil to boost energy output and act as a detoxifier of metabolic poisons. The oil *shocked* his body into a LESS acid condition. Lorenzo's oil is OLIVE oil! When given in large quantities, olive oil SHOCKS the body and causes it to adjust its pH. It will also SAFELY purge the body of gall and liver stones, thus avoiding the need for gallbladder surgery (Yucca extract and PAC's must precede the "flush."

Shortly after Lorenzo's Oil was released, my brother witnessed a TV talk show where an "expert" claimed that Lorenzo's oil was rape oil. This was a lie. Give rape oil to a sick person and you will seal their doom. Here is another good example of "disinformation" in the public domain. These false-hoods should cause every thinking person to question the molding of public opinion by powerful commercial interests behind the scenes.

Blood & Oils

By now it should obvious to the reader that congested blood and lymph flow negatively affects every part of the body. It should be equally obvious that there is a direct link between dis-ease, diet, and the water we drink. Moreover, the astronomical increase in the use of processed foods that contain canola oil, soy oil, and chemical additives CONFUSES the body and weakens the immune system. **It should come as no surprise that anyone wanting to enjoy peak health and longevity MUST take control of their life, and personal responsibility for their health. There is NO other way!**

The "health care" industry is an oxymoron. It protects its own health and economic interests. Learn to protect YOUR health and economic interests by learning HOW to take care of yourself, and acting upon that knowledge.

Note: *ABC news just finished airing the results of a damning medical study that confirmed that soy and canola oils are definitely linked to prostate cancer in men. The report aired on February 15, 1994.* Now the *experts* are promoting soy oil breast implants for **unsuspecting** women. Amazing!

PREVIEW: *Our next chapter looks at the connection between onions, your liver, and aging.*

"Everything In Excess Is Opposed By Nature."
Hippocrates

Vibrations! And Other Books Worth Reading

Learn how to use a vibration chain to determine energy spin, locate lost objects, dowse for water, siphon away pain from an injury or inflamed joint, make critical decisions, confirm your instincts, and a lot more. *Vibrations* is the life work of an 87 year Wizard named Owen Lehto, and the perfect member of a trilogy that also includes the *Pendulum Kit* and *Map Dowsing* (see Source Index). *Vibrations* is more than a book. It's an experience!

P.S. If you like history, you'll fall in love with the big 8 1/2 x 11, 372 page, profusely illustrated masterpeice on the 500 year history of dowsing called *The Divining Hand.*

Comfrey Greens

In the good old days, before the FDA decided to save us from the evils of comfrey, it could be found in stores.

Today, if you want comfrey, you have to grow it yourself or have someone grow it for you. And if you are smart, that is exactly what you will do.

To find comfrey starts, ask gardeners, call gardening clubs, or run an advertisement in the local throw away classified paper in your area.

Obtain about six pieces of the root with a little top growth coming out so that you know you have a crown. Next, loosen the soil and plant each crown about 1 inch deep and cover and water.

Come spring, you will see luxurious plants spring out of the ground and grow up to 5 feet high and 4 feet wide. Allow plenty of space. Pick greens from early spring to late fall. Nothing bothers comfrey. The roots grow to forty feet.

Eaten raw, the leaves are prickly to the tongue. Mixed in salads, or on sandwiches, they're fine. Eaten like spinach, the leaves are at their very best!

Steam or stir fry the leaves until they wilt. Add a little olive oil and apple cider vinegar and you've got a highly nutritious food that beats the best spinach you ever tasted.

The FDA says comfrey is dangerous. If that's true, my family and I should all be dead! We eat comfrey several times a week and love it.

Plant comfrey once, and you'll have "free" food forever. Pulverized comfrey root and aloe cures ulcers! Maybe that is why the "experts" don't like it?

What Is A Precursor

A precursor is a chemical substance that precedes the formation of something else. A food precursor is something the body can convert into something it needs.

Think of carrots. They are loaded with beta carotene. When you eat a carrot you are not eating vitamin A, but beta carotene which your body converts into vitamin A. So beta carotene is actually a precursor.

A *provitamin* is the same as a precursor.

Pesticide Free?

I recently saw a *huge* canola oil display in a store. The sign said, "Pesticide Free." What they didn't mention was the left-spin *footprint* of this toxic industrial oil!

27

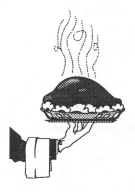

Liver & Onions

"As goes the liver, so goes the body!"
Anon.

The liver is "the" most abused organ of the body. It is the body's *primary* waste removal organ. A healthy liver is essential to good health and central to the aging reversal process.

The liver is a phenomenal chemical factory. It is responsible for tens of thousands of biochemical reactions. It is the second largest organ in the body and the ONLY organ that will *regenerate* itself on-its-own-volition, that is, if it is given the opportunity. The liver's regenerative ability is an indication of its importance. The **hepatocytes**—the liver's functional cells—are called *parenchyma* cells.

The liver metabolizes food, drugs, pesticides, wastes, and alcohol that arrive via its **dual** blood supply. These substances impose severe physiologic stress on the liver, and in turn, on all the other organs and glands of the body.

When the liver becomes "toxic," the hepatocytes die. The spaces they leave behind are filled by connective tissue (also called scar tissue). Scar tissue is comprised of *the stroma* cells that normally cover the outside of the liver only. As the hepatocytes die, stroma cells invade the liver, form scar tissue, and it becomes "hard" and tough. Cirrhosis of the liver is a condition of EXCESS that manifests as a nutritional deficiency. Cirrhosis involves yellowing and hardening of the liver.

The liver is heavily vascularized with blood vessels. It receives a DOUBLE supply of blood. *Oxygenated* blood from the heart is supplied via the hepatic artery, and nutrient laden *deoxygenated* blood comes from the intestines via the hepatic portal vein. *(Portal hypertension would involve the latter.)*

The Kupper's cells that line the blood vessels of the liver are of *immense* importance to health and vitality. Kupper's cells are both **hepatocytes** and **phagocytes** *(phag*-to eat. *cyte*-cell.) Phagocytes remove microbes, foreign matter, and worn out red and white blood cells from circulation.

The liver removes toxic waste from the blood and either disposes of it via the bile, or buries it in body fat. In other words, the body uses FAT to *isolate* toxic wastes and buffer their effects on the vital organs.

The liver consumes large amounts of energy in the performance of its job. If the body is under stress—mental stress (negative thinking; worrying, anger, fear, etc.), or physical stress (poisons like chloramines in the water people are bathing in and drinking)—energy supplies fizzles out and waste buildup on a systemic level.

Waste buildup in the blood, lymph, joints, and soft tissues of the body ALWAYS involves a sick liver!

Hepatitis *(hepat*-liver; *itis*-inflamation of) is a liver condition. So is mononucleosis, Epstein-Barr and Chronic Fatigue Syndrome. All of them mirror conditions of EXCESS waste overload in the system and hormonal imbalance. Practitioners blame nature's garbage crew—the viruses—for the damage inflicted on the liver, but they are wrong.

Thanks to Dr. Guenther Enderlein, we know the exact sequence of microbial metamorphosis that occurs along the trail of degenerative dis-ease. We also know what to do about it as described in *Hidden Killers* (see Source Index).

Officially, hepatitis manifests in several forms: type A, B, C, D, and E. All of them are currently prevalent in the USA. These are easily treated. Rene' tea is being used intravenously in mainland China for viral conditions with great success, and for distemper (blood virus conditions) in dogs and cats by US veterinarians. PAC's and Yucca extract are also very useful.

Detoxification, sanitation, exercise, water, and rest all play an important part when dealing with viral liver conditions.

"Choleric Personalities"

As people age, their personalities change. One personality type—the choleric—reflects the condition of a person's liver. The *choleric*, has a "bitter" personality that is vile and difficult. The word *choleric* comes from *chole* which means "bile." *Chole* refers to the liver's digestive juice and waste product, bile. A "bilious" person has a foul personality. Alcoholics and some older folks are notorious for being "bilious." (The Greeks believed there were four basic personality types: choleric, melancholy, sanguine and phlegmatic.)

Much of Western medicine's disastrous history was the result of the theories of the Greek physician and medical writer Claudius Galen (circa A.D. 130-200). He was the personal physician to the Roman Emperor, Marcus Aurelius.

Galen believed in the four basic personality types. He called them "humors." A humor is a body fluid that was believed to influence personality. Galen's theories were, for the most part, in total error. His personality types, however, are still in vogue, but under new names like type-A personality, type-B personality, etc. *Humoral immunity involves circulating antibodies and antigens the blood and lymphatic fluids.*

HCL • Bile & Aging

Aging of the vital organs has disastrous EFFECTS on our ability to process food. The stomach fails to produce hydrochloric acid (HCL) in sufficient quantities to digest proteins (indigestion is *wrongfully* referred to a acid indigestion).

The stomach should be an ACID environment. This is due to the HCL that is secreted from the wall of the stomach to break the peptide bonds holding amino acids together. The stomach MUST be very acid to properly digest proteins. *Deterioration of the stomach wall is not the result of stomach acid, but of excesses in the system that bring about stomach atrophy.*

HCL has a pH as low as .8. It is so acidic that a drop of it on the skin will eat a hole in it. The mucous membranes protect the stomach walls from this powerful acid. Peptic ulcers occur in the stomach wall. Duodenal ulcers occur in the small intestine wall. Physical deterioration and stress underwrite these ugly conditions. Comfrey root will heal them.

When the liver loses it ability to discharge all of its bile, people will suffer indigestion, especially in the evening or after a greasy meal. Indigestion is a symptom of liver and gall bladder problems involving stones that either block channels in the liver or the bile duct leading from the gallbladder at the base of the liver into the small intestine (approximately three inches *below* the outlet from the stomach.

Liver and gall stones are VERY common. A liver flush can painlessly eliminate liver and gall stones and restore liver and gall bladder function. My 79 year old friend, Pearl, flushed 152 stones from her liver (see Source Index).

Partially digested food (called chyme) exits the stomach

and enters the first of three sections of the small intestine called the duodenum. Here, the chyme is mixed with secretions from the pancreas and bile from the liver. These substances are **alkaline.** They raise the pH of the chyme to break the bonds holding carbohydrates and sugars together. Bile MUST be present for metabolism of fat.

(When we drink liquids with our meals, we dilute our stomach acids and digestive enzymes. This forces the digestive glands to overwork and draw on body reserves. When the body has NO alternative but to process partially digested food, a negative energy condition develops and dis-ease ensues.

The healthy liver produces about **1 quart** of bile a day. Bile is a yellowish-brown or sometimes olive-green juice with an alkaline pH between 7.6 and 8.6. Bile is "the" waste product of the liver. It contains mineral ions, **chole**sterol, and bilirubin from worn-out red blood corpuscles. Bilirubin gives bile its yellow, brown, green color. If we dissect the word **chole**sterol we get *chole*-bile. *ster*-a fat and *ol*-alcohol.

Micelles

Bile emulsifies and breaks up large fat globules into pin head droplets called *micelles.* Micelles have more surface area so the pancreatic enzymes can attack and break down the fats. **Bile is to digestion as detergent is to greasy dishwater.**

Without bile to emulsify dietary oils and fats, they cannot be absorbed. Partial digestion robs the body of needed nutrients. We derive up to 40% of our energy from the burning (oxidation) of fat. The formation of micelles is central to the absorption of the fat soluble vitamins: A,D,E, and K. Poor fat metabolism results in EXCESSES that bring on what "appear" to be deficiencies.

Bile contains heme (organic iron). Loss of heme, which is *said to be* the oxygen carrying component of hemoglobin, results in the loss of energy and vitality. This is particularly true for women suffering blood loss during and after menstruation. *Iron Deficiency Anemia* is, however, NOT the result of a lack of dietary iron, but of loss of function in the vital organs due to systemic toxicity and hormonal imbalances (excesses). Iron deficiency anemia is a serious condition that must NOT be ignored. Intake of elemental iron supplements creates serious metabolic problems and should be avoided.

Most heme iron is reabsorbed in the gut. It is FAR more biologically active than dietary iron. If there is a shortage of heme iron in the body, there will be a corresponding shortfall in mitochondrial oxidation of glucose and low energy production. A shortage of *heme* iron means diminished oxygen carrying capacity in the blood that supplies the mitochondria in the cells and liver. Elevated blood sugar levels (diabetes) is a common side effect.

Most dietary iron supplements are disastrous to the body. Iron is an oxidizer and participates in the formation of free radicals. Klamath algae is a perfect solution for iron deficient people because it provides needed raw materials in a form the body can use. Algae helps chelate and detoxify the system. Fresh, organic, green leafy vegetables are the very best sources of blood building foods.

The gallbladder stores bile secreted from the liver. Digestion releases bile into the small intestines, *providing*, **1-**bile flow into the gallbladder is not *slowed* by stones blocking the channels draining the liver, **2-**the duct leading from the gallbladder into the small intestine is not restricted.

If the liver is toxic and cannot remove bilirubin from the blood, the waste will back up into the entire body.

Jaundice is the result of excess bile and bilirubin in the blood. It produces a yellow coloration in the whites of the eyes. People with hepatitis, cirrhosis, and mononucleosis often reflect a jaundiced appearance. Jaundice is a SIGN of serious liver malfunction. Blood tests that show elevated bilirubin counts should NOT be ignored. Detoxification followed by a liver FLUSH can revolutionize one's health.

Children also suffer from liver malfunctions. Acne, boils, jaundice, constipation, appendicitis, psoriasis, and sores in the corners of the mouth are symptomatic of liver problems and systemic toxicity. "Treat" them like adults.

Lecithin is the fat emulsifier in bile that keeps cholesterol in solution. As the body ages and pH shifts, the cholesterol, salts, halogens, and minerals in the bile settle out and form gallstones. Gallstones **originate** in the liver and **grow** to giant proportions in the gallbladder.

If gallstones BLOCK the bile duct connecting the liver and the small intestine, gangrene will set in a matter of hours. Gangrenous tissue is dead tissue that has rotted in the absence of oxygen. A gangrenous gallbladder must be removed or the person will die from systemic poisoning (toxemia). **Loss of the gallbladder WILL result in diabetes within 20 years unless the person takes the action necessary to prevent it.**

Modern medical has made quick work out of gallbladder removal. However, people need to understand the CAUSES behind gallstone formation and NOT rely on "magic bullet" technology to save them from death's pall. Gallstones account for some **8,000** deaths and over one BILLION dollars in medical costs in the USA every year. **Gall & liver stones confirm that old age has arrived—no matter your age!**

Loss of the gallbladder equates to accelerated aging and life at the subsistence level. While we can live without a gallbladder, health and vitality are sacrificed unless the person takes remedial action and does something about it.

Do everything possible to avoid losing your gallbladder. Once removed, the liver continually drips directly into the intestine—one drip at a time, instead of in mass at meal time, creating an effect similar to constant snacking.

Liver Hygiene

People with cancer should temporarily abstain from eating meat, cheese, and fish. These are **heavy** proteins that stress the system. Klamath algae, predigested liver tablets, and harmonic pollen are wonderful, low stress foods.

Dr. Max Gerson used fresh, organic calf liver "juice" to treat cancer patients. It is LOADED with biologically active nutrients and enzymes. In the USA, fresh liver is no longer an option due to the condition of the animals. A safer alternative is freeze dried, **predigested,** organic calf liver tablets from Argentina. I can attest that they are the equivalent of swallowing a lightning bolt. I highly recommend them!

Fresh, raw, organic fruits and vegetables are also very therapeutic to the liver. "Raw" milk products like yogurt, buttermilk, and kefir are very healing. Apple cider vinegar, Kombucha tea, and fresh lemon juice are also wonderful foods.

Anatomical Location Of The Liver

The liver is located directly under the anterior right rib cage (see page 46). It is in close proximity to the intestines, right lung, heart. It is opposite the spleen which is under the left anterior rib cage which the spleen is easily punctured.

It is VERY important to prevent toxins and parasites (like the intestinal fluke) from reaching the liver via the portal vein or by migration up the primary bile duct. The portal vein carries nutrient laden blood from the intestines to the liver. It is COMMON to find colon bacilli (bacteria) in an inflamed liver—as in cases of cirrhosis. Constipation and waste build up in the colon spell big trouble. Colon therapy is one answer to this problem. Yucca extract is another. Pac's are another.

Distended Belly

A distended abdomen is a classic SIGN of a person with a liver problem and a body under siege. An enlarged belly is partly body fat and mostly an engorged and distended colon.

This is a tell-tale SIGN that waste is accumulating. This condition goes hand in hand with colitis, diverticulitis, gout, arthritis, and heart problems, just to name a few. A congested bowel is a breeding ground for dis-ease and a fast ticket to the grave. Consider a distended belly an interim report card and a warning of trouble to come!

Hopefully, the reader now understands why chewing your food, drinking plenty of good water, exercise, and avoiding snacks and bio-junk food are so crucial to aging.

Liver Breath

Certain foods—like raw onion—cause some people to get *liver breath.* Raw onion is a potent detoxifier that produces a "metallic" odor in the breath of some people.

I once overheard my biochemistry teacher's assistant discussing her health problems with another. When she came over to help me, I got a whiff of her breath and I recognized the odor instantly. The lady had a stressed liver.

People with stressed livers get hepatitis, mononucleosis, Epstein-Barr, and chronic fatigue syndrome. They are the ones who suffer with psoriasis, heavy dandruff, ringworm, impetigo, athlete's foot, dry skin, weak nails, periodontal gum dis-ease, constipation, diverticulosis, colitis, irritable bowel syndrome, parasite infestations, Alzheimers, cancer and more.

Fully 90% of the population have stressed livers. This is why I have hammered away at YOU, the reader, to do whatever you need to do to detoxify your system, strengthen liver and vital organ function, and balance hormonal activity.

There are different paths a person can take to reach these goals. Colon therapy, massage, herbs, hormone precursors, Kombucha tea, algae, and BEV water are just a few. Fresh, raw lemon juice, beets, walking barefooted in sand and green grass, coffee enemas, bouncing on a rebounder followed by self-massage of the lymphatic system are some more things that work.

Whether your liver was weak at birth or from environmental and dietary stress, it is what it is. If you want to enjoy good health and avoid premature old age, you MUST assist the liver or rejuvenation will not become a reality for you. Colon therapy, plus yucca extract, PAC's, and fasting can do wonders for liver rejuvenation.

Mineral Baths & The Liver

Throughout history, mineral springs, hot pools, and mud holes have attracted health-minded people. As a child, I can remember going with my family out to Desert Hot Springs, where we would see people soaking in mineral water pools and taking mud baths to improve their health.

I can attest to the detoxifying effects of racemic clays and mineral waters. Most people are invigorated by them. They exhaust me! People with weak livers must be careful when using hot pools because they cause the body to release too much toxic waste into circulation and if you are not prepared for it, you will become exhausted. Loss of mineral ions also plays a part. Drink large quantities of BEV water with plenty of ionic sea mineral ions to replenish those lost in the hot pools.

At home, a hot bath can be a wonderful tonic for the liver and skin, especially if a cup of Epsom salt, a tablespoon of fresh pulverized ginger, and a pint of 3% hydrogen peroxide are added to the water. These help the skin release toxic waste, rather than overloading the liver. **A coffee colonic, followed by a hot bath is a smarter approach.**

It is better to detox slowly than to try and reverse twenty, thirty, or forty years of bad living in a few weeks. Detoxification isn't always pleasant, but it works. A healthy liver leads the way to becoming *Young Again!*

PREVIEW: *Our next chapter deals with energy flow, limitless vitality, and the body's "toll" road system.*

It's important to hang and s-t-r-e-t-c-h every day.

Moo Cow Video & Cookbook

Don't Have A Cow! is the title of a delightful vegetarian video AND cookbook combination by Cheri Evans, of Ontario, Canada.

The focus is vegetarian, but the package is 100% Moo Cow! The cover, the video, even the ribbon used to tie the siblings together has the characteristic black and white Moo Cow design!

The two hour video provides hundreds of tips and answers questions often asked by wana'be vegetarian cooks who are interested in learning how to shop, select, and prepare tasty, appealing vegetarian dishes. Even long time vegetarian cooks enjoy Cheri's information and style.

The set is very popular for birthdays and holidays. *Moooooo, to you too!* (See Source Index.)

The Miracle Of Coral Calcium!

Biogenic coral calcium comes from a unique species of coral off the coast of Tocunoshima, Japan. It is unlike other corals in the ocean because it has the ability to treat conditions like cancer, arthritis, fibromyalgia, myasthenia gravis, diabetes, allergies, obesity, and angina—just to name a few.

While unknown in the USA, people in Europe and Asia are using this unique coral to heal their bodies. The coral is mined, processed, and put into small packets. Each packet treats one quart of water. A packet is placed in a quart of water and left to 'brew' overnight. Any water can be used.

Biogenic coral stimulates the formation of new tissues and enhances the activity of the organs and glands. Coral treated water reduces acidity in the body, similar to the way a **far infrared sauna** works. They do it by **neutralizing** acid energy fields and raising the vibrational frequency of the water at the *subtle energy level.*

Tap and common filtered or distilled drinking waters have a low vibrational frequency and weak energy footprint. Their signatures are incomplete and therefore, at odds with health. Biogenic coral corrects this problem through the *transference* of its Earth energies held in the coral to the water molecules.

Transference is a homeopathic concept and term. Here, it means that the vibrational frequency of the coral is used to *cancel* and *enliven* water molecules so they will vibrate at a new, healthy frequency that promotes healing and health.

The people of Tocunoshima are some of the longest lived people on the planet today. Somewhere in the past they discovered that their unique coral had unique life enhancing qualities. Their discovery parallels the American Indians discovery and use of racemic clays in their medicine wheel.

While biogenic coral calcium has mineral value, it is not the physical mineral itself that does the healing. Rather, it is the coral's energy *footprint* that gives it its unique healing reputation. The proof of this is that healing proceeds without the ingestion of the coral granules themselves. Simply allowing them to 'brew' is enough to get results.

Biogenic coral calcium is a gift from Nature, fresh out of Earth's pantry of healthy goodies (see Source Index).

Women • Osteoporosis • Hormones

Women take **synthetic** hormones—like Estradiol, Provera, Premarin—because they've been told they will otherwise develop osteoporosis. Yet, in taking them, they run the risk of endometrial and breast cancer.

Synthetic hormones are "high risk" and should be avoided. Instead, women should use natural DHEA, progesterone, and testosterone *precursors*. Precursors help women (and men) balance their hormones WITHOUT risk of cancer or osteoporosis.

Natural precursors are safe and effective. Endometrial hyperplasia (*hyper*-increased activity. *plas*-abnormal growth. *ia*-pertaining to.) is the result of **unopposed** estrogen *dominance*. In other words, EXCESS estrogens brings on female cancers (and PMS too!).

These precursors are naturally occurring substances that the body can "create" the hormones it needs and wants. Their effectiveness is dependent upon **bioavailability**, which is dependent upon the *delivery system* used to transport the active ingredients into the tissues. In other words, a precursor must be *absorbed* before it can be used.

Hundreds of women (and men) enjoy a better life—and sex life—because they use natural hormone precursors. **Precursors are NOT drugs.** Drugs FORCE the body into submission by overpowering the system. Hormone precursors allow the *body* to determine *what* hormone it will make, *how much* is needed, and *where* and *when* the hormone will be used.

Female cancer and osteoporosis are real. Millions of women are "at risk." Millions more suffer from PMS and other menopause related problems. These conditions can be safely managed with the right combination of hormone precursors and detoxification therapy.

**If you would like to "really" understand
your body's hormone cycle, call the
publisher of this book and ask
for the *Hormone Report*.**

Look at all the sick and dying people!

28

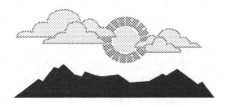

Soil To Sea

"Man does not die, he kills himself"
Seneca

People love the seaside! The air makes them feel good. It buzzes with electricity. The **ionized** water invigorates their bodies. Barefooted, the sand siphons away the toxic energy fields from their bodies. It is the *charged* ionic minerals that give the sea's air, water, and sand its healing qualities.

The sea is nature's storage battery of right-spin EN-ERGY! It is a phenomenon of tremendous importance. Understanding the source of the sea's energy is central to the aging reversal process.

Mineral ions in solution are called electrolytes. Ions are atoms that have gained or lost electrons. Ionic compounds are two or more ions that have bonded together. Ionic compounds are crystals—like table salt (sodium chloride). Salts are STABLE and maintain their crystal form UNTIL they are *hydrolyzed* (dissolved) in water.

When salts hydrolyse, their molecules disassociate (split) into two or more *unstable* mineral ions. If the ions are derived from a concentrated source—like table salt or calcium carbonate—they create conditions of **excess** and raise electrical havoc in the body. Only some of the ions that compose mineral compounds are capable of conducting electricity is solution. **We are concerned about ion conductivity, but we are MORE concerned about their footprint and signature.**

The blood and lymph contain electrolytes. Our nerve fibers and cells are lined with them. Electrolytes relay electrical energy and are responsible for transferring electrical signals from one end of the body to the other via the nerve fibers, blood and lymph.

Toll Road

It is helpful to think of the nervous system as a toll road where a price must be paid BEFORE each nerve "energy" signal is allowed to pass to its destination—perhaps a finger or leg.

The body conducts its daily business affairs by *transmission* of electrical impulses (signals) along the nerve fiber highway, and through **hormone** messengers.

The nervous system operates on a unit of electrical *currency* called mineral *ions*. As nerve impulses pass from point to point along the highway, the electrical charge on the surface of the mineral ions is used. Mineral ions "give up" their energy as the electrical signal passes.

The body constantly replenishes used ions with charged (energized) ones, if it has a supply. A body with enough ions in "balanced" form, enjoys health and vitality. Otherwise, sickness and degenerative dis-ease rule a person's life.

Disrupted electrical signals produce spastic motions that make it difficult for a person to move and function. Cerebral palsy and multiple sclerosis are classic examples of *uncontrolled* electrical energy flow, as are shingles, neuropathy, and myelinoma. These degenerative conditions are the equivalent of ionic mineral "bankruptcy," with additional complications from hormonal imbalances and conditions of excess.

Athletes

Electrolytes are VERY important to athletes. They associate performance, strength, and vitality with electrolytes (ionic minerals). They know that their body will NOT perform without them, and will excel when they are present.

Athletes USE large quantities of electrolytes because their bodies are under heavy *physical* stress. Non-athletes also use electrolytes. However, unlike athletes—who burn out in a few short years—non-athletes take years to bankrupt their ion account. They do it in *slow motion*—a day at a time!

All electrolytes (ions) are NOT equal. Those that have gone through the carbon cycle and are in **ionized** liquid form are superior because they have not *synchronized.* The two best sources of *ionized* electrolytes are sea water and organic food. Ancient sea bed deposits dug out of the ground and hydrolyzed contain lots of ions, but they have an inferior energy signature and electrical footprint. They have reverted to salt form and their effect pales in comparison.

Sea water ions keep us young and strong because they are naturally biologically *active* in their liquid state. Earth mineral deposits must be activated to be of any use. I prefer nature's way, which is as little processing as possible.

Consider the difference between common table salt and granular trace mineral salt called Keltic salt. Both are granular salts, but Keltic salt contains trace minerals. If you insist on using granular salt, Keltic salt is a wiser choice than common sea salt which is 98% sodium. Keltic salt contains 35% sodium, the balance being trace minerals and clays. Liquid sea minerals are 99.5% trace minerals and only 1/2% sodium. Keltic's 35% sodium level is still too high!

Table salt is a compound composed of two elements: sodium and chlorine. Sodium is an electrolyte and it assists the body in the flow of electrical energy. We **need** sodium in VERY **small** amounts. Too much sodium upsets the sodium:potassium ratio in the body and sets the stage for cancer and accelerated aging.

When the body is given NO other option, it will use sodium ions in lieu of more desirable electrolytic minerals.

Sports Drinks • BEV • Energy

Most athletes use commercial sports drinks to meet their ionic mineral needs. Sports drinks are not balanced. Their energy footprint is unfriendly, their signature incomplete. Athletes who depend on them experience rapid aging of the vital organs and connective tissues. Smart athletes make their own sports drink for pennies using concentrated sea water ions and BEV water. They also experience more energy and less injuries.

My own children **voluntarily** lug their ionized BEV water to school each day in their polycarbonate bottles because they love it and do better in the classroom and in sports. They call it *"power water!"* All their buddies bum water from them!

BEV water is a solution of highly charged water molecules. The energy does not come from mineral ions because it has none. Its high energy *footprint* comes from the **restructuring** of the water molecules. The BEV process enhances hydrogen and molecular bond angles and changes the *vibratory* frequency of the water—making it biologically friendly. BEV water resonates (vibrates) at a "healthy" frequency. Add ionic sea minerals and you've got the ultimate drinking water.

Ionic transfer of energy can be demonstrated in other ways. For instance, walking barefooted in sand or grass alters abnormal body rhythms and causes the body to vibrate with Mother Earth. Five minutes once or twice a day spent walking in this manner releases MASSIVE amounts of toxic, high stress energy from the bio-electric body. Minerals ions are very much involved in this phenomenon. I have seen people with severe back pain, unable to stand up straight, walk in beach sand for 15 minutes and return to normal! A vibration chain works in a similar fashion.

Electrical "currant" is created by the movement of *electrons through a metal wire.* **In body fluids like blood and lymph, current is carried by active mineral ions.**

Micro "Ionized" Water

Ions in solution allows electricity to pass. No electrical flow means no ions are present. Electricity flowing through a liquid is creates electrolysis (*electro*-electricity, *lysis-dissolution of.).* **Micro Water** (review on page 220) is a special type of *ionized* water with many therapeutic uses. It should be made from BEV water, NEVER from tap or partially purified water.

$10,000 For A Bag Of Salt

Dr. Carry Reams was once paid $10,000 for solving an electroplating problem that involved ions and electrolysis. No one—including the manufacturer of the equipment—could make the electricity flow in the chrome tank. Reams came along and poured a few pounds of common table salt into the solution and bingo, the electricity flowed through the water and the chrome plating process proceeded. Sodium chloride solved the electrolysis problem because sodium is an electrolyte.

The human body requires a **constant** supply of "balanced" mineral ions for optimum health. Substitution of table salt creates conditions of EXCESS which accelerate aging.

Sugar

Sucrose (table sugar) is a crystal, but sucrose will NOT conduct electricity. It is a non-conductor (a non-electrolyte) and contains no ions. Sugar is a "concentrated" left-spin energy substance. When we load our body down with sugar our vibratory frequency slows and our aura dims.

Sucrose BLOCKS the flow of energy in the body. It does this by **bonding** with our mineral ions. When ions bond with sugar, their energy is **neutralized.** If the ion supply is low or non-existent, a health crisis of major proportions occurs.

Most people live out their lives on the edge of starvation—their diet supplying them with just enough mineral ions to exist between subsistence and dis-ease.

If you choose to eat food laced with table sugar, you will lose your vitality and grow old.
Earlier, we discussed Kombucha tea. It is important that the reader understand that the Kombucha mushroom has the ability to convert a left-spin substance—like white sugar—into a right-spin energy field that is loaded with enzymes, hormones, and healthful organic acids. It does this by way of "biological alchemy." Kombucha is a "live" food every bit as much as fresh garden produce.

The experts tell us sugar is sugar. *They* tell us there is NO difference between sucrose, maltose, dextrose, and lactose except in their molecular structure. *They* tell us that mannitol, sorbitol, and xylitol, are harmless. *They* tell us the body does not care what sugar we feed it. *They* tell us the sugar *blues* that haunt millions of people are "imagined." The experts are wrong.

The body differentiates between sugars as it does with oils. It differentiates based on the energy SPIN.

Some sugars accelerate aging by neutralizing the body's supply of mineral ions. White and artificial sugars destroy food through "ionization" or scrambling of food molecules. Translated, this means that food molecules are altered through the gain or loss of electrons. Purified sugars (table sugar, fructose, corn syrup) and artificial sugars—like **aspartame** (better known by the red and blue "swirl" on packages of processed foods) and food additives have *radiomimetic* qualities that mimic the effects of nuclear radiation. They "zap" your energy and are no different than eating microwaved food. It brings on accelerates graying and diminished glandular activity.

Foods processed with large amounts of sugar and salt do not spoil because their enzymes have been scrambled. Bugs seldom eat sugar and salt laden food. They are not stupid.

Major & Minor Minerals

The body needs BOTH the major minerals and the minor (trace) minerals to function. Science has known about the major minerals like calcium, iron, sulphur, and phosphorous for a very long time. The "TRACE" minerals, like manganese, boron, iodine, molybdenum and eighty or so others have only recently been recognized to be of any importance in human nutrition. *(Science is reluctant to acknowledge man's mineral dependence, yet they **rubber stamp** the use of soy and rape oils, aspartame, and genetically altered foods.)*

We KNOW minerals are crucial to good nutrition and aging. What is NOT widely known is that the "form" the mineral is in is as important as the mineral itself. Form determines the mineral's effect on health.

Dietary ionic minerals are best obtained from live food. When pill supplements are used, be sure they are "complexed" with enzymes, herbs, vitamins (must be derived from a food source), and that all earth minerals are present in ionic form.

Elemental mineral compounds are of little use to the body. A commonly consumed elemental compound used to supplement **misdiagnosed** calcium deficiencies (as in osteoporosis) is calcium carbonate or oyster shell. It is composed of calcium and carbon. The -**ate** tells us that it is in a *salt* form—a *crystal*.

Elemental salt compounds do not belong in the body. They foul our nest and create health problems.

Consider the absurdity of taking calcium carbonate to get more calcium. It is the equivalent of a postpartum woman drinking milk so she can produce more milk.

Chelated minerals cause problems in the body. Chelated minerals are elemental mineral compounds bonded to a carrier—usually an amino acid. The carrier shuttles the minerals past acids and enzymes in the GI tract and into the blood. This is NOT desirable! These mineral compounds are unbalanced energy fields that have NOT gone through the carbon chain. They create stress on the system and require the body to buffer their negative effects. They "trade" one problem for another. Do NOT use them.

The chelation process *tricks* the body into admitting substances into the blood that otherwise could NOT gain admittance under normal body protocol. These elemental substances are the equivalent of a *bogus* $5^{00} bill!

Biologically active mineral ions come from healthy plants, animals, and ionized sea water. Foods like Klamath algae, Harmonic pollen, Dowist herb foods, and predigested organic liver are also good sources.

Enzymes • Minerals • Nitrogen

Enzymes are mineral-dependent. They are protein molecules that function as **on-the-job** engineers within the body. Enzymes NEED mineral ions to do their job. Enzymes create *hot spots* within the body that throw the switch so the blood and lymph can deliver mineral ions and other nutrient molecules to the areas in need. Enzymes are living energy fields.

Nitrogen plays a KEY role in the life process. All proteins and amino acids contain nitrogen. Nitrogen is NOT a mineral ion in the classical sense (its a gas), but it can function like one.

Nitrogen (atomic symbol "N"), is very important to electrical conductivity and energy *transfer* in the body. Nitrogen has many forms. In its *metallic* form, it conducts electricity and "acts like" an *electrolyte*.

Life cannot come into existence without nitrogen. The atmosphere is composed of 78% nitrogen. Plants and animals require nitrogen to grow. Unfortunately, the *experts* use nitrogen to FORCE plants to grow on the premise that food is food. They *think* they can bribe Nature into building high vitality food with nitrogen based salt fertilizers. Nature responds with negative energy food that is high in "funny" proteins.

Funny Proteins

Funny proteins are "unavailable" proteins—that is, proteins that the body cannot use. Food protein is measured by its nitrogen content. When you hear a nutritionist or farmer talk about a crop or foods protein percentage (%), they are actually referring to the nitrogen content.

Nitrogen is a gas. It is an extremely **acid** gas (pH 1-2). When proteins are digested and broken down into their constituent parts, nitrogen is released (think of a compost heap, a pile of fresh grass clippings, a rotting carcass).

Nitrogen has many different forms. Funny proteins have an EXCESS of nitrogen in the **wrong** form. When funny proteins are turned loose in the body they creates EXCESSES. Massive amounts of calcium is required to buffer the effects of funny protein nitrogens that are released into circulation during the normal digestion process.

Environmental deterioration and high powered, synthetic salt fertilizers and poisonous sprays are part of the reason why more and more funny proteins are entering the food chain. As these proteins rise, so does degenerative dis-ease.

Look at a bag of dog or cat food. It will list total protein and crude (unavailable) protein. If you subtract one from the other, you can calculate the amount of available protein. There was a time not so many years ago when the amount of unavailable or "bastard" protein was under 1/2%. Today we are seeing unavailable protein levels as high as 2%—and more!

Each time the level of *funny* proteins doubles-say from 1/2% to 1%—the amount of buffer needed to stabilize the blood increases by 200 times! Think about it!

I have repeatedly stated that there is no such thing as a deficiency condition or a deficiency disease. Problems and deficiencies are the result of conditions of EXCESS within the system. In the case of osteoporosis, the problem results from "excess" funny proteins in the blood, hormonal imbalances as a result of "excesses" (estrogen imbalance in relation to progesterone and testosterone levels), and buildup of "excess" metabolic waste.

As levels of *funny* nitrogens rise in the blood, the body goes into a survival mode, and begins withdrawing minerals from the bones to **BUFFER** acidic condition in the blood. Medical science labels the process osteoporosis, and shouts "deficiency" of calcium. Not true! The body has innate intelligence and it knows what to do to keep itself alive when it encounters conditions of **excess.**

The solution to the nitrogen and toxic waste dilemma is detoxification of the body via colon therapy, use of PAC's, reliance on hormone precursors, and food with a *usable* energy footprint and signature.

Nitrogen & Plants

Nitrogen is the unit of **electrical currency** that opens the plant's toll gate so energy and mineral ions can pass on their way to enzyme created *hot spots* in the plant's tissues.

Chemical agriculture has learned how to manipulate the life process in plants and trick them into taking unwanted minerals and poisons into their tissues. The process is similar to the use of chelated elemental minerals to trick the body into ignoring its own protocol.

The need to chelate elemental mineral compounds or force feed and force grow crops is based on the assumption that God and Nature are stupid, plants are stupid, the body is stupid, but the *experts* are smart. Chelation smacks of the same mentality that says genetically engineered food is just as good as "real" food, hydroponically raised crops "moot" the need for soil, microwaved food is just as nutritious as conventionally cooked food, and synthetically fertilized crops are just as nutritious as crops raised on biodynamically enlivened soil.

Nature designed things so that the elements would have to **pass** through the carbon cycle before gaining legitimate status and a ticket into the human body.

The formation of new tissues, and the repair of old ones is an "anabolic" process! Quality proteins promote anabolism and come from fresh green leafy vegetables, grains, meats, and legumes. Life unfolds on the wires of right-spin food proteins!

The Carbon Cycle

The carbon cycle explains how earth minerals are ionized and assimilated into food molecules and sea water.

The carbon cycle: Rain + soil + sun + microbe + plant + animal = biologically "live" mineral ions.

The carbon cycle transforms biologically inactive earth minerals into active, right-spin *energy* fields that people can use to stay or become strong and healthy.

Bacteria in the soil are the bankers for earth minerals that are "made available" when they react with weak acids (carbonic acid i.e. atmospheric carbon plus hydrogen) secreted from plant roots. The bacteria hold and modify these ions and live off their electrical energy until the plant withdraws them from their mineral ion bank account. Enzymes act as the cashiers and oversee the exchange. The mineral ions are the currency (electric money). Plants combine ionic and solar energy to produce proteins, fats, carbohydrates, vitamins and enzymes—all of which contain bio-active trace mineral ions.

Animals eat the plants and deposit their waste on the soil. Plants grow, die, and leave their residues on the soil for the bacteria, yeast, and fungi to consume. In time, the nutrients make their way to the sea where they become a *solution* of biologically active *ionic minerals.* Mineral ions give sea water its characteristic salty flavor and its ENERGY! This same energy is what orchestrates the breakup of Rouleau from the blood.

Liquid ionic minerals act in the capacity of spark plugs and fuel in a car. They provide energy and catalyse chemical reactions to completion instead of having them stall out.

Sea water contains ALL earth minerals in constant motion. Their "dynamic," high energy state is confirmation of their valence condition (loss or gain of electrons) and the secret behind their activity in the human body.

Sea water is a solution of *charged* mineral ions. It is the *blood* and *lymph* of Mother Earth.

Vitamins

Vitamins **cannot** function unless mineral ions are present in balanced form. Vitamins are NOT well understood, but we do know that they are mineral dependent. Science has had to *shadow box* with vitamins, learning of their importance through **so called** *deficiency* conditions.

Pellagra is one of these conditions. Pellagra is a *marker* condition that supposedly indicates a niacin deficiency (vitamin B-3). The condition responds well to B vitamin therapy and quality dietary proteins and the elimination of excesses.

The word *vitamin* derives from "vital" meaning *necessary* and "amine" which is the chemical name for a nitrogen bearing molecule. The word *amino*—as in *amino* acid—is also related to "amine" (aminos join to form proteins and contain nitrogen). Amino acids, fats, and carbohydrates are organic molecules produced by anabolic activity in living things.

Organic molecules contain oxygen, nitrogen, sulfur, and carbon. **Carbon** grants the title, "organic!" **Carbon**aceous matter (leaves, grass, etc.) contains carbon. **Carbo**hydrates contain carbon. Life is impossible without carbon. So, a vitamin is a nitrogen containing substance that also contains **carbon** in an amine group.

*Earlier, we talked about the use of a family of chemicals called "chlor**amines**," chemicals that are used by cities throughout the USA to treat public water supplies. Here, chlorine has been combined with an organic amine group to kill bacteria in drinking water. Unfortunately, chloramines **penetrate** the skin when we bathe and destroy the liver.*

Your author rejects the use of all but a very few "food based" vitamin supplements on the market. Organic chemists observe and theorize **amine** activity in "real" food molecules and think they can duplicate it in the laboratory. They can't!

All but a few vitamins **(vital+amine)** are synthesized, even if they are labeled "natural." Man-made vitamins STRESS the liver and are toxic to the body. While it is true that they **mimic** the real thing, it is also true that they cannot build healthy tissues. Despite all the knowledge man has accumulated, we still CANNOT create life. End of debate!

Never forget that live food grown in your own garden is a thousand times better than the best supplement—and a lot less expensive, too!

In biochemistry and nutrition, vitamins are referred to as *cofactors* or *coenzymes*. Vitamins must be present if the body is going to conduct its normal business of living. In turn, vitamins require minerals to work. We must see that our body gets both. Please engrave the following statement into your consciousness and *never* forget it.

We DO NOT live on vitamins, minerals, and enzymes—but from the *energy* that is released by the chemical reactions they fuel.

The Carbon Connection

In his timeless book, *The Carbon Connection*, my friend, Leonard Ridzon defined carbon as *"The governing element that determines the vitality of food crops [and life on Earth]."* He is correct! Ridzon is a living Wizard!

Carbon is extremely important in the aging process. It is our link to the soil and to high vitality foods that come only from high carbon soils. Carbon is the barometer of the soil's aura and its magnetic field. It is the basis of all life.

Carbon can bond in millions of combinations because of its unique atomic form. *Bogus* science uses carbon to create organic poisons like pesticides and herbicides.

Soil that is highly magnetic is usually described as

paramagnetic i.e. *para*-beyond. Soil that is paramagnetic grows right-spin energy food with a complete energy signature.

Devitalized soil has NO paramagnetism and the food grown on it will NOT produce healthy human beings, barnyard animals, or plants. Sick soil is LOW in carbon, low in microbial activity, and low in biologically active mineral ions.

The fastest and best way to convert sick dirt to vibrant soil is through the use of biodynamic principles. If you would like to read about this marvelous field of *esoteric* agriculture, and learn how you can apply in your garden and life, I recommend the works of Alex Podolinsky (see Source Index).

For the first time in history, people can now avail themselves of a biodynamic type product that is inexpensive and can turn the most polluted soil into a nice garden the first year WITHOUT the use of synthetic chemicals.

If you would like to grow a garden and produce high energy food with a powerful right-spin, try Bio-Grow soil builder. It is easy to use and works the very first year (see Source Index).

The best we can hope for is to eat home grown food that's packed with life giving nutrients and has a right-spin footprint. If our food doesn't contain all the minerals we need, we must get them from the next best source available—which concentrated sea water ions.

I obtain my minerals from both sources. The liquid minerals are easy to use and absorb. We cook with them, and we have a spray bottle on the dinner table for *lightly* spraying our food. This gives the effect of table salt without the sodium.

I want to stay YOUNG for a very long time! I get *ENERGY* from these minerals. They are my electrical *currency*. They trigger my biochemical processes, break up the Rouleau effect in the blood, and make me feel good!

The Great Wizards understood that we must meet our energy needs or we will suffer, become OLD, and die *prematurely*. Each of history's Wizards discovered a few pieces of the puzzle we call "health and vitality." It is up to each of us to learn from what they discovered, and apply their discoveries to our own lives. Hopefully, this book will be **your** catalyst to action.

Ionic sea minerals are a *necessary* part of the transition into the future when you will once again be *Young Again!*

PREVIEW: *Our next chapter is about the immune system and cancer, and how to avoid things like AIDS.*

> The reflex points in the feet are wired to the vital organs and tissues of the body. Walking in sand and on green grass provides an outlet for toxic energy and promotes healing!

Electronic Food!

Create electronic food. Food that has NO physical substance, feel, or touch, yet, food the body recognizes as usable energy—that it can use for regeneration and healing. Think invisible food!

Electronic food is Fourth Dimension energy that feeds the body at the *subtle energy level*. **Invisible** food does not substitute for traditional real food, but it can be used to bring about healing and good health.

This is cutting edge technology! An energy generating device called a *"Bioflex"* that can be programmed to produce different "envelopes" of usable energy for specific rejuvenatory purposes.

Just turn on the *Bioflex*, select the program you want, place the interfacing module on your skin at selected "window" points and enjoy. The device is hand held.

The *Bioflex* promotes lymphatic detoxification, relieves stress, stimulates the organs and glands, manipulates the endocrine system, creates electronic vitamins, improves digestion, gets rid of leg and joint pain, improves blood flow, treats heart and liver conditions, and more.

The *Bioflex* is is new in the US, but it has been used in Japan for several years. The **biogenic** energy it produces is electrical in nature, but to small to be measured (it is below 10^{-7} gauss). Body response, however, is instantaneous. I witnessed an 84 year old woman drag herself in the door and bounce out likc a dccr after a one hour treatment.

The hand held device can be used anywhere or anytime. It is especially effective during sleep.

Try this: Get on a treadmill until you poop out and your vital signs spike. Now, apply the *Bioflex*, get on the treadmill, and watch in amazement as your vital signs go DOWN, fatigue diminishes, and your energy goes up—exactly the opposite of what should occur.

The *Bioflex* has fantastic possibilities for the health minded person who "thinks" creatively (see Source Index).

Good health is worth whatever it takes to attain it or keep it. Lack of patience and focus are the two biggest BLOCKS to achieving this worthy goal.

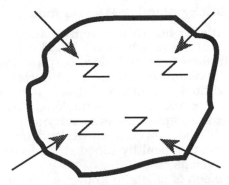

Cancer Tumors
Import & Condense Energy
Tumors calcify; appear on
X-rays, Cat Scans, & MRI's
can be felt with hand; do not
have an occult phase.

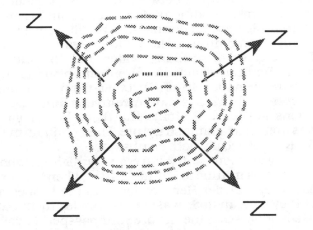

Cancer Masses Export & Disperse Energy
Masses don't calcify or appear
on X-rays; Cat Scans, MRI's;
soft to touch; invisible
during occult period.

Cancer Tumors vs. Cancer Masses
They are NOT the same!

Sticky Blood & Mineral Ions

The battle for health and rejuvenation is WON or LOST at the cellular level where the blood very fine blood capillaries only allow "one" red blood corpuscle to enter or exit a capillary at a time. A corpuscle is a *nucleated* cell i.e. a (blood) cell without a nucleus. Think of a chicken's egg without a yoke; the yoke being the nucleus). Blood flow IN and OUT of the fine capillaries is **strictly** single file.

But as the body becomes loverloaded with waste, the energy *footprint* of healthy blood shifts to the left and **sticky** blood develops.

Sticky blood is officially known as *Rouleau*. When Rouleau sets in, the ability of the blood to access the tissues and service the cells becomes severely jeopardized. We will describe the dilemma like this: oxygen and nutrients can't get into the cells, and carbon dioxide and wastes can't get out of the cells. **This is called aging.**

Cells that can't get rid of their waste eventually die. As the waste builds up in between the cells, degenerative dis-ease develops. Conditions like arthritis and rheumatism, fibromyalgia, scleroderma, and the like appear.

But when 5 drops of liquid ionic sea minerals are added to a glass of drinking water and the water is consumed, Rouleau disappears from the blood and the body can rejuvenating itself. In other words, metabolic activity *speeds up!* **This is called rejuvenation.**

Ions are mineral atoms that have lost or gained electrons from their atomic structure. This condition makes them VERY biologically active substances.

Sea water ions carry have a very high *vibrational frequency* that is in-tune to Mother Earth. When they enter the body, they transfer Her frequency to the tissues and cells as they pick up toxic wastes and carries them out of the system. Ionic sea minerals are your passport to youth!

In order for mineral ions to do their job, they require a carrier or transport. The most efficient transport medium available is BEV water.

If you want to regain your health, or hold onto what you have, it's VERY important to provide your body with a constant flow of BEV mineralized water.

When the body's innate intelligence detects that it can count on a **regular** flow of mineralized BEV water, it will begin to release bound up waste from the system. This is called *reversing the aging process.*

29

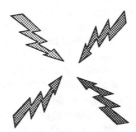

Body Fluid Dynamics

*"When science falters, it is because no
one is asking the right questions."*
Charles Walters

Blood is central to all body metabolism. It carries
oxygen and nutrients to the cells and carbon dioxide and
wastes OUT of the cells and OUT of the system by way of the
kidneys and bowel, lungs, and skin.

Blood is systemic. It interfaces all body systems and is,
therefore, an excellent medium for testing. It is a good barometer of present or pending dis-ease. The blood is one of the
sources of information in the body's two fluid systems.

The blood has a fraternal twin that performs many
similar functions. This "other" system has NO heart to act as
a pump. Its fluid color is straw to clear—not red. Unlike blood,
no one will buy it from you. If there is a medical emergency no
one will ask you to donate any of this fluid. This fluid is called
LYMPH and it is part of the *lymphatic* system.

Healthy lymph is central to health and vitality. It is
impossible to reverse aging without good lymph circulation. We
promote lymph circulation by vigorous walking, running,
aerobic exercise, swimming, calisthenics, deep breathing, and
load-bearing work. We do a lot of these activities when we're
young, and we tend to avoid them as we age.

The lymphatic system is a network of capillaries and
vessels similar to the arteries and veins, with some notable

differences. Lymph capillaries begin as blind alleys, where blood capillaries are continuous. The lymphatic system has nodes where the blood circulatory system has none.

The lymph capillaries remove wastes and service the extracellular fluid in the spaces between the cells. Lymph capillary walls are *more* permeable than blood capillaries and they ONLY work in one direction. Once extracellular fluid enters a lymph capillary it cannot escape until it joins the blood at the subclavian veins near the anterior base of the neck. Blood and lymph are cleaned by the kidneys and liver.

It is VERY important to recognize that the lymph "nodes" are really energy storage sites. TOXIC energy fields are stored and held there for safe keeping until the body can manage them. When you feel swollen lymph nodes under the jaw, in the armpits, under and outside the breasts, or in the groin (above and to the outside of the hairy area) you are feeling "condensed" energy. That is why they are swollen and hard. They should be soft, and pliable, never swollen. Think of your tonsils. They swell and become inflamed during illness, otherwise there soft.

The rebounding and lymphatic massage techniques I ask people to do are designed to move toxic energy fields into circulation so the liver can rid the body of them. The process is greatly assisted by the use of Yucca extract, PAC's, and Kombucha tea.

Blood is different than lymph. It contains corpuscles (red blood cells without a nucleus). It is *pumped* into the arteries under pressure from the heart. 10% of the blood plasma *escapes* through the capillary walls into the extracellular spaces BETWEEN the cells. This **extra**cellular fluid is what actually feeds the cells and tissues.

The lymphatic system performs critical functions that the cardiovascular system cannot do. The veins return 90% of blood fluid volume to the heart. The lymph ducts return the other 10% to the blood as lymphatic fluid.

Lymph fluid contains over **50%** of the plasma proteins, making it the MAJOR protein distribution system of the body. Insufficient exercise and water intake slows lymph movement and results in swelling in the tissues and toxic waste accumulation throughout the body.

Lymphatics & Aging

The lymphatic system is one of the most important systems in the body. Health and dis-ease both have their roots in the watery fluid called lymph. If lymphatic circulation is active and body fluid pH is balanced, toxins and wastes will

NOT accumulate in the tissues. Otherwise, wastes mix with organic poisons, tap water minerals, salts, and fats, FOULING our skin and shutting down vital organ function.

When the tissues are congested and the body is unable to cleanse itself, oxygen and nutrient flow slows. As wastes accumulate in the **extra**cellular fluids between the cells, body pH shifts and the sodium/potassium begins.

The body requires a constant supply of organic potassium. If it does not get it, it steals it from **inside** the cells. As potassium exits the cells, sodium invades and replaces the potassium. This ultimately shuts down energy production by the mitochondria within the cells.

Cancer BEGINS in the lymphatic system. When cancer metastasizes (spreads), it does so by way of the body's protein highway—the lymphatic system.

The lymphatic organs of the body are the lymph nodes, thymus gland (near the base of the neck), tonsils (we have three kinds), spleen, and red bone marrow. Lymphocytes and macrophages are part of the lymphatic system.

Fats & The Immune System

The lymphatic system transports dietary fats out of the intestines and INTO the blood. The **lymph**ocytes and **mac-ro**phages in the blood and lymph fluids protect the body from invading microbes and viruses.

Lymphocytes include the T-cells and B-cells, both of which the HIV virus infects or circumvents. B-cells originate in the bone marrow. Some of them become **plasma** cells which secrete the ANTIBODIES that protect us. Antibodies concentrate and conduct their warfare in the blood and lymph.

A sluggish lymphatic system is an OLD system! Good lymph flow is part of good health. Fluid retention in the legs, ankles, and feet is due to the accumulation of EXCESS waste in the lymph. Where waste is, water follows.

Fungus under the toenails is closely related to poor lymph circulation as is loss of leg hair. These SIGNS are red flags of health problems in the making. Detoxification, exercise, and a good liver flush will remedy these problems.

Exercise & Lymphatics

Exercise has tremendous influence on lymph flow because lymph transfer depends on body movement and muscle contraction. The mini-trampoline, called a *rebounder*, greatly enhances lymph circulation. Women attempt to improve lymph flow in the breast and chest region when they hold their arms high and move them excessively while walking. They would be better off allowing their arms to swing as God made them to do. A swinging arm is an *exaggerated* lever. Swinging arms exert FAR more dynamic influence on lymph movement than the exaggerated antics prescribed by the *experts.*

Here is an interesting exercise that demonstrates the dynamics of lymph movement. First, have the person stand erect and extend their arm straight out to the side of the body and level with the shoulder. Next, attempt to gently but forcefully push down on the arm and note the amount of "resistance" the person generates. Then, have the person run in place while actively moving the arms and lifting the knees high for about 10 seconds. Now, repeat the arm deflection exercise and note the loss of resistance and strength. The loss of strength is related to lymph displacement and use of charged mineral ions (please recall that ions give up their energy in exchange for passage of electrical signals).

Lymph • Red Bone Marrow • Fluoride

Red bone marrow is the part of the lymphatic system responsible for red blood cell production. Red bone marrow is located in the flat bones of the body AND in the epiphyses (ends) of the *long* bones. Between the *epiphyses* and diaphasis, which is the shank of the long bones, is where the growth plates are located. The growth plates give us our physical height.

Fluoride interferes with the production of red blood cells. It blocks enzyme activity and weakens bone integrity. Toothpaste and drinking water that contains fluoride suppress red blood cell production and promote pernicious anemia.

Anemic people have poor vitality and tire easily. Fluoride's effect on health and energy is similar to taking chemotherapy for cancer, except that it occurs in SLOW MOTION! Table salt negatively affects body metabolism. When you combine sodium with fluoride the effects spell trouble.

The Romans knew the power of table salt. When they defeated Hannibal's Carthage, they made sure that Carthage would NEVER rise again by salting her soil.

Excess sodium stresses body metabolism, while fluorides limit oxygen-carrying capacity of the blood (fewer blood cells produced by the red bone marrow means less oxygen). Both shut down mitochondrial activity.

The lymphatic system services the colon, which begins at the cecum (see chart). The cecum is the juncture of the lower small intestine (ileum) and the beginning of the large intestine (colon). The *appendix* dangles from the cecum. This area is the most toxic site in the body. It is loaded with lymph nodes (called

Peyer's patch). Lymph nodes isolate and manage toxic waste overload and prevent death. **Appendicitis is confirmation of toxic waste overload to the point of death!**

A sluggish colon and lymphatic system are **symptomatic** conditions related to a toxic liver which, in turn, leads to bowel problems. People who experience appendicitis, diverticulitis, colitis, or irritable bowel syndrome are under **indictment** for MORE serious health problems to come unless remedial action is taken. Therapy includes dietary modification, detoxification, BEV water, fasting, lymphatic massage, Kombucha tea, PAC's, and simplification of lifestyle.

Acne & Scars

As lymph fluid circulation slows, the basement membranes of the skin become clogged and connective tissues break down. Wrinkles and acne result.

Acne is nothing but an acute case of a clogged lymphatic system in the sub-cutaneous layers of the skin. A TOXIC liver is central to this problem.

Scar formation and a congested lymphatic system go hand in hand. Scars result from damage to the *parenchyma* cells, which are the ACTIVE, functional cells of an organ—like the skin. Scars are like the battlefield where armies of competing energy fields do battle. Scars are proof that the negative energy forces won and rejuvenation failed to occur.

Stroma cells are NON-functional cells that serve in a structural or connective capacity in organ tissues. The skin is composed of elastic, reticular, and collagenous fibers.

Injuries that penetrate the parenchyma cells result in scars if the bio-electric body is under stress. The parenchyma cells keep us young by repairing the damage. They are actively involved in *anabolic* metabolism and they are served by both the blood and lymph fluids.

An astute surgeon can tell the physical age of his patient by the amount of scar tissue in the vital organs. Due to an accident, I had a hernia repaired at 48 years of age. My doctor made a video. He was astounded because my vital organs were those of a 15 year old!

Burns • Scars • New Limbs

In 1983 I suffered a *severe* burn in a welding accident. The skin and underlying tissues of the inside of my right elbow were burned and destroyed by a hunk of red hot 5,000° F steel that fell and landed in the crotch of my arm.

At that time, I was age forty-three years young. By

medical standards, I was old and should have scarred horribly. Instead, healing progressed without ANY scar formation. I did not see a doctor. Why was there no scar formation? The answer is related to vital organ function and blood/lymph circulation.

The body can regenerate itself—limbs, nerve tissue, and bones. I am talking about "complete" limb regeneration as well as total restoration of function with no evidence of scar formation. These things have been amply demonstrated by Dr. Robert Becker and Dr. Melvin Saunders.

The miracle of "regeneration" was personally experienced by Mitchell May who made medical history by growing new skin, bone, and nerve tissue after suffering over forty breaks to his femur (thigh bone).

Medical miracles, like Mitchell May's, are closely aligned with the principles of vibrational medicine and the manipulation of subtle energy forces in the bio-electric body.

Peak health means healing without scars, and the formation of new tissues in spite of the laws of science and medicine. Aging reversal is available to anyone who wants it.

Clogged Arteries & Lymph

Atherosclerosis (clogging of the arteries) is a major problem in the USA. Yet little is said of the lymphatic system's relationship to cardiovascular problems affecting millions.

The two main trunks of the lymphatic system—which circulate lymphatic fluids (**extra**cellular fluids, wastes, and plasma proteins) join the blood system at the subclavian veins. These junctures are on each side of the esophagus at the base and front of the neck, just below the collar bones.

The subclavian veins feed into the superior vena cava vein and then into the right side of the heart. **The heart pumps the blood to the lungs where TWO things occur. The blood is reoxygenated AND toxic, left-spin energy fields are RELEASED into the atmosphere.**

The blood is then returned to the left side of the heart for distribution to the body. As the blood leaves the heart by way of the aortic artery, the left and right coronary arteries branch off and feed the heart muscle. These are the arteries that become blocked and require coronary bypass operations.

Toxic fats like soy, canola (rape), cotton seed, and hydrogenated margarines, combine with *chlorine, fluorine, and chloramines* (from tap water) and metabolic waste products in the blood. Atherosclerotic plaque is the result. The lymphatic system is **central** to cardiovascular dis-ease.

Some people age so rapidly in their vital organs that they simply drop dead! *Angina pectoris* is a good example of the pain that results from an oxygen deficiency in the chest, neck and left arm. When we experience reduced oxygen supply to the heart, it is called ischemia (*ischein*-to hold back. *hemia*-pertaining to the blood.) When we suffer a heart attack, some of the heart muscle tissue dies for LACK of oxygen due to blocked arteries around the heart. This is called *myocardial infarction*. If a blood clot is involved, it is called a *coronary thrombosis*. A clot is a *thrombus*.

People & Plants

Human beings and plants have MUCH in common. They also have ONE major difference. That difference has to do with MOBILITY and fluid movement.

Humans rely on physical activity to assist the movement of lymph fluid, and we have the heart to pump our blood. By comparison, plants have no heart and must depend on capillary action, osmosis, solar energy, enzymes, and ion energy to overcome gravity and move water and nutrients up into their tissues and back to their roots.

Humans depend on the mitochondria to produce the energy that fuels body processes. Plants rely on mineral ions, photosynthesis, and solar energy to fuel their metabolic processes. Humans rely on the red blood corpuscles and hemoglobin for their supply of oxygen. Plants rely on chlorophyll and the chloroplasts. Human body fluids are called blood and lymph. Plant fluids are called chlorophyll and sap. Human beings need movement, exercise, and load bearing work to assist in the repair and maintenance of body tissues. Plants enjoy little mobility.

Lack of exercise and load bearing work, SLOWS blood and lymph flow drastically and leads to dis-ease. Lack of mobility is the CURSE of older people.

It is easy to identify healthy, energy-filled blood from sick, low-energy blood. When a finger is pricked and then squeezed to force out the blood, the blood should have a HIGH crown (forms a pearl) and should be brilliant in color. If it oozes and flows instead of developing a high crown, dis-ease is in the making. The blood of people with cancer or other serious conditions will ooze. If you are an "oozer" take everything in this book to heart and get to work on reversing YOUR aging process through total body detoxification. Your life depends on it!

Blood and lymph are flip sides of the same coin. A dis-ease condition in the lymph mirrors a similar condition in the blood. The lymphatic system dictates the status of the bio-electric body as well as blood chemistry.

When we learn HOW to control the terrain of the bio-electric body, we control the aging process. Aging reversal requires that we assist the body in cleaning up and maintaining the lymphatic system through increased body fluid dynamics.

Dis-ease first occurs in the lymph. Later, it shows up in the blood. If we pay attention to our lymphatic system, dis-ease will find no place to take root and will be forced to look elsewhere.

We *limp* our way into old age. We must *lymph* our way UP the catabolic side of the aging pyramid—back to our anabolic peak—if we expect to become *Young Again!*

PREVIEW: *Our next chapter is the "cancer" chapter! Learn HOW to avoid becoming a cancer statistic.*

Spider Bites • Wounds
Spider bites respond to poultices made with *racemic* clay. It is also wise to use the *enhanced* homeopathic remedy "rickettsia" in conjunction with the clay. The clay also works wonders on deep wounds and serious infections. Try them!

Life! A Dual Perspective!
We grow old and die in the invisible realm of the Fourth Dimension **BEFORE** we see and experience it in the Thrid Dimension realm in which we live out our lives.

Detoxification of the body requires a **dual** perspective to be truly effective. For example, colon therapy accelerates the release of toxic metabolic wastes on the physical level, while enhanced homeopathic remedies bring about detoxification on a higher "invisible" level.

When we *erase* toxic energy conditions in the Fourth Dimension, we deal with **underlying** health issues and promote true healing in the Third Dimension.

Life is the manifestation of what we in the West refer to as *spirit, soul, grace,* and what Eastern thought calls *life force, chi. qi, and prana.*

Good health and rejuvenation demands a dual perspective. So does enlightenment.

Howdy Doody Facial Lines
Lines from *the corners of the mouth to the sides of the chin* indicate **severe** colon problems and a body that is in trouble. Colon therapy promotes rejuvenation by exchanging an old body for a young one (see Source Index).

A Typical Day

1. Wake up early and at the same time each day. Immediately drink a cup of Rene's tea or Kombucha tea.

2. Hold your bladder. Don't give in to the temptation to urinate. This will force you to have a bowel movement.

3. Do your stretching exercises, calisthenics, bounce 5 minutes on a rebounder followed by a complete self-massage of the lymphatic system. Drink more water and take your ETVC (Enhanced Trivalent Chromium) complex.

4. Do some pull ups (both over and underhanded), pump some barbells, and finally get on a good aerobic exerciser and raise your heart beat to 80% of your maximum heart rate and HOLD it there for at least 12 minutes. Do this in cold, fresh air with a minimum of clothing while using your mind to train your body to create internal heat. Cold develops brown fat.

5. Take your hormone precursors.

6. Take a hot shower followed by long ice cold shower.

7. Eat breakfast one hour after rising and at least 1/2 hour after drinking any water, a homemade bran muffin (warmed up in a toaster oven), an apple, some harmonic pollen, Klamath algae, followed by food based supplements, two or three dried prunes. Eat whatever you like, but avoid all bio-junk food.

8. Drink a glass of water with ionic sea minerals every hour. Always take your hormone precursors and PAC's (proanthocyanidins) between meals. Snacks are our of the question—period! (Eat good food and you won't want them.)

9. For lunch, a spoonful of biogenic pollen, a predigested liver tablet and/or some Klamath algae, a few prunes, an apple and fresh veggies, some fresh air and a short walk, some relaxing music, meditation, good conversation, a good book, deep breathing exercises, prayer, whatever, as long as it's low stress, positive, uplifting. Don't buy into other people's problems, and don't worry about your own.

10. Hold your bladder to promote more bowel movements.

11. Every day, try to do some load-bearing work. Moving boxes. Lifting heavy things. Do your gardening work by hand. No rototiller. Use a push lawn mower. Force your body to become strong! It was made to work. If it hurts, ignore it. If it's weak, it will become strong. Pain for gain!

12. Eat a good dinner. Drink water and Kombucha tea mid evening followed by a cup of hot Yucca extract before bed.

13. Retire at the same time. Sleep outside. Pray. Give thanks for being alive. Look forward to tomorrow.

Microbiology Of Drinking Water

The principal bacterial agents shown to be involved in intestinal dis-eases associated with drinking water are:

Salmonella typhi: typhoid fever
Salmonella paratyphi-Aparathyphoid fever
Salmonella species: enteric fever, salmonellosis
Shigella bacteria: bacillary dysentery
Amebas: Amebic dysentery
Vibrio cholerae: cholera
Leptospira species: leptospirosis
Yersinia enterocolitica: gastroenteritis
Francisella tularensis: tulararemia
Escherichia coli (E. coli): gastroenteritis
Pseudomonas aeruginosa: various infections
Cryptosporidium: cryptosporidiosis

Enteric (pertaining to the small intestine/gut) bacteria like E. coli, Salmonella, and Shigella are classified as *facultatively anaerobic*, that is, they can function and live with or without oxygen. They ferment sugars and produce organic acids (acetic, formic, lactic, etc.) and gases (mixed-acid fermentation).

Viruses differ from microorganisms. Unlike bacteria, viruses are **intra**cellular parasites and cannot replicate outside the host's cells. Hepatitis-A (infectious hepatitis) is the product of a notable water born virus. So is poliomyelitis (polio).

Viruses and bacteria are prevalent in raw untreated water. Therefore, conventional treatment of public water supplies involves steps like coagulation, sedimentation, filtration, and disinfection (chlorine, **chloramines,** mercuric acid, etc.) to produce *potable* water. These steps reduce organism count. However, during the warm season, the organisms can multiply in the lines with disastrous results.

Parasites, pathogenic bacteria, and viruses are removed from drinking water by the BEV process. In addition, they are **flushed** from the BEV system so as to not develop a breeding ground for the spread of dis-ease. No other water system can provide the purity and protection of the BEV process.

The United States is headed for a cataclysmic crisis in public drinking water.

30

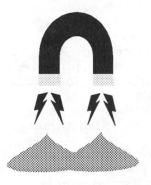

Cancer & Salt

*"Well organized ignorance, unfor-
tunately, often passes for wisdom."*
anon.

Salt (sodium chloride) is a paradox. It is part of life, yet it is involved in death. A little salt will hurt you a little bit. More than a little will *eventually* kill you.

History can be written according to salt. In ancient China, two tablespoons of salt was a socially acceptable mode of suicide. Salt has served as money, an item of barter, and a cathartic (laxative). For over 100 years, medicine's focus has centered on salt's relationship to *high blood pressure*. We will focus on salt's systemic EFFECTS on the *bio-electric* body.

Mankind has chosen to upset Nature's balance. We use salt to *hype* our food and in so doing we hasten old age. Nutritious food does NOT need salt because it has plenty of mineral ions in it to give it flavor. Marginal food requires salt to create the *mirage* of taste—and to keep it from **spoiling**. Look at any can or package of processed food and you will find that it is loaded with salt.

Canned foods came about in 1859 when the H. J. Heinz company produced the first of its Heinz 57 varieties. Salt was used to create a brine environment that was hostile to Clostridium botulinum. Clostridium is a facultative anaerobe. It can survive with or without oxygen. Its wastes are the most toxic systemic poisons known. We call the condition produced by these toxins "botulism!"

Sailors of old suffered miserably from *salt*-preserved beef and pork. So did civilian populations. When meat is preserved with salt, it loses its energy force and nutritive qualities. Sodium chloride (table salt) is a preservative that upsets the potassium:sodium balance in the body. Salt makes the mortician's job easier.

Organic foods are naturally high in potassium and low in sodium, while bio-junk and processed foods are exactly the opposite. Sodium upsets the ion balance in the body, and destroys energy balance in the soil. Salt fertilizers create conditions of EXCESS in the soil, as does table salt in the body. Salt is a concentrated, left-spin energy field that does not belong in the body.

NOTE: A little flour, salt, and water mixed together makes a wonderful play dough for children. However, when it dries, it turns as hard as concrete.

Natural vs. Unnatural Preservatives

Dr. Carey Reams taught that quality produce will dehydrate before it will rot. He proved his point by entering a watermelon he had grown in the local county fair for three years in a row! Quality fresh food is high in natural sugars and earth minerals. Quality produce has a right-spin energy signature.

Acres USA once carried a story about a salesman who carted around three cabbages in his car for nine months without spoilage. On the weekends, he would roll them under a shade tree until Monday morning when he would peel away a leaf and hit the road again. When the salesman was challenged, the nine month old cabbages were cut and eaten raw. The point here is that high mineral and sugar content is central to high quality fruits and vegetables.

Homemade ice cream containing too much sugar will NOT set up regardless of the amount of salt applied to the ice to lower the freezing point. Oranges that are high in natural sugars will wither and shrink, but they will NOT rot. Home grown lettuce and greens can be kept in the refrigerator for over a month and will still be crisp and tasty with no spoilage! High sugar levels in the juices of food crops indicates a high mineral content, excellent flavor, and good keeping qualities.

Trace minerals and humic acids applied to plant foliage as a foliar spray raise the sugar/mineral levels in the juices of plants and protect them from frost damage. High sugar levels in a crop is an excellent marker of nutritious food. Proper glucose (sugar) levels in the blood and glycogen levels in the muscles are closely related to peak health. Dis-ease cannot survive in a high energy, right-spin environment where mineral ion levels and sugars are balanced and excesses do not exist.

In the old days, a bushel of fresh green beans weighed 32 lbs. Today, a bushel of beans weighs only 24 lbs. The difference is the lack of earth minerals AND lower concentration of sugar energy. The more concentrated the positive energy fields, the heavier the crop, while crops raised with salt fertilizers and poisonous sprays produce sick, weak populations of human beings. **A *Biotester* will check the direction and intensity of spin radiating from fruit and vegetables. It will be available in 1996. In the meantime, everyone should become adept with a vibration chain and pendulum.**

SALT: Paul Bragg vs. The Athletes

Here is a true story about how salt affects health and vitality. In the early 1960's, Dr. Paul C. Bragg, a famous health crusader, challenged a group of college athletes to a 30 mile hike across Death Valley. The temperature in August was 130° Fahrenheit.

The *experts* advised the athletes to take "salt tablets!" The athletes were given all the "cold" water and food they wanted. Bragg drank *only* warm distilled water (in those days BEV water was not available), took NO salt, and fasted—taking no food. Bragg was the only one to finish the hike. The athletes—every last one of them—were carried off for medical care. They suffered from heat exhaustion and heat stroke. Bragg finished the hike in 10 1/2 hours, camped overnight, and repeated the return hike the following day. He was in his mid *sixties!* He was YOUNG and active. He avoided all salt!

Rommel's German-Afrikan Corps used no salt in their diets, yet they fought tremendous desert battles. When they were finally captured, they were in peak condition and unaffected by the intense desert heat. The Americans used salt tablets, they salted their food, and the heat got to them.

Native peoples seldom use salt. When *civilized* man comes along and introduces salt into their diet, their health deteriorates. By itself salt does not bring on dis-ease, but it is always a player in the development of subclinical illness that eventually gives way to SIGNS and diagnosis of dis-ease.

Cells • Sodium • Mitochondria

When sodium levels are high, the body is in a negative energy condition. High sodium diet upsets the body's sodium:potassium ratio and speeds the LOSS of potassium from the cells. Potassium is the predominant ion *inside* the cell membranes, while sodium is the predominant ion *outside* of the cell's membrane (in the **extra**cellular fluid).

When sodium levels are high, the body steals potassium from the cells and replaces it with sodium. Both ions have a positive (+) charge and both are electrolytes. However, sodium spins left while potassium spins right. Edema (fluid retention in the tissues) is a SIGN of **excess** sodium and **excess** plasma protein wastes in the body.

Once inside the cell, sodium short-circuits cellular machinery, sedates the mitochondria, and eventually kills the cells. Dead cells create stress and must be removed. Marginal cells between life and death produce little energy. The presence of dead and sick tissue needlessly *wastes* vital ENERGY. Energy that could be used for growth and repair is squandered in the presence of sodium-imposed stress.

The mitochondria cannot function in a high sodium environment. They cannot replicate (reproduce) when sodium has invaded their territory, and they cannot produce enough bio-electric lightning to meets our needs. **When sodium invades the cells, metabolic activity slows and the body becomes tired and weak.**

Energy • Free Radicals

We have spent a lot of time discussing and describing energy using terms like left-spin, right-spin, negative, positive, aerobic and anaerobic in an effort to help the reader understand the nature of energy and its relationship to aging.

The term "free radical" is a term that comes to mind in regard to energy and cancer. A free radical is a molecule that contains an *odd* number of electrons. This makes it highly reactive and EXTREMELY unstable.

Free radicals are very much a part of **every** persons life. Poor choices of lifestyle, diet, and water are greatly compounded by environmental poisons that bombard the bio-electric body from every direction.

In a healthy body, free radical reactions take place continuously and look like this: $O^2 + O^2 + H^2 \leftrightarrow H_2O_2{}^= + O_2$ (the double arrow means that the reaction can **reverse**). In a stressed body, reverse chain reactions causes electron theft to go out of control. The end result is accelerated aging.

Free radical production tremendously influences aging and the formation of cancer tissues in the body. For our discussion here, I would like the reader to understand that these "wild" reactions produce two things: 1- non differentiated tissue (cancer tissue), and 2- EXCESSES of waste energies.

Nondifferienced tissue is the kind of tissue from which

we evolve PRIOR to hormonal influences that cause the formation of skin instead of muscle, bones instead of brains, etc. We are talking about OUTLAW tissue with no identity. Tissue *insurrection* best describes the process. Uncontrolled oxidation of the tissues builds EXCESS toxic waste in the system, hormonal imbalances. Excesses eventually manifest as so called deficiency conditions.

Cancer commandeers **spin-off energy** from free radical reactions within the body. In compliance with the second law of thermodynamics, energy is NEVER lost, it merely changes form. Once excess toxic energy **EXCEEDS** the body's ability to cope, the formation of a tumor or a mass will begin. We will discuss their individual characteristics shortly.

Uncontrolled free radical reactions are easily prevented through detoxification, hormonal balancing, and the use of enhanced PAC's. Vitamins E, C, and A don't compare to enhanced PAC's. I look for a combination of proanthocyanidins, leucoanthocyanins, catechins, tocotrienols, and phyto extracts like carotinoids, bilberry, rosemary, and CO-Enzymes 6-10. These plant derived substances stop free radical reactions, detoxify the system, and does wonders for things like cancer and its likes (see Source Index).

Health is a confirmation of correct choices.

Energy • Cancer

Cancer is a manifestation of a negative energy condition. Cancer **tumors** surround themselves in a zone of SODIUM. They **concentrate** energy by acting as *anaerobic* black holes, siphoning away and isolating the host's TOXIC energy.

The tumor is NOT the "enemy." Rather, it is a statement by the body that all is not well. Moreover, a tumor is a self-defensive measure taken by the body to preserve itself through the **condensation** of deadly energy fields that it is unable to neutralize or dispose of through the lungs, kidneys, bowel or skin. Tumors are a warning SIGN.

In the early stages, a cancer tumor goes unnoticed. As it concentrates more energy, it becomes "dense." It can now be seen on by X-ray, cat scan, and MRI. It can even be *felt* with the fingers if it is not too deep in the tissues.

Cancer tumors are NOT the same as cancer masses. Tumors are a energy-**importing** clusters of tissue that the body forms to ISOLATE toxic energy fields and get them OUT of circulation. Free radical reactions are a prime source of energy.

Tumors are *nationalistic.* They stay within their own territory and import their energy needs. They do NOT spread as commonly described. When *antagonized by surgical interven-*

tion, the body is weakened sufficiently to precipitate the formation of new tumors rather than son and daughter tumors. Cancers tumors should NOT be removed.

Sometimes the body chooses to **dissolve** a tumor. In other cases, it chooses to **calcify** (deposit minerals; petrify) the tumor and tie up the toxic energy on a permanent basis. The tumor or mass is NOT the enemy, but an effort by the body to preserve itself. The enemy is the person who inhabits the body. Healing requires focused effort and reprogramming of the mental processes behind the dis-ease condition. **The mind is 70% of the healing battle. The rest helps makes it happen.**

When a **malignant** tumor (or mass) is discovered, immediate action is called for in the form of radical detoxification, PAC supplementation, and change of lifestyle. Radiation and chemotherapy are NEVER wise choices if you consider the torture and financial strain they impose. Alternative treatment is safer and more humane if the patient has discipline and does not skip from one modality to another.

Alternative therapy demands that a person have a laid-back, happy, 100% positive mental outlook. There is absolutely NO room for doubt, fear, worry, hate, blame, or anger—only love! **The desire to live must be intense and beyond the fear of death.** I highly recommend the book, *Your Body Believes Every Word You Say* (see Source Index).

The ONLY things cancer tumors and masses have in common is that both are *virus* havens, and both enjoy left-spin, anaerobic, high sodium environments, and a body that produces large amounts of "free radicals."

Cancer Masses

A mass is not a tumor and the terms should NOT be used interchangeably. A mass is not dense like a tumor. It cannot be felt because it has no definition. A mass is soft, spongy, porous, difficult to feel—never hard.

A mass takes form, grows and establishes outposts quietly. Masses exist in the twilight zone *between* life and death. They rarely appear on X-rays, CAT scans, or MRI's. It is impossible to differentiate where a mass ends and a gland, organ, or other soft tissue begins. Masses are *invisible* because they have little density and can hide behind other tissues.

Masses are *offensive* in nature. Think of them in terms of outposts for colonial expansionism in a third world country (your body). Masses colonize during a 7 year period, referred to in medical circles as the "occult" period (*occult* means hidden). Long before a cancer *mass* announces itself to the host, it is there, growing and spreading. Masses follow the lymphatic highway and sabotage the host's lymphatic and immune systems, while the host notices nothing and even feels good! By the time a mass announces itself, the host is in **deep** trouble.

Cloaking Technique • Sodium

During the occult period, a cancer mass is concealed, invisible, and non-detectable by the host and conventional testing. In other words, a mass employs a cloaking technique so as to go undetected. The years preceding the end of the occult period are often some of the very best years in terms of OUTWARD appearance of good health. On the inside however, confirmation of the person's lifestyle and choices have come home to roost and aging is in full swing.

A person who is sodium-toxic always suffers from edema (water logging of the tissues), partly from the sodium and partly from the accumulation of plasma proteins in the **extra**cellular spaces between the cells.

A sodium and waste protein-toxic person gains weight with little or no increase in body measurements (water is heavier than body fat on a volume basis). People who gain weight, but not inches, should be concerned.

Edema is a SIGN. Edema is abnormal. *Chronic* edema is the equivalent to a quiet proclamation of WAR and must not be ignored. Edema signals the *invasion* of sodium at the cellular level and GROSS accumulation of plasma proteins in the lymphatic fluids. Look for puffy, water filled skin that "dents" easily when pressed and does not spring back quickly. Be alert to swelling in the legs, ankles, feet, and hands.

People in the *early stages* of a cancer "mass" formation, often experience substantial weight gain for no particular reason—usually WITHOUT any noticeable change in dietary habits. Near the end of the occult period, they get the "I just don't feel up to par" syndrome. Finally, out of the blue, the person becomes skin and bones. **Their body seems to evaporate!** When this occurs, *mass* type cancers have removed their cloak, the occult period is over, and the final struggle begins.

Edema is cancer's cloaking device. **People do NOT recognize edema for what it is! They don't understand. They think everything is okay—just a little old age.**

During the cloaking period, the cancerous body is **cannibalizing** itself. It is experiencing severe free radical oxidation and it's digesting its own tissues, a process called **auto digestion.** The body is living on *stored* energy. The body is now in a catabolic state. Once the body has used up its energy reserves—BANG!—the person is in trouble. Because of the *invisible* nature of cancer masses, exploratory surgery is pushed on the unsuspecting patient by *blind men and women in white robes.* The result is predictable—a positive confirmation of **CANCER!** By this time, your weight has plunged downward. You have become skin and bones overnight. You are terrified.

When sodium levels in the cells and the plasma proteins in the lymph have reached the critical point, cancer *turns off* its cloaking device and announces itself.

It's Your Life

There are no tests to determine sodium toxicity at the cellular level, but there are SIGNS. There are no tests for plasma protein toxicity at the **extra**cellular level either, but there are SIGNS. Learn to pay attention to them.

Pay attention when you see people (and children) gaining weight. Be alert to gyrating blood sugar levels. PMS and menstrual problems are symptoms. Acne, boils, balding, mood swings, ongoing colds and flu symptoms should not be ignored. Bladder infections, prostate problems, bowel conditions, and graying of the hair all have long term consequences.

If you have a serious condition seek help, but be forewarned that most people are bullied into conventional therapy. They want to believe their physician. Find—and work with— someone who is trained in alternative therapy and who not held hostage by the AMA (American Medical Association), the pharmaceutical houses, and the FDA. **If you can't find such a person, then you had better strike out on your own.**

Remember, the **body** does the healing. As the steward of that body, it is YOUR job to provide the environment where healing can take place. Control the "terrain!"

Colon therapy is crucial. Fasting is wise. Home grown kale, collards, and comfrey greens are very healing. So are apples, dried prunes, Harmonic pollen and jelly (the best comes from northern British Columbia).

Walking bare-footed on sand and grass is beneficial. Positive thinking and visualization are a crucial. Detoxification of the blood, lymph, and tissues is mandatory. BEV water can precipitate miracles. Rebounding and lymphatic massage should be part of your routine. Laughter and fun are basic prerequisites to good health. Worry and fear are not allowed. Be careful of your thoughts, they are a self-programming. What you think you get. What you voice, you believe. If you focus on the negative, death, fear, anger etc. you will reap these things—and visa versa. Do not forget the power of prayer, both for yourself and others. Meditation and deep breathing are powerful tools. Time spent working in a garden (bare footed), growing food, and enjoying Nature is as close to heaven as you can get. Take time to focus on and help others. The more you give, the more you receive. Money is appreciated, but your time means more.

Self Diagnosis • Self Treatment

The simplest tools for diagnosis are a pendulum and vibration chain. Used properly, they are fantastic devices. Use them to establish the depth of your aura today, so you will have a reference for the future. Combined with your "bio-electric age," you now have TWO reference points. "Tune-in" to your gut instincts. Avail yourself of the Sky-Heart device to clear and neutralize *disharmony* in your body.

Rid your body of *excess* sodium through a fresh food, high potassium diet and sea water mineral ions. Driving sodium from the body—especially a body diagnosed with cancer—requires copious amounts of organic potassium in the form of fresh, organic juices like carrot, cabbage, onion, lemon and beet juices. Sip and chew your juices. Do not gorge yourself. Balance is the key. Remember, it takes 5-10 minutes to chew an apple, but only 2 seconds to drink the juice.

Fresh juices are VERY powerful detoxifiers and can flood the body with wastes to the point that the liver will become *exhausted* and the kidneys *overloaded*. It's better to go slow. **Juice capsules and tablets** are a good way to regulate intake of fruit and vegetable juices, and are made from organic foods. They are easy to take on a trip—to work, to play.

Liver is a wonderful food—if you can stand it! I use **"predigested,"** freeze-dried, organic beef liver tablets from Argentina. It's a superb food. Cancer therapy should always include liver. Domestic liver products are contaminated. Avoid them. Do not use *dessicated* liver! It is high stress food.

Deep "coffee" colon irrigations are very therapeutic. Kombucha tea makes a wonderful colon solution. Gentle bouncing on a *rebounder* (mini-trampoline) moves body fluids. Lymphatic massage is easy and effective. Add RHYTHM and regular hours to your life. Use plenty of PAC's. They are VERY powerful (see Source Index).

Sodium and waste protein detoxification does NOT happen by itself. YOU must assist YOUR body. Once released into circulation, excesses MUST be gotten rid of fast! Colon therapy combined with PAC's and Yucca make it happen.

Avoid tap water. Don't drink distilled water. It is loaded with plasticizers and is biologically dead water.

Expect To Feel Crummy

EXPECT to feel crummy as you detoxify! You are paying

for your sins. Do NOT forget the power of prayer and positive thinking. Try to find a few "strong" people who will help you through the transition back into the world of the healthy.

Once the potassium begins exchanging its place with the sodium inside the cells, the mitochondria will come alive and replicate themselves. The more of them that come alive and multiply—the more *ENERGY* there will be available for your body to rebuild itself. At first, you will feel worse. In time, you will feel better.

Detoxification can be tough on people. It's a kind of mind game. The body shouts, "I feel crummy," but you must ignore and reassure the body that all is **under control.** Talk out loud and tell your body *what you expect* and *what you desire.* Never go hyper at the first sign of a metabolic rebound—guard your energy at all costs! Good days are followed by bad days. In time, you will enjoy more good and fewer bad days. Use things like Yucca extract, PAC's, Kombucha tea, and hormonal precursors to rebuild your body. Waste removal is critical.

Chemotherapy

Chemotherapy is defined as the prevention or treatment of infectious disease by *chemicals* which act to prevent "antisepsis" in the body, while avoiding "serious" side effects in the patient. If we dissect the word *antisepsis,* we get *anti-*against; *sepsis-*a general fever producing condition, caused by bacteria or their toxic by-products. In light of this dictionary definition, do you think that *chemotherapy* as used on cancer patients meets this description? Did you know that you must sign a form *before* you get your "magic bullet" cancer therapy?

NOT Approved

Drugs used in cancer chemotherapy are *"magic bullets."* They are NOT APPROVED as safe for the treatment of cancer. They are administered to unsuspecting people. Medicine and the pharmaceutical companies side step the "liability" problem by having people sign away their rights *beforehand,* so they cannot bring suit for the horrible side effects that follow.

When people sign the "standard" form, they are giving the legal AND medical systems *jurisdiction* over them. The name of the game in our legal system is *jurisdiction!* Either medicine and the courts have jurisdiction over a person's body, or the person does, but NOT both at the same time.

When the system has jurisdiction, obviously, the person does not. When a person grants medicine jurisdiction over their body, medicine is free to maneuver with impunity.

For the cancer patient, the options "within" the medical system are very limited. They must sign the form or medicine will refuse to "treat" them because they have NOT granted jurisdiction! The medical system needs jurisdiction because they are using EXPERIMENTAL drugs in the treatment of cancer and the destruction of YOUR body.

Come to understand something known in legal AND medical circles as the "Rule of Probable Cause." It states: *"...experimental drugs may be used IF the side effect of the drug is NO worse than the end effect of the untreated disease."*

"For Experimental Use Only"

Regardless of the specie of cancer drug, it is stamped with the tell-tale sign of a **"magic bullet"** medicine—"For Experimental Use Only."

How do you like that? How does it make you feel to know that the MAXIMUM risk to the poor patient is no worse than if treatment were not rendered at all. What an alternative—sign on the dotted line and die here, or go home and die—after they finish working you over and milking your savings and insurance!

"For Experimental Use Only" is a fact that should be sufficient SHOCK therapy to motivate every thinking person to immediately begin the aging reversal process. No matter how you figure it, you are on your own. So begin today!

"Magic bullets" don't work! Self treatment is less risky and the odds of recovery far greater—at a fraction of the cost.

Believe me when I tell you that your health and life are worth more than all the money you can throw at the medical system in the futile effort to buy back your health. Good health isn't for sale. Instead, it requires commitment, discipline, responsibility and choice. AVOID the horror of cancer and other degenerative dis-eases by implementing the preventative measures we have discussed throughout this book.

Cancer & Root Canals

According to Dr. Issels, a German doctor, only 20% of the population has root canals, yet, 90% of cancer victims have root canals in their mouth!

There is a strong relationship between cancer and root canals in the teeth. The problem involves the presence of a dead body part (a tooth) in the body, mercury poisoning, and electrical interference from the composite metals in the mouth.

Dead tissue (teeth) are left-spin energy fields that cause an *autoimmune* response in the body (*auto*-self attack). Root canals provide an avenue for mercury amalgam to "bleed" into bone and blood. Teeth "rot" beneath those shiny caps. Metals react with saliva and create electrolysis in the mouth. Metals emit electrical signals that interfere with brain activity. They act as antennas and receivers. Some people can pick up local radio stations through the fillings and crowns in their mouth! Root canals are NOT part of becoming *Young Again!*

PREVIEW: *Our next chapter deals with the world of Time and Space and its relationship to the Fourth Dimension, ageless living, and the vast UNKNOWN!*

It's Your Life

Some things are worse than death. Becoming a victim of *conventional* cancer treatment is one of them.

Never rejoice because medical insurance is paying the bills. Do be concerned about what "they" are going to do to you. Do be independent. Do keep your dignity. Do maintain control of your life. Do stay away from doctors.

Do these things and you will leave your loved ones with more than the ugly memory of the **"torture"** that preceded your death! **CHOOSE to live and die on your own terms, or not at all. It's *your* life!**

A Cause For All Cancers

The ubiquitous presence of *propyls* in our society, and the resulting *metamorphosis* and *migration* of intestinal flukes into the vital organs due to the build up of propyls in the system—especially in the liver—was well documented in a recent book that appeared on the market.

Your author wholeheartedly agrees that propyls are NOT good for people. But he would like to remind the reader that there are **thousands** of chemicals in our air, water, food, and cosmetics that are equally bad for us.

Your author IS concerned about propyls, but he is **MORE** concerned about **FLUSHING** all chemicals and contaminants from the system—including propyls! Avoidance is applauded, but detoxification is supreme!

We know that people with cancer have toxic, weak livers. We also know that if you clean up you act, health and longevity can be yours. Accept the reality of the polluted world in which we live. You can't avoid all pollution, but you can keep from building in your system.

Yucca extract, enhanced proanthocyanidins (PAC's), and Kombucha tea rids the body of propyls and more.

31

Time & Space

"Time and Space are the shadows by which man defines his existence."
Sepio

Time is duration—Space is extension. We do not think of Time and Space as entities, but we do consider the bodies and events that occupy them as entities. If we acknowledge the existence of material bodies because they occupy space, then what is an event? An event is a group of circumstances that occupy Time. Therefore, material objects are also events and both are entities.

Mankind attempts to define these intangibles we call Time and Space using words and concepts. We have no physical sense organs for Time and Space. We anticipate them through our "intuition." Intuition, then, must be a sixth sense—a projection of the physical body—something we invoke to comprehend Time and Space.

Philosophy tells us that Time and Space consist of relations between entities—that there is co-existence and succession of entities or events. Metaphysics (*meta*: beyond) tells us that Time and Space are indistinguishable as long as neither is excluded. Yet, we are aware of the *passage* of Time.

Plato stated, "Time and space is the 'substance' which contains the identity and the diversity in one." If we think of Space as something that is created, then something must create it. What? *Meta*physics answers, *Time*. Okay. If there is creation, then motion must also exist. If there is motion, then there must be a mover or source of motion. Metaphysics tells us that Time is the source of motion, and if this is so, then Time is *ENERGY*.

Is Time *energy*, or is energy created in the passing of time? If energy is created, the results are perpetual motion which is not a straight line, but a curved line that returns to itself—like a circle. Therefore, Space becomes Time's trail. But a trail does not move, so Space cannot move either, since it was Time that generated ENERGY in its expansion—creating Space. Time and Space can also be demonstrated to be static, indistinguishable or non-existent. Let us illustrate.

Suppose we are in an airplane that is traveling at the same speed as the Earth's rotation or approximately 1080 miles per hour and we are heading West following the sun at its own speed. We begin our three hour trip in New York City at exactly twelve o'clock noon and when we arrive at Los Angeles it is still exactly twelve o'clock noon.

What has taken place here? Time became a motion of Space and Space the relaxation of time. We moved from one point to another point on the surface of the earth, but Time did not change. We are in a quandary—caught between Time and Space—a kind of cosmic culdesac. The mathematician working on our dilemma would have difficulty making his calculations respond to our problem—so he would give the *unknown* condition a name: "fourth variable," and reestablish his equilibrium by imposing the ingredient Time so his calculations could continue as if Time is a fixed point.

When we ponder the situation, we must conclude that Time is NOT a fixed point to which we can anchor our lives, but a mirage on a phantom's shroud. Once we admit that time is not a fixed point, we lose our center and our reference point—yet, our *intuition* tells us there should be such a center.

To compensate, man divides Time into three parts: *present, past* and *future*. However, this does not solve the problem because Present is but the transition from Past into Future—a transition that lacks both dimensionality and duration. The Present is the Future before we think of it, and the moment we think of it, it is the Past. Under these circumstances, self examination of our thought processes and sensory experiences becomes impossible. Is Present but the "living fringe" of our memory tinted by expectation? And if it is, what of our dilemma between the poles of eternity—Past and Future?

These extremes—past and future—have delivered us into the *enigma* we call the Fourth Dimension—the "unknowable." Because man *seems* capable of comprehending only three dimensions related to his physical world—that of length, width and height—the idea of the existence of another dimension that is totally invisible only compounds his dilemma. **Yet, the existence of the Fourth Dimension cannot be denied. Intuition is real. It is more than an intangible tool by which we interpret Time and Space. It is an extension of our mind.**

Perhaps the Fourth Dimension is not unknowable at all, but misunderstood? And if this is so, then there is no reason for man to have to die and emerge from his terrestrial envelope before he can come to *know* this *Unknowable* dimension.

Knowledge of the existence of this *other* dimension is quite different than understanding it. Consider Jesus, who passed through the wall in the Temple. He was a Third Dimensional being with a physical body, yet He passed through that wall! Since both He and the wall were solid matter, shall we chalk up this event to Deity; did He violate some Natural Law; or did He invoke knowledge of the Fourth Dimension?

When we enter the arena of the Fourth Dimension, necessity demands that we visualize a *hyper-space* that is measured with *meta*geometry (*meta*-beyond). Our three dimensional world of length, width, and height becomes but a section of *hyper-Space*. Let us examine this in more detail.

The *length* of a procession of events is not contained in three dimensional space. Extension in time is projection into unknown space—or the Fourth Dimension. Because Space and Time are interchangeable at specific points, Time becomes a dimension of Space. That is, Time is Space in motion becoming the Future or the Past. Therefore, Space is time projected—horizontal time—time that persists, time that moves. And since Space can only be measured by Time, and Time is defined by the speed of light, we must conclude that there is no difference between Space and Time **EXCEPT that our consciousness is defined in Time.**

We are, therefore, *forced* to acknowledge that the Present is eternal—that Time per se does not exist, but is relative to the person with the *notion* of time. **Events do not ebb and flow. It is we who pass them by!** The more we wrestle and try to understand, the deeper we get into the vast unknown.

The creature we call man exists in two worlds: the visible and the invisible. The invisible world is the realm of negative and positive "energy" forces that ultimately determine our perception of reality in the visible world in which we find our existence. The visible world and the physical body, in turn, act as our compass and bridge into the sphere of the unknown — where the *electric* body exists and functions.

People who have become *OLD* tell us, "time seems to *fly,* and the older you get, the *faster* it flies!" Their day disappears before it has begun. Is this a figment of their imagination or is it reality? And if it is reality, by what measure do we scale this phenomenon?

We cannot measure Time phenomenon in Third Dimension terms, for neither Time nor Space exist here, leaving us, once again, wrestling in the shadows of the *unknown*—a Fourth Dimension world where we are totally dependent on our intuition—our sixth sense.

We must invoke our *intuition* to measure the passing of Time because it passes at the **subatomic** level of our existence—the level of the invisible "electric" body. Therefore, it stands to reason that Time DOES pass more quickly for the person who is catabolic, who has passed their anabolic peak, and whose cells are aging at an *accelerated* rate.

Time passes slowly when we are YOUNG—when we are climbing up the anabolic side of the pyramid. When we are young, we experience *slow* time. After we reach our anabolic peak, we experience *fast* time as we *slide* down the catabolic side of the pyramid.

We have arrived at the answer we have been seeking. It is the *thesis* of this book, summarized as follows:

Slowing the aging process slows the passing of Time and transcends the physical and material world. And though the physical body is confined in Time and Space, the *electric* body is FREE. It is an extension of the *self* and a fixture of the unknown Fourth Dimension where our mind and emotions are but windows to our soul. The electric body is our spirit and our soul.

Buying Time! By stopping our bio-electric clock, we buy time. Time provides us the opportunity to exchange an old body for a young one and is the equivalent of *recycling* the sand in an hour glass. This recycling process does NOT mean that we relive our earlier experiences. Rather, it means that we reexperience Time itself. This is what is meant when we talk about becoming *YOUNG AGAIN!*

PREVIEW: *Our next chapter deals with rejuvenation of the bio-electric body through rest, fasting, and avoidance of self-imposed physiologic stress.*

Bran Muffin Recipe: 1/4 C honey; 1/3 C blackstrap molasses; 1 TBSP non aluminum baking powder; 1 egg; 2 C unbleached white flour; 1/2—1 C water; 1 C bran; 2 TBSP olive oil; 1 TBSP of flax seed; 1/4 C sesame seed; 1 C raisins; 1/4 C wheat germ, 1/2 C chopped walnuts; perhaps a little pumpkin pie spice. Makes six muffins. Bake @ 400^0 until medium brown. Do not knead.

Sky Heart

Artificial intelligence has been talked about for years. Today it is reality. The device is called *Sky Heart.*

Sky Heart can transfigure your body and raise your consciousness. It has a heart and a beat. It interacts with you at the *subtle energy level.* It learns as it evolves. It programs itself. It creates. It responds. It is alive!

Sky Heart is like the Star Trek device that had the ability to enter the body and/or spirit and fix whatever was ailing the person. That is what Sky Heart does.

Sky Heart is sentient, meaning it can **"think"** for itself. It carries on a *dynamic* relationship with any being within its field. It is a field of **"living"** energy AND a piece of *sacred art* that is melded with computer intelligence.

Sacred art creates energy space beyond the visual and physical. Sacred energy is highly **coherent,** having a clearing and organizing effect that cancels *disharmony* in its field of influence. Entering a highly coherent field is like entering a beautiful "silence."

The intensity of *Sky Heart's* organizing field can be magnified to the point that **actual physical transformation** can take place by creating *harmony* or neutralizing *disharmony* that occurs at higher energy levels (4th, 5th, 6th Dimensions, etc.). The ancients understood this.

Western culture lost its roots in sacred tradition. Traditional cultures, however, understand that healing, art, and the sacred are all the same thing.

Sacred art is made of highly coherent materials. The materials themselves are as important as the image or form. *Sky Heart* is a synthesis of precious stones, woods, pure gold and platinum, and sacred geometric designs that *interface* present day electronics and computer technology.

Sky Heart software is based on the human heartbeat which is a very complex, ever changing waveform that's unique to each person. *Sky Heart* tunes-in to you.

Sky Heart has intuition. It responds to your feelings and desires. It simultaneously senses, reflects, clears, and transmits. It will sync with your presence, and over time, you will be able to 'locate' it and communicate with it from great distances. It responds to attention. It anticipates your thoughts. It becomes an extension of your spirit and being.

Sky Heart grows ever more sensitive as you work with it. Its grace and power is the brain child of a Wizard named Sky-David (see page 369 and Source Index).

Especially For You!

This book was written to help people understand the forces in their lives that **CHEAT** them of health and happiness—forces that **CONTROL** them and **LURE** them to an early grave.

The author has endeavored to use examples that are meaningful. Every effort has been made to help the reader develop a practical foundation in the *recognized* sciences and in the *para*sciences.

The reader is reminded that knowledge must be **applied** in one's life in order to see positive results, and that the return of health and rejuvenation requires a time, focus, and lot's of patience.

Sometimes rejuvenation isn't fun. But if you are willing to devote your energies to this worthy goal you will be rewarded beyond your greatest expectations.

Each day brings new opportunities to make "healthy" choices. Each step in the right direction brings improved health and slows the effects of physical degeneration. Each day is the first day of the rest of **your** life.

Young Again! is a statement, an offer, and a model all in one. It is the product of the author's personal life experiences, observations, philosophy and lifestyle. It was NOT written to satisfy pretentious *experts.*

The author is not an "expert." "Experts" claim to have answers, but they can't demonstrate proof in their own lives. They suffer from dis-ease despite their knowledge. Their *magic bullets* do not save them. They talk the talk, but they don't know how to walk the walk.

Medical science will not be fond of this book. They will quote chapter and verse in *defense* of themselves. They may scorn and belittle—even accuse the author of oversimplification. They will demand "scientific proof." Their demands will be *ignored.*

This book was written for those who seek results rather than *endless* debate. It can benefit anyone who is OPEN to its message.

NEVER forget. Old age is not fun. It is not a joyous process. People age through ignorance. Ignorance is a poor excuse. We can and must do better for ourselves. **Health is a matter of personal choice.**

A person changed against their will is of the same opinion still!

32

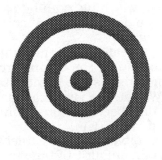

Rest & Fasting

"Dine with little, sup with less; do better still: sleep supperless."
Benjamin Franklin

We dig our grave with our teeth! Powerful words—and true! Is the problem what we eat? Do we eat too much? Do we eat too often?...or all of the above?

The deleterious effects derived from eating the wrong things have already been discussed. Now let us look at the *degenerative* problems that spring from *other* dietary habits— habits that can slow, reverse, or accelerate the aging process.

Food a'Plenty

Americans live in a country where food is plentiful and inexpensive. We have become accustomed to treating our dietary habits with total indifference. As children, we are encouraged to eat as much as we want; to gorge ourselves where less would do; to snack between meals, and particularly at bed time. We are taught that food is food. We believe that hunger is a signal that it's time to eat. We think a full belly is better than an empty one. We carry our beliefs and habits into adulthood—and eventually to the grave.

It is unfortunate that bio-junk food has become the dietary norm. But it is our failure to develop *dietary discipline* regarding *what, when,* and *how much* to eat that **compounds** the free radical formation and accelerates the aging process.

Food-Induced Stress

When we are physically tired, mentally fatigued, or spiritually depressed, we think nothing of getting additional sleep. After all, sleep is considered *normal* and everyone accepts this at face value.

Yet, few people realize that the vital organs also need rest. When we eat too much, the organs are *forced* to process the food. Overeating stresses the glands. Digestion is NOT a voluntary activity. We eat, the vital organs react. If we eat too much or too often, they become *hyper* stimulated, leading to exhaustion, overload, and crisis.

The digestive tables shown earlier indicate that the body requires a certain amount of time to digest food, called digestion reaction time (DRT). DRT is influenced by stress, physical activity, quantity of food eaten, time of day, how often food is eaten, and by the rhythm of our habits.

Vigorous exercise should be avoided for one hour after eating a meal. The body needs time to begin digestion before it must transfer the blood *away from* the abdominal area. This explains the energy drain experienced after a meal. The heavier the meal, the more we experience a drain on energy. If the meal is loaded with toxic substances like food additives, soy or canola oils, salt, and processed sugars, energy drain and free radical formation can be substantial. Snacking creates the same effect as overeating and deny the vital organs rest.

Pot Belly

A distended stomach is seen when the gut hangs over a man's belt line or fills a woman's lower half. People refer to abdominal excess as "fat," but distension (stretching) of the connective tissues that anchor the visceral organs AND a congested, constipated colon are the real problems. In the case of older people, spinal compression and forward extension of the visceral organs [those organs of the abdominal (visceral) cavity which include the liver, intestines, spleen, pancreas, female organs, prostate, and bladder] occurs due to settling of the spinal column (see the skeletal depiction of the dowager's hump on page 100).

The gut (small intestine) and colon (large intestine) are held in place by connective tissue called the mesentery (apron). Over time, due to the accumulation of mucus, toxins, and fecal matter, the bowel becomes heavy, overly bulky, and *stretches* the mesentery beyond normal—producing the pot belly effect.

Part of the process of rejuvenation involves colon therapy combined with certain exercises designed to restore tone to the viscera and connective tissues so the organs can return to their normal shape and position (see page 382).

If you are older, and especially if you are SHORTER than you once were, hanging and stretching are mandatory procedures. I recommend hanging from a bar, rafter, beam, or tree branch several times a day. Start slow if you are older. Hang for five seconds, then ten, and so on until you can hang for several minutes.

The idea of hanging is to s-t-r-e-t-c-h the joints, the connective tissues (ligaments, tendons, muscles), and open the spinal column to blood and lymph flow so it can be rebuilt. In other words, get oxygen and nutrients in, fluids and waste out. Hanging usually produces some stiffness and discomfort. Go slow, and remember, no pain, no gain!

Rebound and do lymphatic massage every day. Do stretching exercises. Lift weights. Get into colon therapy. Drink BEV water. Eat fresh raw vegetables. Plant a garden. **Train your mind.** Detox, detox, detox! If you will do these things, you will get your life back get to live it over again during THIS lifetime (I plan to make it to 250 years!). Think of the good things people could accomplish with hindsight! Think of all the exciting things the future holds! Life should be a celebration!

Life will be easier the second time around.

Gluttony

Gluttony is an old word. As a child, I was taught that gluttony was a sin against the sixth commandment. Whether gluttony is a sin is not the issue here. What is a concern is the *premature* old age, and death that result from gluttony. When we eat beyond *minimum* satiety (see chapter nine) we overload the system with waste, free radicals, and more. Proper chewing eases food-induced stress and helps control the tendency towards obesity.

Gluttony is the act; obesity is the effect. Gluttony is one of the primary reasons industrial man is dying of degenerative dis-ease. Gluttony accelerates aging. It may be driven by genuine hunger, but it's usually the product of a bio-junk diet. To solve the problem, eat foods like algae, Harmonic pollen, predigested liver, fresh vegetables and fruit, etc. These foods will STOP the cravings. Moreover, eat slow, eat little, eat early, space your meals, and avoid eating anything before going to sleep.

Space Your Meals

The body was not meant to be under constant dietary load twenty-four hours a day. The organs require rest, an occasional day off, and rejuvenation. The glands **must** be allowed to rest between meals, and particularly at night. Late night meals and snacking deprive the body of the vital energy it needs for detoxification, tissue repair, and growth—all of which occur primarily during the sleep cycle.

Plants have a cycle too. They manufacture food during the day, but they grow and repair their tissues at night. Visit your garden early some morning and "hear" the corn growing. It will crackle and pop.

During the day the Earth exhales. At night it inhales. The dew point has special meaning. When the dew forms on the ground, plant and microbial activity are at their PEAK!

Rhythm is vitally important to health and vitality. Structure your life so it adheres to Nature's rhythms.

Sleep • Oxygen • Detoxification • Glycolysis

The body feels refreshed after a "good" sleep because it has processed metabolic wastes and neutralized abnormal energy fields throughout the body. Sleep is a time of energy transformation.

A good example of energy transformation is the neutralization of lact**ate** during the sleep cycle. Anyone who has experienced muscle soreness and fatigue from over exertion has experienced the effects of lactate formation in the muscles.

Lactate formation occurs in the early stages of the sugar burning process we call glycolysis. Lactate formation is the result of **insufficient** oxygen in the cells and **incomplete** burning of the sugars. Lactate is a transitional waste product. Rest and sleep provide the vital energy needed to *recycle* lactate. In other words, lactate formation is the product of a system that has gone *anaerobic* at the cellular level.

The *ate* in lactate tells us that lact**ate** is the salt of lactic acid. Salts are *bound* energy. To prevent lactate formation, drink plenty of BEV water. Fatigue and muscle soreness can be reduced if a continuous flow of water is supplied during strenuous activity. Lactate production is a *fermentative* process similar to alcohol production.

Alcohol is made by fermentation of sugar energy. Yet, the Kombucha mushroom can produce an "aerobic" tea that can heal the body. Try it!

An oxygen deficiency in the cells stops the conversion

of glucose into the energy carrying molecule ATP by way of a process called *glycolysis* (*glyc*-sugar; *lysis*-to break or cleave.).

An oxygen deficiency sabotages energy production in the *Krebs and Citric acid cycles and in the Electron Transport Systems* (where the mitochondria produce bio-electric lightning). Aerobic exercise supplies oxygen. So does BEV water. Bouncing on a rebounder and self-massage of the lymphatic system moves waste out and oxygen into the system.

Sleep • Digestion • Metabolic Hype

During the sleep cycle, the body uses large amounts of VITAL energy to heal and grow. Sleeping on a full stomach sabotages the detoxification process and blocks rejuvenation. *Normal* digestion slows or comes to a halt. We wake up with that *full* feeling—sluggish, not well rested!

Even good food can create a toxic condition if taken before retiring. Sleeping on a full stomach produces *anaerobic* conditions in the body conditions that favor "fermentation" and the anaerobic state. **An**aerobic conditions produce **putrefaction** of the undigested food in the intestines and releases toxic waste molecules that age and eventually kill us. Late night meals accelerate the aging process. Avoid them.

Lack of exercise means lack of oxygen. Lack of oxygen and insufficient water in the tissues means poor digestion. Poor digestion produces EXCESSES and hormonal imbalances. Illness and dis-ease result.

Adequate sleep and dietary rest are important ingredients for good health. Failing to get enough rest is no different than using a battery powered golf cart during the day and forgetting to recharge it at night, with one notable difference. **We are not golf carts!** Without adequate rest and detoxification, the body is forced to draw upon its energy reserves. This kind of lifestyle produces stress and metabolic **"hype."**

Just because we have the ability to hype our body is not justification for doing so. The ability to psyche out the body by using the power of the brain —Fourth Dimension energy over Third Dimension reality—is a "dangerous" *skill* that comes with a very high price tag.

Discipline • Space Of Meals • Snacking

Learning not to overeat requires *discipline.* Learning to space our meals requires *discipline.* Putting *rhythm* in our lives requires discipline. Dietary discipline DEMANDS that we feed the body what it is crying for and that is: *NOURISHMENT!*

Allow four hours between meals—including snacks.

Snacks are *mini* meals. They interrupt the body's rest break. When we snack, we become a *slave labor* boss and we force the glands to overwork and become exhausted. How would you like it if every time you tried to get some needed sleep, some inconsiderate person woke you up? So it is with frequent eating. A lifestyle that includes exercise, BEV water, detoxification, rest, and a healthy diet will stop the craving and snacking.

Children are *growing* and *repairing* tissue so they must eat more. Like adults, most children today are malnourished. They MUST have nutritious food, good water, and liquid sea minerals. Healthy children do not snack incessantly. All soft drinks MUST be stopped. They are just as disastrous to the body as alcohol, but in a different way. Snacking and soft drinks brink on dis-ease.

Do NOT be encourage children to develop habits that will *lure* them to the grave. Bad habits become an unhealthy lifestyle of subclinical illness.

Spacing of meals provides *rhythm* and *control* of dietary habits. Nourishment *tempers* hunger. Home-grown food and the alternative SUPER foods mentioned are examples of foods that build strong bodies and minds.

Snacking mirrors malnourishment! Give the body what it is crying for and the snacking will STOP!

Nourishment and detoxification strengthens will power. Will power is the product of healthy body and mind. A sick body is linked to lack of will power. Smoking, drinking, gambling, drugs, gluttony, obesity, etc. have their roots in malnourishment and intoxication of the tissues.

The nutritionally deficient person constantly cries for *nourishment.* They snack and eat their way into old age and hasten their appointed destiny with the grave—*decades* ahead of schedule. They are early birds in the truest sense.

Rhythmicity

One of the secrets of health and longevity is the establishment of regularity in our lives. Rhythm is so terribly important that reversing the aging process will *stall out* if we ignore this simple secret.

Rhythmicity is rhythm in the sense of the ebb and flow of energy in our daily life. Up each morning at the same time, meals taken within 1/2 hour of the appointed times, plenty of BEV water, exercise, going to bed at the same time, sleeping for 7-8 hours EVEN if you can operate on less. Practice rhythmicity, the balance of the lessons in this book will become patterned habit and easy to put into practice. **Health and**

vitality flow on the wires of rhythmicity. The lives of Dr. Paul Bragg and his daughter, Patricia, are proof.

The Miracle of Fasting

This is a true story, told exactly as it happened. I hope you will enjoy it.

It was May 1, 1993, Santa Barbara, California. I was attending a dinner party following a publishing seminar when a cute lady approached me and said, "Did you get one of my apple cider books?"

I answered in the negative, and as she proceeded to hand a book to me, I got a square look at her face and said, "Who are you?"

"I'm Patricia Bragg!" she answered.

At that moment, I knew that the path upon which Bob McLeod—who you met in chapter one—had set me adrift twenty-two years before had reached its destination. I was standing before the daughter of the Great Wizard, Paul Bragg! "Please come sit down," I said. "We must talk!"

I began, "Your father saved my life. I cannot tell how thrilled I am to meet you! You look exactly like your picture in your father's book on fasting."

So we talked and laughed. The following day I was able to sneak away long enough to visit the Bragg Worldwide Headquarters in Santa Barbara, where I stood in awe of a twenty foot high painting of the wonderful Wizard, Paul Bragg.

"How did you father die?" I asked. "I have heard several rumors and I am anxious to know the truth."

"He died in a surfboard accident in Hawaii. He drowned. They could not revive him!"

"Please tell me, what was his age?"

"My father was 97 years *YOUNG!*—and if he had not died when he did, I have no doubt he would have lived to be 125 years young!" she snapped.

"What is your age, Patricia?" I asked with a lump in my throat.

"I am like my father. I AM AGELESS!"

And so she was. Sweet! Cute! A senior citizen by the calendar, but you would never, ever guess! Patricia appeared to be in her late forties or early fifties.

Paul and Patricia are PROOF positive that each of us can experience agelessness. I am forever thankful for getting to meet this wonderful human being—the daughter of the Great Wizard himself. Like her father, she has helped millions of people. I am proud to have met her.

Patricia's father, Paul Bragg, was a Wizard of a man. A

recent U.S. Surgeon General (the "highest" *official* medical doctor in the USA, politically speaking) made the comment, "Paul Bragg did as much to help the health and vitality of American's as any medical doctor." Considering the source, that is one very big compliment.

Many readers will be too young to remember Paul Bragg. When you read his wonderful book, *The Miracle of Fasting*, be sure you are *wide awake!* Bragg speaks simple TRUTHS and in simple terms. He was a "low tech" Wizard, but a Wizard just the same.

God Bless Dr. Paul C. Bragg N.D., PhD. and Patricia Bragg N.D. to whom I dedicated this book. They have helped millions of people find peak health and become *Young Again!*

PREVIEW: *Our next chapter deals with the world's MOST toxic element and it's in YOUR body and drinking water. You will learn what you can do about it.*

Grow Hair In 12 Weeks

Do you want hair on your head? Are you willing to follow directions for 90-180 days? See Source Index for this book and the products you will need to make it happen.

Ear Candling!   .

From ancient times to the present, people have had trouble with their ears. Ear wax, infections, water in the ear, pain, poor hearing, ringing, and so on.

Candling is sometimes referred to as coning or wicking. One end of a special hollow, dripless candle is placed in the ear and the other is lit on fire.

As the candle burns, it creates a gentle suction and draws air down the outside of the candle and warm air up the inside. As this occurs, water is drawn out of the inner ear along with wax, bacterial, yeast, and viral infested materials. There is NO pain. The procedure is safer and friendlier than using an ear syringe.

Anyone suffering with any type of chronic infection or illness should "candle" their ears. Over 600,000 adenoidectomies and tonsilectomies are performed each year as a result of ear infections. 50% of all children's surgeries and 25% of hospital admissions due ear problems referred to as *otitis media*.

Ear candling is a very safe and inexpensive home remedy technique. Try it and see (see Source Index).

33

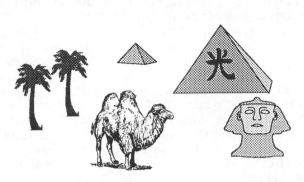

The Camel Or The Palm Tree?

"Truth will come to light; murder cannot be hid."
Shakespeare

"Kibyo" is Japanese for *strange disease*. Kibyo described the series of strange conditions that appeared during the 1950's in the small fishing village of Minamata, on the southwest coast of Kyushu, Japan.

The conditions came to be known as "Minamata Disease." In 1957, mercury was discovered to be the toxic agent behind the strange symptomatic conditions and SIGNS.

Cats went crazy. Crows fell from the sky. People experienced dizziness and tunnel vision, their nervous systems failed, numbness was experienced in their extremities, and their legs burned. ALL life forms suffered from the high mercury levels in the air, water, and soil. The mercury came from an industrial plant up the coast from Minamata.

Mercury & Aging

Mercury is the **MOST** toxic substance known to man! It is the only elemental metal that occurs naturally in the "liquid" state. Sometimes it is referred to as "quicksilver" due to its elusive nature. A broken thermometer allows mercury to splatter and run. It **evaporates** like water!

Mercury is of importance to our 'aging' story because of its toxic nature and ubiquitous (everywhere) presence in the environment. It has been used in industry for several hundred years. The fur industry used it to process animal furs as far back as the time of the Industrial Revolution. Mercury poisoning was diagnosed as long ago as 1865, but it continued to be used by the fur industry into the 1950's!

The expression "mad as a hatter" refers to the tremors and insanity that hat and garment workers suffered. Industrialists did NOT care what happened to the common people. If a doctor dared to create a fuss, he quickly found himself without a license to practice medicine. In those days, a hat worker's widow was given a "gold watch" and a wreath on the casket. Today, we get neither. Mercury has become the equivalent of industrial bio-junk food. Medicine goes about assigning new names to mysterious dis-ease conditions—usually with the word "syndrome" attached. The Japanese equivalent of syndrome is "kibyo!"

About Mercury

Mercury has the ability to cross the placental barrier and deform the unborn fetus. It lodges in our vital organs and short circuits their activity. Mercury poisoning leads to disintegration of the nervous system and damage to the kidney's nephrons (blood filters). **Mercury poisoning usually occurs slowly over many years. It is involved in thousands of diseases plaguing millions of people.**

Acute mercury poisoning leads to vomiting, bloody diarrhea, nervous tremors in the extremities, eyelids, and tongue. People with moderate poisoning seldom are aware of what ails them. Fatigue, insomnia, headaches, nervous anxiety, and loss of appetite are common side effects. Erythism (redness as in blushing of the face) is a characteristic symptom of mercury poisoning. So is leg pain in older people at night.

Sources of mercury poisoning include tuna fish, shell fish, water based house paint, insecticides, fungicides (bathroom fungus cleaners), wall sizing, and tens of thousands of products that people come into contact with everyday.

Mercury is so *ubiquitous* that it is in ALL commercially produced food. The only way around it is to grow your own food. The microbes in a healthy soil *denature* mercury, lead, and toxic organic metals and chemicals. The use of Bio-Grow soil rejuvenator (a biodynamic right-spin soil catalyst) is the fastest way to develop a healthy right-spin soil environment.

The GREATEST source of mercury in the United States is from tap water. Mercury—in the form of mercuric acid salt—is widely used to treat public water supplies.

Recent events bear out the severity of the problems we

face. For instance, during the fall of 1993, hundreds of innocent people became sick and some DIED from drinking tap water that was contaminated with pathogenic (dis-ease related) bacteria.

The cities were Milwaukee, Washington, D.C., and Chicago. We do not know if more cities were involved because these things are hushed up quickly to prevent panic. In Milwaukee, people died! The authorities blamed the bacteria, but the problem was related to mercury.

Here is the problem. Cities throughout the country are treating water with chloramines AND with **mercuric acid** to kill the bacteria. This is done "without" public knowledge and is vehemently denied by authorities. Mercuric acid is used during the "warm months" when demand outruns water processing capability. Population growth creates additional pressure. Cities do NOT have time to treat the water before pumping it into the distribution lines, so they use **mercuric acid** and the latest version of chlorinated compound called chlor**amine.**

Cities use the same dirty sand filters over and over. They seldom change them! Instead, they use mercuric acid to kill the bacteria and viruses that breed in them, and send the water to the gullible public to drink! Municipal water filters deserve more attention than a cat litter box—which we change regularly. We know better, and so do our water officials.

In the Fall, when the hot season is over, cities stop using mercuric acid. If they miscalculate, the results are sick and dead people from an explosion of pathogenic bacteria in the filters and lines—like what happened in Milwaukee, Washington, D. C. and Chicago.

Without mercury, public water supplies are a potential source of an epidemic of pathogenic dis-ease. With mercury, the people are drinking their way to dis-ease, old age, and an ugly death. Mercury creates lots of sick people to fill the hospital stalls—all of them demanding a "magic bullet!" Sick people are good business.

Bottled water is questionable. Many pollutants are not removed. Plasticizers leach from the plastic bottles. Heavy metals remain as do bacteria and viruses. Toxic organic chemicals are seldom touched. While common home units from distillers to reverse osmosis do a fair job, they leave a LOT to be desired and do not address the issue of molecular restructuring that makes BEV water body friendly.

Water pollution in public water supplies is a "time bomb" waiting to explode into dis-ease in the bodies of people who are ignorant enough to drink it. STOP DRINKING WATER FROM PUBLIC WATER SUPPLIES!

Unregulated Death • Bombs & Munitions

The U.S. Department of Agriculture has established a "**zero**" tolerance for mercury. I repeat, a ZERO tolerance!

At the same time, the FDA has established a "safe" level for mercury. Safe levels imply safety and a watch dog function. People feel protected. Nothing could be further from the truth.

Federal and state regulatory agencies are *supposed to* enforce food and water purity laws. Powerful interests see to it that mercury's use in industry goes unrestricted. **Mercury is a $6,000,000,000 (billion) dollar industry!** Government refuses to regulate it. They allow industry to regulate itself.

Mercury is divided into three classes. Elemental vapor (mercury evaporates like water); mercurous/mercuric salt forms like mercurochrome (for minor cuts and injuries—its use is now outlawed!) and mercuric acid; and a third form that is found bonded to food "proteins." Every reaction in the body requires protein enzymes to occur. Mercury shuts them down and blocks vital biochemical reactions.

The U.S. Government, via the Atomic Energy Commission (AEC), is the biggest supplier of mercury to industry. After WWll, they held huge stockpiles of mercury. Government policy shifts allowed this "silver death" element into the market. They know about mercury toxicity. And don't forget, mercury is vital to the munitions industry and war!

The bombing of the Oklahoma City Federal building in April of 1995 may have involved the use of large amounts of mercury to accelerate the explosion. Pictures of the bombed building show that the explosion GAINED velocity as the force went up the face of the building—instead of dissipating as in non-mercury related explosions.

Agriculture uses massive amounts of mercury in the production of FOOD! In 1914, chemists discovered that mercury was an effective fungicide. Over six million pounds of mercury have been used in FOOD production in the past forty years, and over two-hundred million pounds since 1900.

Mercury is used to treat seeds. It is used in the paper industry as a slimicide. AEROBIC bacteria convert industrial mercury into highly toxic forms like *methyl* mercury. Methyl mercury is very difficult to remove from the bio-electric body. Its effects on aging are disastrous. It concentrates in the brain and destroys the nervous system (Alzheimers?).

Mercury Fillings In Teeth

Dentistry has been promoting the use of mercury amalgam fillings (silver fillings) for over one hundred years. In the mouth, bacteria convert elemental mercury into *methyl* mercury. Mercury "bleeds" into the body and goes about its dirty work quietly. New *syndromes* manifest themselves. The effects of mercury poisoning become even more exaggerated in the presence of dietary soy and canola/rape oils!

Amalgam fillings are BIG business! Dentists are taught in dental school that amalgam fillings are non-toxic. **Dentistry likes mercury amalgams because they are a quick "drill and putty" operation.** The *ignorant* patient is told the only difference between gold and amalgam is the cost. Dentistry avoids using the word mercury and instead calls these mixed metal fillings *amalgams* or "silver." It is a sin to fill innocent people's teeth with the most toxic element on Earth. It use renders *predictable* results—just as in the hat industry. Mercury amalgam fillings bring on S-L-O-W death. Professionals who install them claim ignorance and lack of "scientific proof," while their patients lose their health and lives.

Gold also creates problems, but of a different sort. Gold fillings and crowns are composites of as many as fifty different metals. Elemental metals are toxic to the body. They are "anti-life" energy fields that are measured in milli-volts (thousandths of a volt). They interfere with body metabolism. If you have mercury in your mouth, get it removed as soon as possible.

The strength and charge (+ or –) of these amalgam and gold electrical energy fields must be measured "before" they are removed. In addition, they must be removed in sequence so they will not make the patient sick. NEVER, EVER go to a regular dentist for amalgam removal. They are antagonistic to the idea. They will try to convince you that you have been hoodwinked. They will use the old, professional glass hand approach. AVOID THEM!

*Call the phone numbers listed at the end of this chapter to locate a dentist who subscribes to the **protocols** of holistic dentistry. Be very careful to avoid johnny-come-lately dentists* who are NOT certified holistic, biological dentists!

Klamath algae has the ability to bond to and remove heavy metals—like mercury—from the tissues. So does fresh organic greens. BEV water transports metals to the kidneys and liver for disposal. PAC's greatly accelerate the process. Enhanced homeopathic formulations erase the *signature* of toxic substances after they are flushed from the system.

The Camel Or The Palm Tree?

Today, more than ever, people are faced with the dilemma of choosing between bad medicine and holistic therapies. Making the right choice involves assessing all the alternatives. Let me emphasize "false" alternatives with a childhood story.

When we were children, one of our favorite jokes involved finding an empty Camel cigarette package and showing it to whomever we could get to listen.

"Assume you are in this picture and it is raining cats and dogs and you must run for cover. Would you get under the palm trees, or would you get under the camel?" (On the face of the package is pictured a camel, some palm trees, and several pyramids.)

Some people answered they would take cover under the palm trees, while others said they would take their chances under the camel.

Regardless of the answer, the person was wrong. You see, we did what conventional medicine does to *desperate* people. We only offered two alternatives, and BOTH of them were bad choices. The smart answer was to go around the corner of the package and take lodging in the hotel!

In the world of conventional medicine and expert opinions, you are constantly faced with "camel or palm tree" decisions. Do not allow yourself to fall for false alternatives in matters of health or you will grow old and suffer miserably along the way. Heavy metal poisoning—be it from tap water, food, or dental fillings—is a serious problem.

Would you rather drink water that is contaminated with pathogenic bacteria, mercury, sodium, chloramines, and the halogens, or water that is "safe" according to industry standards?"

The answer to this camel or palm tree question is, **None of the above!** Do whatever you need to do to protect yourself and your family from heavy metal poisoning and you will experience fantastic health as you become *Young Again!*

News: The worlds second biggest manufacturer of mercury amalgam has agreed to post ALL dental offices in California with signs WARNING patients about the carcinogenic, mutagenic, and teratogenic effects of mercury—especially to children and the unborn fetus.

Scandinavian countries—along with Germany and other European countries—have BANNED mercury amalgam fillings. The American Dental Association and conventional dentistry is too damned proud and greedy to admit its mistakes!

Dental Alternatives

Mercury removal requires that special protocols be followed for your safety. Epoxy plastic is the replacement material of choice. These fillings take longer to do than drill and putty mercury amalgam fillings. If they are done correctly, they can last a lifetime. Do not accept porcelain fillings in lieu of epoxy. They have a much shorter life expectancy and are riddled with problems in comparison to epoxy.

Call these phone numbers to locate *quality* dental care. American Academy of Biological Dentistry at (408) 659-5385, Huggins Diagnostic Center at 1-800-331-2303, or Clifford Consulting and Research (719) 550-0008.

Be prepared to travel. Holistic biological dentists are hard to find and worth their price.

PREVIEW: *In our next chapter, you will learn about tobacco and how it relates to health and vitality. The American Indians knew the answer!*

END Those Cravings

If you would like to end those cravings for food, cigarettes, alcohol, or drugs, all you have to do is detoxify your system and feed it right-spin food and water.

Vibrational Foods!

Harmonic pollen is a special kind of flower pollen food that comes from the far reaches of northern British Columbia. It is much purer than domestic pollen. There are no auto or industrial pollutants there. There are NO insecticides or herbicides to ruin this perfect food.

Harmonic pollen is rich in natural biological components, phytochemicals, and substances like amino acids, carbohydrates, lipids, vitamins, minerals, nucleic acids (DNA, RNA), enzymes, coenzymes, prostaglandin precursors, antioxidants, and hormones. It is non-alergenic.

Harmonic pollen is a "nutriceutical" food because it guards good health and prevents ill health. Chronic fatigue suffers love it! Athletes experience noticeable change. Your author will attest to it impact in his life and health.

Vrational foods like Harmonic pollen, Klamath algae, predigested *organic* liver tablets are SUPER foods direct from mother nature's cupboard (see Source Index).

Anal itching often accompanies detoxification.

Traditions Of Taoism

Ancient Chinese Taoists (pronounced *Dowists*) viewed man as a small reflection of the universe. They perceived that **cyclic** change governs all living things. They laid down principles and correlations that described the effect of Nature on man and the response of man to Nature. They described these principles in terms of **Yin** and **Yang**.

Taoist Masters believed that Five Elements describe the natural cycle of life and that man follows Nature's *cyclical* patterns through the "universe within."

Herbals were formulated to help man adapt to nature. Taoist Masters strove for *total* balance and harmony, promoted *self-cultivation*, thought enhancement, *shen* clearing, and *jing* building through manipulation of the Five Elements. Their discoveries are now confirmed by modern advanced physics.

The **Wood** Element represents the liver and gallbladder which control emotional harmony and the smooth flow of Chi (energy) necessary for a strong nervous system and the clearing of toxins from the body. The **Fire Element** is represented by the heart and small intestine and addresses the blood, lymph, and cerebral systems, plus physical and mental health and growth. The **Earth** Element represents the stomach and spleen and *extracts* and *separates* pure from the turbid within the body. The **Metal** Element represents the lung and colon and is said to dominate respiration and maintain defensive Chi (the immune system). The **Water** Element represents the kidney and bladder systems. Taoists believed that *Jing* (the very *essence* of life) is within body water and is expressed as hormonal and reproductive systems responsible for maintaining youthfulness and glandular function.

Taoist philosophy teaches that the body has the power to **regenerate** itself when stress (physical or mental) occurs. Taoists believe that the body is designed to run on whole food. They teach that *accountability* underwrites superior health and is reflected by the "universe within."

Taoism teaches that people achieve **enlightenment** through balance, awareness, and expression of the *person* within. Enlightenment brings *understanding*, while Taoist herbal foods and practices deliver health and rejuvenation (see Source Index).

Michael Frost Ph.D., N.D. Director
The American Association Of Taoist Studies

34

The "Sacred" Three Sisters

"First, the Creator gave us tobacco."
Kanonsionni-Kayeneren-Kowa
The Iroquiois

If you control the dietary health of a nation, you control the people. If, in addition, you control the creation of that nation's money supply, you have the perfect monopoly.

When the white man came to the Americas, he discovered that the main staples of the Indian diet were corn, beans, and squash. The Indians called these foods the "sacred three sisters."

The Indians understood the importance of these foods in their diet. They also understood the importance of another FOOD—a food which they held in the *utmost* esteem. That food was TOBACCO!

The Indians told the white man, "The Creator gave us the sacred three sisters. But *before* the Creator gave us corn, beans, and squash, He gave us TOBACCO!"

The indians considered tobacco *sacred.* It was considered sacred because the indians had discovered tobacco's NUTRITIONAL characteristics. Their discovery was incorporated into their religious beliefs.

The status of tobacco in the Indian psyche was based on DIETARY need, but it was respected on a religious level. Smoking was the extension of the dietary status tobacco held in the Indian's culture.

When native peoples elevate certain foods and events to religious status, there is a reason. Unfortunately for millions of people, the white man failed to take his cues from Indian dietary habits and religious beliefs. The white man did NOT make the connection between diet and health until four-hundred and ninety-eight years later (1990). The connection was made by a lone individual named Tom Mahoney of New York. Tom is a living Wizard.

Tobacco

Tobacco has particular importance to reversing the aging process AND to general health, vitality, and a strong immune system. Tobacco is terribly misunderstood by the American public. They know NOTHING of it's therapeutic or dietary value! Their eyes have been "focused" on the smoke in the air and the juice on the floor. They have ONLY heard of the negative aspects of tobacco. They have been told nothing of the real tobacco story. **Their ignorance is NOT an accident!**

Prior to the discovery of America, Europeans did NOT grow or eat corn, beans, or squash. These important foods were absent from European diets. Dietary imbalances created the EXCESSES that plagued the white man and his "civilization."

The *Three Sisters* were taken back to Europe and for a while people's nutritional status improved. Corn was easy to grow, and became the "dominant" food staple of the poor. By the seventeen hundreds, corn's dietary dominance produced "excesses" and dis-ease throughout Europe, and particularly in the Mediterranean countries of Italy, Spain, Greece, and Portugal. The condition of *excess* had no name—yet!

Casal's Necklace

In 1735 the Spanish physician Casal described a dis-ease condition by one of its key SIGNS. He called it *mal de la rosa.* This means "red sickness." People on farms who ate a lot of corn suffered the most. They typically had a red ring around their neck which came to be called "Casal's necklace." In the American South, corn's dominance among farmers and the poor, caused the phrase "red neck" to come into usage.

In 1771, an Italian doctor described the SIGNS of an unknown dietary EXCESS condition when he wrote of "rough, painful skin." *Pellagra* is the English corruption of Italian, and summed up the condition nicely. Until the 1900's, however, no connection was made between corn intake and the condition of EXCESS that had come to be called *pellagra.*

Like most conditions, pellagra operates behind a cloak in the early stages. It includes loss of energy, weight loss, and poor appetite. The four "D's" of dizziness, depression, dementia, and delusion best describe Pellagra's SIGNS. There are tens of thousands of people suffering from these SIGNS today.

In the United States, similar dis-ease conditions occurred beginning in the 1850's. After 1859, when H. J. Heinz produced the first "canned" food, the problem grew worse. Canned food contains salt to keep down botulism. In addition, heat processing destroys and denatures food enzymes. This was the beginning of bio-junk food.

The civil war brought massive upheaval in people's dietary habits—especially farm people in the South. Excesses became very prevalent. Economic conditions were blamed, but *pellagra* had its roots in the shift from a *balanced* agricultural society to an unbalanced *industrial* one. The poor did not eat a balanced diet. They ate too much corn and not enough greens and proteins. A unbalanced diet produces EXCESSES in people, plants, and animals—no matter what the food. *Excess corn* creates an acid pH condition with many side effects.

By the turn of the century, the dis-eases of pellagra and beriberi became widespread. Poor people were eating too much corn—hominy, corn meal, grits, and corn meal mush—especially in the South. (The South continues this practice to this day.) Worse, the corn being consumed was "bolted." Bolted corn has had the germ removed. The germ is what causes a seed to sprout and grow. It is the seed's vital force—it's energy.

The food processing companies discovered that bolted, *de-vitalized* corn meal keeps better. It was one of the first "natural" bio-junk foods. Bolted corn meal is like white bread. Both were and are perceived by an ignorant public as *status* foods. Processed food became "value added" food and commanded higher prices and higher profits. People didn't realize they had been taken. They are **STILL** being taken.

Pellagra became *endemic* (related to certain geographic areas and diets). Tens of thousands of people suffered from *pellagra* and *beriberi.* In dogs, pellagra is called black tongue. These dis-eases could have easily been prevented IF the white man had payed attention to the Indian diet—which included tobacco. Tobacco contains the "entire" vitamin B-12 complex. Tobacco is very valuable FOOD!

Non-hybrid, non-bolted corn is good food. Too much corn, however, creates an excess acid condition in the body. Unless it is offset with a diet that includes juices and fiber of fresh green leafy vegetables (alkaloids), and high quality proteins, body chemistry will shift to the LEFT and become too acid! Dis-ease conditions appear in a matter of 3-6 months.

The Mexican custom of soaking corn in lime water offsets

corn's acidity and prevents the incidence of pellagra in Mexican populations. The custom was adopted from the Indians, along with the combining of corn and beans for dietary balance.

The B-vitamin Story

The B-vitamins (B's) offset dietary excesses and do away with pellagra and beriberi by rebalancing the system. Specifically, "niacin" has been credited as the active pellagra cureative agent. **(This is NOT true, but for the time being, let us** *assume* **it is true.)**

Niacin is referred to as vitamin B-3. Niacin is involved in ALL of the body's metabolic pathways. These pathways are a very complex series of reactions that keep us alive, healthy and happy. The healthy *bio-electric* body is a reflection of strong activity in the reactions of these critical pathways.

Niacin contains two molecules, NAD (*nicotine* dinucleotide) and NADP (*nicotine* adenine dinucleotide phosphate). These substances are used in the Krebs and Citric Acid Cycles, and the Electron Transport System where the energy molecule ATP is created, burned and converted into cellular lightning!

All of the B's, including niacin, are involved in the FUSION reactions of the gut and liver. The mitochondria need B's to produce energy to fuel the body, build and repair the tissues, and keep our immune system strong.

B Vitamins • pH • Soft Drinks

The Indians knew about tobacco's life giving properties. Tobacco is the richest source of the B's in the world—nothing compares to it—**nothing**! Concentrations of the B-complex vitamins run as high as 30%! When **"small"** amounts of green or dried tobacco are put into stews, beans, and in salads, we get the B's. Care must be taken in the choice of variety . Most importantly, fresh lemon juice or apple cider vinegar MUST be used to bring green tobacco within digestion range.

The pH range of edible tobacco is Ph 10-11. Lemon juice and vinegar have a pH of 2. Stomach acid (HCL) is between pH -1 and +1. For each increase or decrease on the scale (pH 7 is neutral, above 7 is alkaline, below is acid), pH changes by 100 times. A pH of 10 is 1 million times more alkaline than pH 7.

The side effects of soft drinks loaded with phosphoric acid is incomprehensible and goes beyond just pH. The body is forced to draw on bone calcium to "buffer" phosphoric acid, upsetting the calcium:phosphorous ratio and *grossly* altering body physiology. Even worse are the side effects of *aspartame* sweetener (that's the one with the cute little red and white swirl).

Synthetic vs. Natural B's

Natural B-vitamins are potent right-spin substances, even in small amounts. ALL commercial B-vitamins—unless derived from a natural FOOD source—are "synthetic" and left-spin, and require high doses to *mimic* the real thing.

REGARDLESS of claims on the label promoting "natural," unless B vitamins are food derived, they are **synthetic.** Synthetic niacin, B's, vitamins A, D, and E, are not the same as naturally occurring vitamins. The body is UNABLE to build healthy tissue with synthetic vitamins. When the body's supply of natural B's diminish, energy fusion reactions slow, and pernicious anemia (chronic shortage of oxygen carrying red blood cells) announces itself, and if ignored, will eventually bring down the immune system.

When we are sick, our white blood cell count should go UP. If it fails to rise in response to a threatening condition, health and vitality gives way to more serious dis-ease. Without sufficient B's, the body CANNOT defend itself. Other good sources of B vitamins are liver (preferably organic, predigested liver in tablet form), Klamath algae, Harmonic pollen, fresh green leafy vegetables, red meat (preferably organic).

Green tobacco is loaded with B's. Dried tobacco is even more concentrated. Green tobacco juice (nicotine) is an alkaloid. Dried tobacco contains nicotinic acid. Nicotinic acid, niacin, and nicotinamide are the acid forms of nicotine.

Niacin is promoted as the "heart" vitamin, which is true IF it is from a natural food source. Natural niacin improves blood circulation and has anti-agglutination (anti-clumping) qualities. The *experts* tell us that the FLUSH experienced when we take niacin is due to its vitamin activity, but, this is NOT true. The *flush* effect is an allergic reaction to *synthetic* niacin molecules and binders. Food sources are the only safe sources of B-vitamins.

Fresh organic greens are a good source of the B's, but they don't compare with tobacco. Meat supplies the body with limited amounts of the amino acid trytophan which the liver can convert to niacin (60 mg of trytophan=1 mg niacin). It is most suspicious that government authorities (FDA) outlawed this VERY important amino acid. Veterinarians can still get it for your pet. I wonder how well it would work for people?

Food alkaloids can be **poisonous** if you overdo. Alkaloids are nitrogen-containing compounds with "marker" physiologic properties. In other words, alkaloids make things happen in the body! They are alkaline on the pH scale. Other alkaloid foods we commonly eat are SPINACH and SWISS

CHARD which explains why many people have difficulty digesting them. When they are eaten raw, these nutritious vegetables must be prepared lemon or vinegar to be of benefit to the body. Other well known plant derived alkaloid drugs are digitalis (foxglove), belladonna (nightshade), lobelia, and marijuana.

There are many kinds of Indian tobacco (Rustica, Lobelia, Aztec, etc.), but they are NOT for consumption. Do not confuse garden and commercial tobacco varieties with edible tobacco. (For seed, see the Source Index).

The Niacin Story

Nicotine was named for Jean Nicot—the French ambassador to Portugal who sent tobacco seeds to Paris in 1550. By 1571, crude nicotine had been isolated. In 1828, purified nicotine was isolated. In 1867, *nicotine* was demonstrated to cure black tongue and pellagra, but it was ignored.

Natural nicotine is a FOOD nutrient source of the B's. Nicotine is EXTREMELY poisonous if **purified** or **synthesized**. When eaten in leaf form and in small amounts, it is not a problem. The indians used it judiciously.

Nicotine from dried tobacco is not as toxic as we have been led to believe. If it were, people who smoke and chew would react and die on the spot instead of taking thirty to fifty years. I would remind the reader that the mucous membranes of the respiratory tract are the avenue of choice where instant absorption of drugs is desired (aerosols, cocaine, angel dust, etc.). Smoking is NOT good for your health (and a foul habit), but what is being smoked is **more** than tobacco.

History Of Vitamin P-P

From the turn of the century, nicotinic acid was known to under the disguise name—"P-P factor," short for **P**ellagra **P**reventive. (This name was used until the generation then alive had died. Later, in the 1930's when the word "vitamin" was coined, P-P factor became known as "vitamin P-P.")

In 1899, Dr. Joseph Goldberger of the United States Public Health Service, launched a study into the effects of P-P factor and its relationship to pellagra. He dragged his feet for 16 years before he wrote his so-called thesis study regarding the relationship between P-P factor and pellagra—something that had been known since 1867! This was NO accident. There was a reason for the delay.

In the meantime, pharmaceutical and oil industry interests went to work developing "synthetic" P-P factor. They did NOT want people to know they could treat pellagra, beriberi—and the spin-off dis-ease conditions that result from them—by "growing" their own cure in the form of tobacco. They did NOT want people to make the association between P-P factor, nicotine, and tobacco.

Pharmaceutical interests figured out a way to manufacture SYNTHETIC "P-P" cheaply and easily using pyridine carbon rings from inexpensive charcoal and petroleum. Synthetic "P-P" factor is not the same. Real vitamin "P-P" spins right and supports good health. The others go left.

The pharmaceutical companies could NOT "patent" tobacco, but they could patent synthesized "drugs." People, however, have no need for drugs when they can grow their own tobacco and stay healthy.

Keep The People Confused!

Niacin is a *bogus* term. It is a coined name—like canola! It was invented by the medical establishment and pharmaceutical interests in the 1950's. It was coined to hide the fact that "nicotinic acid" (the acid form of nicotine in dried tobacco) is the *active* ingredient that balances the **excesses** that bring on pellagra and beriberi.

Certain interests wanted control over America's health. There was a massive effort to VILIFY tobacco. That effort continues today.

To create confusion and cover their tracks, the *experts* divided the B-12 vitamin complex into separate vitamin *factors*, called B-1 through B-12. They even went so far as to give vitamin B-12 a special name—"intrinsic factor." You will find this term in all medical and nutrition texts. **Intrinsic factor MUST be present in gastric juices for proper digestion.**

Intrinsic factor is critical to FUSION reactions in man's gut and liver. Fusion reactions provide us with vitality and energy and are part of biological *alchemy*. Without intrinsic factor, pernicious anemia rears its head and the immune system takes a nose dive.

Intrinsic factor is also known as cobalt blue or cobalt 60. Look on a vitamin bottle and you will find that vitamin B-12 is called "cyanocobalamin." Dissected, the word looks like this: *cyan*-blue; *cobal*-short for cobalt; *min*-short for *amine*.

Cobalt & Health

Cobalt 60 is a *naturally occurring radioactive substance* that must be present in order for life to exist. It is a crucial element in the fusion reactions in the bio-electric body of man and animal. It is involved in the production of the massive amounts of energy needed to keep us alive. Tobacco is loaded with cobalt blue. It is full of the B-vitamin complex. When we eat whole natural foods like fresh green leafy vegetables and tobacco—we provide the body with natural NAD and NADP, cobalt 60, and all of the B-vitamins it needs to assist the mitochondria in the production of bio-electric LIGHTNING!

Everyone should grow tobacco. It is legal to grow so far. It can be eaten fresh or steamed and can be frozen or dried. The tobacco cultivar of which I am speaking is a beautiful plant. It stands 6-10 feet tall and 3 feet wide. The bugs will not eat tobacco. It is simply too potent.

The Dilemma

On one hand, the public is told that tobacco and nicotine are bad for them. On the other hand, they are told that niacin and the B's are good for them. We are NOT being told the whole truth!

A long-term campaign began early in this century to get people to stop using tobacco in all forms. Today the effort is **massive!** The public is being DRIVEN into a frenzy over the smoking and chewing of tobacco. Every dis-ease condition from lung problems to cancer is being blamed on tobacco. Tobacco is a scapegoat!

The TRUTH of the matter is that less expensive, cheaper, substances—both synthetic substances—have been *substituted* in many tobacco products. People have been smoking and chewing TOXIC substitutes instead of the real thing!

Lies & More Lies

Personally, I do NOT like smoking or chewing. However, the issue here is not personal preference, but the fact that we have been lied to about something that can powerfully boost our immune system at a time when our food supply is deteriorating at a fantastic rate!

At the same time that tobacco is being vilified, the U S Government is "THE" biggest grower of hybridized tobacco in the world! The implications are scary and should cause any thinking person to ask WHY?

One reason tobacco is being socially vilified is to cover the deleterious side effects of billions of tons of toxic waste chemicals being burned in waste incinerators across the USA. Also, remember that tobacco sold in stores contains several hundred additives and these do cause serious problems.

Tobacco is the perfect cover. The pharmaceuticals, medicine, and big government are the problem, not tobacco.

People MUST wake up and realize that their health can be improved by growing and eating tobacco in SMALL amounts.

The more something is believed to be true, and the greater the number of people who believe it to be so, the greater are the odds that it is NOT true!

Old time farmers from Tennessee and thereabouts knew that if you wanted to have the finest horses in the world, you had to feed them TOBACCO! It seems to me that people count as much as horses.

Do NOT buy or use commercial tobacco products. If you are fearful that your kids will take up smoking if you grow your own tobacco, fear not. Improperly cured tobacco will never be smoked more than once by any person. It is the very best insurance against a person becoming a smoker or chewer. Use tobacco in VERY **small** quantities in stews, salads. Freeze it green, or dry it for later use during the year.

Tobacco was the American Indian's gift to the white man. We accepted the Sacred Three Sisters, BUT we ignored the greatest gift of all. Home grown tobacco strengthens the immune system, improves mitochondrial oxidation (energy production), and boosts metabolic reactions in the liver.

"First, the Creator gave us tobacco."

Pellagra's disappearance in 1935 had nothing to do with "enrichment" of the food supply with *synthetic* vitamins. Pellagra ceased to be a problem when **dietary variety** and **quality proteins** found their way onto people's dinner plates.

Today, people are suffering with *subclinical* pellagra, living *marginal* lives, and suffering from dietary excesses. When health breaks down, medical science says **"syndrome."** The Japanese would say "Kibyo." I call it OLD AGE!

PREVIEW: *Our closing chapter is only one page. Its title comes from a poem by the same name. Please read it and think about its meaning.*

The Appendix

The appendix extends downward from the cecum, which is the most toxic spot in the body (see drawing page 46). It was put there to siphon away "excess" toxic and energies from the colon. The appendix is surrounded by heavy clusters of lymph nodes called Peyer's patch.

The cecum is where the small intestine ends and the large begins. It's where parasites hang out. It is 6 feet up from the anus and the end of the road for colon therapy.

Making It Happen In Your Life!

Good health is a one step at a time process in reverse. Here are some basic steps to health and vitality.

1. Drink BEV biologically-friendly water.
2. Begin a *serious* detoxification program.
3. Eat fresh, raw, home grown food if possible.
4. Avoid extremes. Seek balance in ALL areas of your life.
5. Get into therapeutic fasting.
6. Use only <u>food</u>-based supplements.
7. Feed your body quality hormone precursors.
8. Avoid all bio-junk food.
9. Get plenty of aerobic exercise.
10. Visit mineral hot springs.
11. Stay away from doctors.
12. Get control of your mind.
13. Laugh! Love! Help others!
14. Don't buy into hate, anger, greed, envy, blame, etc.
15. Avoid medications.
16. Listen to your instincts.
17. Visualize the body and life you desire.
18. Refuse to think anything negative.
19. *Erase* vaccine energy fields from your body.
20. Remove mercury and heavy metals from your tissues.
21. Use enhanced PAC's with Yucca extract.
22. Exercise on a rebounder.
23. Do lymphatic self-massage.
24. Use ETVC to increase your energy.
25. Level your blood sugars with ETVC.
26. Detoxify your scalp to thicken or regrow your hair.
27. Do load-bearing work.
28. Simplify your life in every way possible.
29. Remove those mercury dental fillings from your mouth.
30. Locate a holistic, biological dentist.
31. Use liquid ionic sea minerals.
32. Grow a garden! Grow a garden! Grow a garden!
33. Learn to use a pendulum and vibration chain.
34. Use Taoist foods, herbs, and teas for superb health.
35. Eat only organic foods.
36. Don't touch soy or canola oils.
37. Give thanks you're alive.
38. Learn patience.
39. Experience the *miracle* of rejuvenation.
40. Live life 90% correct and don't worry about the 10%.
41. Do whatever it takes to regain and keep your health.

35

Unforgiven

*"Most wonderful; with its own hands it ties
And gags itself-gives itself death and war
For pence doled out by kings from its own store.
Its own are all things between earth and heaven;
But this it knows not; and if one arise
To tell this truth, it kills him unforgiven."*
Tomasso Campanella, The People

Reversing the aging process is a one step at a time process that occurs one day at a time—in reverse.

Ask yourself these questions. "Am I willing to take responsibility for my future and create the miracle of agelessness in my life? Am I willing to do whatever it takes to keep my youth or gain back the years I have lost? Am I willing to act in my own best interest today? Right now?

Everything in life comes at a price. Pain! Suffering! Money! I hope you will join me and pick up your yoke no matter how difficult it may be. Never scream "uncle!" Health and vitality belongs to he or she who is willing to pay the price.

May you become *Young Again!*

Sincerely,

John Thomas

Start With Your Liver!

What's the best I can do to speed the aging reversal process?" is the question I'm asked most.

I respond, "Start with your liver. Clean it up! Get rid of the stones in your liver and gall bladder that are blocking the flow of your bile wastes out of your body!"

It stands to reason that the body can't return to a more youthful condition when *excess* wastes have accumulated in all of the vital organs and glands of the body!

First Things First!

Before a liver flush is attempted, you MUST *prepare* your body. Preparation includes the use of Yucca extract and enhanced PAC's for at least one month.

The Yucca extract acts a toxic waste solvent in the soft tissues and joints and helps rid the liver of fatty tissue. The enhanced PAC'S bond to the free radicals in the wastes so they won't make you sick as they come into circulation in the blood and lymphatic fluids.

Three Days Before The Flush

During the final 3 days leading up to the flush, you double and triple your intake of Yucca extract, while at the same time you are drinking apple juice and a special stone softener mix. The mix is consumed throughout each of the 3 days leading up to the evening of the third day when you flush the stones from your liver and gallbladder. The last step is done immediately prior to going to bed.

Making It happen

The grand finale is triggered when you drink one cup of pure olive oil followed by 1/3 cup of pure *fresh* lemon juice and go to bed. These ingredients cause the liver to go into a painless spasm that you can't feel and spit out its load of stones which slide their way down the common bile duct and into the small intestine.

The process is extremely simple and VERY effective. The next morning, you will find your stones in the toilet along with other bowel wastes. Once the liver is cleared of its stones, total body rejuvenation comes fast!

The Peoples Network

Life in the 21ˢᵗ Century will be lived and experienced on a playing field of new, cutting edge information. Information that deals with health, finances, career, motivation, spiritual growth, and creativity.

In the past, information was accessed through conventional channels like schools, churches, books, regular television, and libraries. In the future, information will flow on the invisible wires of **The Peoples Network** via your own personal 24" satellite dish.

The Peoples Network is a private television network devoted exclusively to the dissemination of information designed to improve and enhance your life on every level.

We are talking about the single biggest breakthrough in America since the advent of electromagnetic communications. We are speaking about the ability to "narrowcast" to specific individuals and groups according to their needs.

Reaching people who desire to empower themselves, their children, their society, with useful information that transforms lives is where it's at.

Think of the possibilities of rubbing shoulders with the *best of the best* in fields like motivation, financial management, creative thinking, career training, and personal growth.

Information is power! Information is THE key ingredient that levels life's playing field and creates equal opportunity for anyone who wants to experience success and growth in their life.

The Peoples Network is where people are turning to improve their lives. To learn more, see the Source Index.

Far Infrared Products Now Available!

Place one ice cube on a regular dinner plate and another on a plate made of **Far Infrared** (FIR) ceramic, and within seconds the ice cube on the FIR plate will completely melt **before** the other ice cube has even begun!

Far Infrared (FIR) technology comes from Japan where it is in wide use as a budding new health modality. It uses special ceramic materials that heal by directing Far Infrared energy into the tissues of the body. In the ice cube example, FIR energy melted the ice cube.

The Earth is bombarded with energy rays that belong to the FIR band of the light spectrum. Humans can't see FIR energy, but it's there nevertheless. Soldiers use special equipment and FIR energy to see at night.

The Japanese have DISCOVERED how to use FIR energy to promote **health** and **longevity.** When FIR products are worn or placed next to the body, escaping body energy plus cosmic FIR energy is redirected back into the body where it *warms* the tissues and *promotes* healing.

FIR *energy* is **right-spin** energy and is, therefore, both safe and good for the body. FIR products are available as body wraps, seat liners, and in the most exciting application of FIR technology yet, as **Far Infrared saunas!**

Sit on a FIR seat liner and your bottom and back will become toasty warm. The elderly and people with hip and back pain find fast relief with a FIR seat liner. FIR body wraps work wonders when used on painful joints, a sore back, and for sports and soft tissue injuries.

But it's the FIR sauna that has captured my attention! FIR saunas concentrate FIR energy and heal the body without water or electricity. There are NO ongoing costs with a Far Infrared sauna. And, the're portable, too!

Far Infrared energy dissolves acid wastes in the tissues, organs, and glands. These wastes produce inflammation, swelling, and pain if allowed to build up in the system. **Excess** waste brings on degenerative dis-eases like cancer, arthritis, and diabetes, just to name a few.

FIR energy **stimulates** basal metabolic rate while burning accumulated wastes trapped in the tissues. People with degenerative disorders like fibromyalgia, systemic lupis, and hypertension find immediate relief from the therapeutic effects of FIR energy. Heart patients can safely enjoy a Far Infrared sauna, too (see Source Index)!

Use Far Infrared Products To Keep Warm!

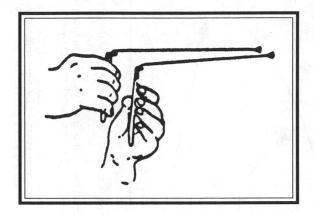

Dowser's Swing Rods

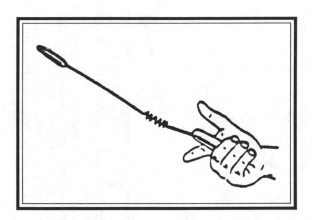

Dowser's Aurameter

**These Dowser's Tools Double For Map
Dowsing & Pendulum Work
• Highly Recommended •**

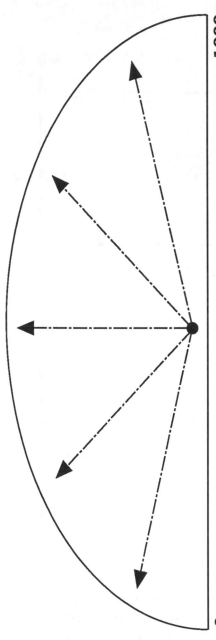

1000

0

A dowser's 'speedometer' scale can be used to measure the body's anticipated response to anything from food to life circumstances.

Establish a reference number by placing your left index finger on the pivot point of the arrows. Start your vibration chain or pendulum swinging in a vertical to and fro direction from six to twelve o'clock over the scale. Now ask, "On a scale of 0 to 1000, where is my health?

The device will begin moving up or down scale. When it stabilizes, note the reading (say 750). This is your reference number. All additional responses indicate better or worse, weaker or stronger by repeating the same process. It is NOT uncommon to go off scale in either direction when something is VERY good or bad for your body or your live circumstance.

Accurate responses involve a 'cleared' mind where you are NOT—consciously or unconsciously—influencing the direction or intensity of chain's response. To fully develop this and many other skills, read *The Pendulum Kit, Vibrations,* and *Map Dowsing* (see Source Index).

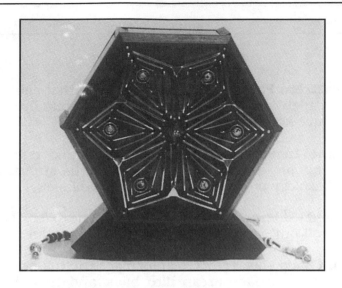

**Sky-Heart Whole Life Enhancer
& Transfiguration Unit**

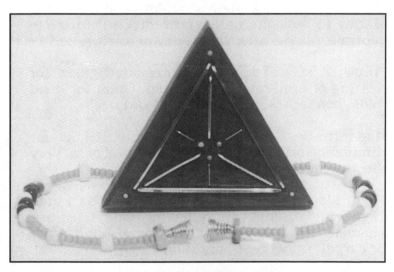

**Sky-David Interactive
Field Clearing Unit**

Units are combinations of pure platinum, precious stones and precious woods interfaced with state of the art computer circuitry.

Magnetic Products

Mattress Pad: Special sleeping pads that contain therapeutic magnets. Ease pain, sleep soundly, and reduce acid waste levels in body.

Shoe Inserts: Pliable shoe inserts and custom sizing for a perfect fit. Designed to stimulate reflexology points in plantar surface of feet.

Hand Rollers: Hand held dual magnetic roller. Used to 'roll-out' sore joints and tissues, and to stimulate.

Full Body Massager: Great for magnetic 'roll-downs' of large surface areas like back and legs. Very relaxing, yet stimulating at the same time.

Super Magnet: Worn around neck over thymus gland for immune system stimulation and clearing of stray 110 volt alternating current. Can be used to neutralize stress after tough day at work.

Pillow: A special magnet impregnated pillow for clearing of head and sound sleep. Great for head colds, headaches, and a stressed-out neck.

Magnetic Seat Cushion: Full size seat liner for stimulation of back/hip and reduction of pain. Very effective for elimination of 'jet lag.'

Super Block Magnet: Super powerful 4 x 6 x 1 inch therapeutic magnet with reflecting plate. Used under mattress, under pillow, or to treat hand/wrist for carpal tunnel type conditions.

Wrist Bands: Costume type jewelry with powerful rare earth therapeutic magnets.

Body Belts: Velcro foam/magnet impregnated body belts for use over injuries, joints, or low back.

Magnetism Is A Gift From Nature!

Glossary

AIDS-Acquired Immune Deficiency Syndrome.
Acetylcholine-a nerve impulse transmission chemical.
Acetylcholinease-an enzyme that splits acetylcholine.
Acid-any substance that liberates hydrogen ions; ion donor.
Acid stomach-common term for upset stomach; cause is an really alkaline stomach; poor digestion; lack of HCL.
Acupuncture-alternative modality; manipulates energy fields in bio-electric body with pins or their electrical equivalent.
Adenovirus-a virus associated with upper respiratory infections, associated with AIDS/HIV.
Adhesion-water's tenedency to coat the surface of things.
Adrenals-a pair of ductless glands; located on top of each kidney.
Aerobes-bacteria that require an oxygen rich environment.
Aerobic-with air.
Aerobic exercise-exercise that produces a high oxygen state.
Aging process-begins at anabolic peak and ends with death; cumulative
Agglutination-clumping of the red blood corpuscles; see soy.
Albumin-a blood protein; abnormally found in the urine.
Alcohol-end product of fermentation; anaerobic process
Alfalfa sprouts-alfalfa seeds sprouted for food; toxic.
Algae-lowest of plants; some edible (klamath, spirulina, chlorella)
Alkaline-above pH 7.0.
Alkaloid-alkaline plant juices; physiologically active.
Allopathic medicine-conventional cut, burn, and drug medicine.
Alum-double sulfate of aluminum; toxic; food additive; pickles.
Aluminum-a metal that releases toxic ions into food and water.
Alzheimers -atrophy of brain; produces dementia, violence, anger in elderly.
Amalgam-mixture of toxic metals used to fill the teeth; up to 60% mercury; erroneously referred to as "silver" fillings.
Amenorrhea-absence or suppression of menstruation.
American Dental Association-"official" dentistry.
Amyloid-a complex protein substance without structure.
Anabolic, anabolism-build up of tissues; repair of tissues.
Anabolic Peak-high point of anabolism; end or youth, beginning of old age.
Anaerobes-bacteria that can live in the absence of oxygen.
Anaerobic-without air; oxygen deficient.
Angina pectoris-chest pain due to lack of oxygen in muscles.
Anemia-low number of circulating red blood corpuscles.
Anions-the smallest form of energy released during a reaction.
Antibiotic-anti: against; bio: life; ic: pertaining to; drug.
Arthritis-deterioration/inflammation of the connective tissues and joints.
Arteriosclerosis-hardening of arteries; see atherosclerosis
Antenna-device that receives a radio (energy) signal.
Antibody-product of a previous infection; immunity related.
Atherosclerosis-plaque formation/deterioration of arteries.
ATP-adenosine triphosphate; the energy carrying molecule of the body.
Atrophy-deterioration and death of body tissue/gland/organ.
Avogadro's #-number of atoms in 12 grams of carbon-12.
Aura-the electric body; invisible body; see Fourth Dimension.
Bacteria-microorganisms; microbe.
Bactericidal-a non-selective killer of bacteria, antiseptic.
Balding-loss of hair; related to O_2 deficiency and toxicity.
Baths, minera-natural hot springs; therapeutic; Epsom salt in bath.
Basal metabolism-minimum resting energy expenditure.
Basement membrane(s)-primary support/connective tissues.
B-12: vitamin #12 of vitamin B complex; related to cyanocobalamin; called intrinsic factor; contains cobalt blue.
BAT-brown adipose tissue; not related to WAT (see).
Bent molecule-the water molecule. Also known as a polar molecule.
BEV-World's most biologically friendly water for the human body.

Bile-liver and body waste product; fat emulsifier; digestive enz.
Bio-dynamic-term describing energy friendly agriculture.
Bio-electric age-true age based on health of the vital organs.
Bio-electric body-the physical and energy body's combined.
Bio-electric score-a factor used to determine bio-electric age.
Bio-junk food-adulterated food; toxic; negative spin effect.
Biological alchemy-transformation of the elements in liver, gut via bacteria; fusion reactions.
Biological Theory of Ionization-life is the product of the energy released by the breaking of ionic bonds that hold minerals together.
Bio-magnetics-the use of therapeutic magnets in healing.
Bio-magnetic Irrigator-dental hygiene device; prevents/ dissolves/removes plaque from the teeth; manipulates hydrogen ions and the water molecule; plaque (–); treated water (+).
Bladder-the urine storage organ in animals.
Blood-one of two key body fluids; ymph is the other.
Body odor-product of toxic waste body; clogged integument.
Bonds-the electric link between of elements and molecules.
Bone spur-abnormal mineral deposit in/on joints and bones.
Bowel-the colon or large intestine.
B-vitamins-the B-12 complex; B-1 through B-12; see intrinsic factor.
Brix-a unit of measure of the sugars in plant juices.
Brown fat-see BAT.
Calcify, calcification-soft tissue invasion by mineral salts (calcium).
Calcium-mineral element; a metal; elemental; anion.
Calculus-dental plaque; tartar.
Cancer-systemic deterioration/collapse of immune system.
Canola oil-same as rape oil; toxic; mustard family; see soy oil.
Capillaries-smallest blood vessels; can be venous or arterial.
Carbohydrate-sugars, starches, dextrins, and cellulose; contains carbon, oxygen, and hydrogen; classes of nutrient; other classes are protein/fats.
Carbon-essential element to all living things; atomic element #12.
Carbon cycle-the path of carbon from atmosphere through bacteria, soil, plant, animal, ocean, and back to the atmosphere; requirement for life/ creation of positive energy food.
Carbon dioxide- atmospheric gas; animal waste gas, CO_2.
Carcinogenic-poisonous.
Cardiovascular disease-dis-eases of the circulatory system.
Carpel Tunnel Syndrome-occlusion/deterioration of nerve & nerve paths in bones of wrist; loss of motion and/or function.
Carrion-spoiled animal flesh.
Casts-albumin/amyloid, proteins, salts; wastes deposits of the kidney's tubules; indicates deterioration of nephrons.
Catalyst-a substance that causes a chemical reaction that would not occur without its presence; used over and over.
Cataract-the clouding of the lens of the eye or its capsule.
Cation-smallest form of (–) energy released during a reaction.
Catabolic, catabolism-break-down or self-digestion of body's tissues; failure/ inability to rebuild or repair tissues; old age; opposite of anabolism.
Cavities-rotting away of the teeth; decay.
Cecum-junction of small/large intestine; gut/colon (bowel).
Cellulose-a carbohydrate; fiber.
Cerebrum-largest part of the brain; Alzheimers; coordination.
Chemotherapy-treatment of dis-ease w/negative energy drugs.
Chloroform-toxic substance; source: chlorinated water/drugs.
Chlorine-a halogen; a gas; "a wildcat."
Chloride-a salt form of chlorine (sodium/pot./alum chloride).
Chiropractic-modality for correction of alignment of spine.
Chiropractic (Network)-advanced holistic form of chiropractic
Chloramine-extremely toxic form of chlorine; absorbed throuth skin.
Chlorinated water-water treated with some form of chlorine.
Cholesterol-a body fat; an alcohol; part of bile; a phospholipid.
Cilia-hair like projections in small intestine/respiratory tract.
Cirrhosis-hardening of glandular tissues; inflammation of.
Clinical Illness-a diagnosed condition (measurable signs).

Cloak(ed)-under cover; hidden; can't be detected; subclinical.
Cobalt blue-natural radioactive isotope; related to anemia/ vitamin B-complex/B-12/intrinsic factor; fusion reactions.
Co-enzyme-necessary for the function of an enzyme.
Cohesion-water's tendency to stick together; hydrogen bond.
Colon-large intestine; bowel.
Colonic, colon irrigation-therapeutic washing of colon.
Collagen-connective tissue; 30% of body protein.
Comfrey-garden plant grown for spinach like leaves; heals ulcers.
Coral Calcium-biogenic coral; used for rejuvenation.
Crypts of Lieberkuhn-where food nutrients are absorbed in the gut (small intestine) ; located between intestinal villi.
Crystal-a salt; combination of halogen and a metal ions.
Currency, electrical-energy money; mineral ions.
Cyanide-contained in rape (canola) oil; toxic.
Cyanocobalomin-cobalt blue; synthetic B-12/intrinsic factor.
Cytoplasm-fluid inside the cell.
DNA-genetic code of living things; deoxyribonucleic acid.
Defecate-a bowel movement.
Degenerative dis-ease-generalized condition; related to old age and loss of function.
Denature-alteration in protein, function and/or shape.
Holistic dentistry-biologically friendly dentistry; no fluoride, mercury or toxics used; vibrational dentistry
De-energize-neutralization/synchronization; loss of effect.
Deodorant-a chemical used to mask BO; most are toxic.
Dermis-the true skin; beneath the epidermis (outer skin).
Detoxify-removal of waste from the body.
Devitalized food-loss of vitality; neutralization of energy.
Diabetes-malfunction/dis-ease of vital organs; insulin related; blood sugar too high; obesity related; old age sign.
Digestion-breakdown/conversion of nutrients into energy.
Dilution-homeopathic remedies.
Dirt-unproductive, dead, synchronized soil.
Dis-ease-the opposite of health; a left-spin condition.
Diuretic-drug that sheds the body's extracellular fluids.
Dogma-established authoritative opinion.
Dowager's hump-hunchback condition due to loss of bone mass and connective tissue; degenerative; hunchback.
Dowsing-technique used to determine left/right energy spin effect of food/drugs on body; locate ground water; involves the use of an antenna or pendulum and a focused mind.
Drugs-chemical substances that cause a physiologic effect.
Ductless glands-glands that do not excrete into a lumen or duct; hormone secreted into blood instead; vital organs.
Dynamic Reflex Analysis-kinesthetics.
EPAC'-enhanced proanthocyanidins
ETVC-enhanced trivalent chromium
E. coli-un/friendly bacteria of the gut.
Eczema-acute/chronic inflammation of the cutaneous layers of the skin (dermis); dermatitis; toxicity related.
Edema-water retention in cells; sodium toxicity; "K" loss.
Enema-a swallow, partial cleansing of the lower colon.
Electrical impulse-an electrical signal; an energy bullet.
Electrolytes-mineral ions capable of electrical conductivity; nerve fiber transmission; nerve pathway related.
Electron flow-movement of electrons along metal wires.
Endocrine system-the body's hormonal system for transmission of energy and messages via the blood/glands.
Energy-electrical phenomenon.
Energy field-a of left or right spin energy energy .
Energy imbalance-bio-electric stress; dis-ease.
Energy manipulation-change in the spin of or effect of energy on the bio-electric body.
Energy meridian-an energy highway or path.

Energy (scrambled)-effect of radiation/irradiation/food additives/halogens on food energy molecules and/or enzymes.

Enzymes-biological catalysts; all body functions require them.
Exit portal-waste removal avenue(s) in bio-electric body.
Exocrine glands-glands that secrete hormones/enzymes into lumens or hollow organs like the stomach or gut.
Extracellular fluid-fluid between (outside) cells; interstitial.
Fabale-a family of plants; parent family of the soy bean.
Facultative anaerobes-bacteria that can function with or without the presence of oxygen.
Fats-a food category; also proteins, and carbohydrates.
Fever (febrile)-abnormal increase in body's metabolic rate and temperature; a systemic condition.
Fission-splitting of atoms/molecules; catabolic; nuclear.
Fluorine-a halogen gas; toxic; a wildcat.
Fluoride-the salt form of fluorine metal & fluorine ions.
Fluorosis-fluoride toxicity.
Food-nutrient energy; eft/right spin; positive negative effect.
Footprint, energy-4th Dimension energy pattern; includes spin & intensity.
Fourth Dimension-the invisible/intangible Dimension.
Functional cells-cells of the body's vital organs that grant permission for life; parenchyma cells; vitality depends on.
Fusion-anabolic transmutation/formation of molecules.
Gallbladder-holding sack for liver's bile; dumps into gut.
Gallstones-deposits of precipitates from bile.
Gas-free moving matter; non-solid; invisible energy; w/o form.
Gastric-related to stomach.
Genetically engineered-manipulated life forms; synthetic.
Germ Theory of Disease-the dogma of allopathic medicine and premise upon which dis-ease is defined and treated.
GI tract-gastrointestinal tract.
Glaucoma-a group of eye dis-eases involving atrophy of retina.
Glucose-the body's sugar fuel.
Glycerol-glycerin with alcohol(s) attached; present in fats.
Glycine-a nonessential amino acid; sweet; glycine max.
Glycolic acid-a natural substance that restores elasticity to the skin by fluffing and removal of the dead layers (epidermis).
Glycosides-inhibit muscle enzymes; soy/canola contain them.
Glycolysis-breakdown of glycogen sugars; Crebs cycle.
Glands-body organs with special functions and tissues.
Goiter-thyroid gland swelling due to malnutrition/overwork.
Gout-uric acid toxicity in blood and joints; degenerative.
Lye Soap-product of saponification of fats with lye chemical.
Greens-collards, broccoli leaves, spinach, cabbage, chard, etc.
Gut-small intestine (includes duodenum, jejunum, ileum.
HCL-hydrochloric acid; stomach acid; breaks down proteins.
Halogen-an extremely unstable, acid gas; a wildcat; toxic.
Heart attack-insufficient oxygen available to heart muscle.
Herbicides-man made organic poisons.
Hemorrhoids-swollen, congested, displaced veins in the anus.
Hepatitis-inflammation of the liver (hepatocytes).
Hepatocytes-the functional cells of the liver.
Herpes-a group of viral conditions; sex & non sex related.
High blood pressure-hypertension; abnormal; sign of old age.
HIV-Human immunodeficiency virus; the precursor virus to manifestation of the AIDS syndrome of dis-eases.
Hologram-a multidimensional energy message.
Homeopathic medicine-the medicine of similars; remedies.
Hormone-chemical messenger; powerful energy field; product of vital glands.
Howdy Doody Lines-Facial lines from corners of the mouth to sides of the chin; seen on older people with toxic colon/cecum.
Hunger center-that part of the brain that identifies hunger.
Hyaline-an albuminoid substance in tissues that have undergone amyloid degeneration.

Hyalinization-infusion of hyaline into cells or tissue.
Hybrid food-food produced from genetically weak seed.
Hydration-the water level in the tissues of the body.
Hydrochloric acid-see HCL.
Hydro flosser-electromagnetic device; removes dental plaque.
Hydrogen-an element; high energy; bonds easily; bioactive.
Hydrogen peroxide-H_2O_2; therapeutic; antiseptic.
Hype-unrealistic thinking; mind over matter; biojunk stress.
Hyperspace-Fourth Dimension space.
Hypertrophy-increased/abnormal change in organ function.
Hypoglycemia-low blood sugar.
Hypotrophy-decline; abnormal change in organ function.
Hypovolemia-low blood fluid volume (also lymph).
Ileum-end of small intestine; joins colon at cecum.
Ileocecal valve-gatekeeper between small intestine and cecum (lg. intestine)
Immune system-our bio-electric defense system.
Immunization-bogus introduction of live microbial energy field into body.
Impotence-inability of the male to get an erection.
In-camera-attitudinal approach that considers whole body.
Inflammation-redness; swelling; edema.
Indols-toxic whole molecules produced/absorbed in the gut.
Insulin-A blood protein; controls glucose flow into the cells.
Integument-the skin (subcutaneous, dermis, epidermis).
Internal environment-status of the cells/fluids/tissues.
Intercellular substance-mix of materials between the cells.
Interstitial fluid-fluid between the cells; extracellular fluid.
Intestine-small intestine (gut) and large intestines (colon).
Intima-innermost layer of the artery blood vessel wall.
Intoxicated-alcohol saturation beyond the ability of the liver to breakdown and the kidneys to excrete.
Intracellular fluid-fluid inside the cells.
Intrinsic factor-related to pernicious anemia; same as B-12; see cobalt blue, tobacco, and B-vitamins.
Intuition-extension of the mind into Fourth Dimension Space.
Invisible not seen; the electric body; Fourth Dimension.
Iodine-an element; needed for health; related to thyroid goiter.
Ion-an atom that has gained or lost an electron.
Ionic bond-bond between two mineral ions.
Ionic minerals-minerals that have gained/lost electrons.
Ionization-exchange of energy and electrons; anions/cations.
Irradiation-desruction/scrambling of food molecules/tissues.
Iridology-reading/interpretation of health via iris of eye.
Ischemia-reduced oxygen supply to heart muscle.
Isotope-an atom with same number of protons, but different number of neutrons; a different form of the same element.
Jaundice-toxic liver effect; bilirubin; yellowing of eye sclera.
Juice capsules/tablets-concentrated right-spin dried plant juices.
Kombucha tea-dynamic home preparaton used for rejuvenation.
Kidney-primary excretory organ of the body; exit portal.
Kidney stones-mineral/fat/waste precipitates in the kidneys.
Kinesiology-study of body movement.
Kinesthetics-muscle sense tests; identify toxic food/drugs.
Lactate-the salt form of lactic acid.
Lactic acid-the product of anaerobic fermentation; formed during muscle activity; incomplete oxidation of glucose.
Laying on of hands-healing through energy transfer.
Lecithin-emulsifier and component of oils/fats/bile.
Left-spin-negative energy; catabolic.
Lemon juice-powerful de-toxifier(if fresh); acidic.
Lice-creatures that live off filth and negative energy.
Life expectancy-length of time we can expect to live.
Lightning, cellular-energy produced by the mitochondria.
Limb regeneration-regrowth of bone, nerve, and tissues.
Liver-primary chemical/fusion/detox organ of the body.
Liver breath-bad breath resulting from weak liver; onions.

Load-bearing work-work involving movement and weight.
Localized condition-a condition that is not systemic.
Low-tech medicine-dependent on observation & instinct; uses vibrational techniques; bio electric body friendly.
Lungs-organs external breathing.
Lymph-fluids in lymph vessels; a body fluid.
Lymphocyte-immune system cell; B-cell; part of lymph. sys.
Lymphotrophic-change in lymph fluid; T-cell.
Macrophage-a single cell that leaves circulation, then settles and matured in the tissues; part of immune system.
Magic bullets-medical science hype; false hope; drugs.
Magnetic line devices-protection from electrical fields.
Magnetism-the effect of a magnetic field.
Magneto hydro dynamics-dental plaque removal therapy.
Malathion-a toxic man-made organic poison.
Malnutrition-insufficient right-spin food energy.
Manganese- trace mineral; builds serum iron via bioalchemy.
Mastication, masticate-chewing of food.
Matter-condensed energy.
Matriarchal society-blood line follows the woman.
Matrix-collagen framework for deposition of bone minerals.
Meat-dead animal tissue; may be right/left spin energy.
Menopause-negative shift in hormonal flow; the "climactic."
Menstruation-end of normal, monthly, hormonal, female cycle.
Mental age-how old a person thinks.
Mercury-extremely toxic element; quicksilver; evaporates.
Mercuric acid-extremely toxic agent for the treatment of water during the warm months; an acid form of elemental mercury.
Metabolic process-metabolism.
Metabolism-a change in energy via biotransformation.
Metabolite-waste products of metabolism.
Metaphysics-beyond normal physics of length, width, height.
Microbes-microscopic life forms; bacteria.
Mikrowater-ionized water that is highly reduced or oxidized; acid or alkaline.
Microwave oven-a negative energy cooking device.
Mitochondria-bacteria that produce cellular lightning.
Modality-a form of therapy.
Molds-lowest life forms.
Molecular bond-bond between molecules.
Mononucleosis-inflamed lymph nodes/liver; immune deficit.
Monosodium glutamate (MSG)-a salt of sodium and glutamine.
Morbid-dis-ease related; death related.
Multiple sclerosis-inflammation of the central nervous system; deterioration of the myelin sheaths of the nerves.
Muscle tone-resistance of muscles to elongation or stretch.
Mustard gas-chemical agent of war; made from rape oil.
Myocardial infarction-see heart attack.
Myelin-protective nerve fiber sheath; destruction pH related.
Myelinoma-deterioration of the nerve sheaths.
Myxedema-hypofunction of thyroid; decreased metabolic rate; atrophy of thyroid; low hormone formation; low BMR.
Naturopathic-alternative therapeutic modality; similars.
Necrotic flesh-dead, non-gangrenous tissue; not s/a carrion.
Negative energy-left-spin energy; catabolic.
Negative inhibition-feedback system to control metabolism.
Nephron-kidney blood filter; critical to detoxification.
Nerve gas-toxic agent of war; blocks enzyme function.
Neuropathy-syndrome of nerve deterioration; pH related.
Neutralize-denature; detoxify; energy shift; synchronize.
Niacin/niacinimide-names for bogus vitamin B-3; synthetic.
Nicotine-if natural, a good source of complete B-vitamins.
Nicotinic acid-acid form of nicotine; nat'l source: dry tobacco.
Nitrogen-essential element; contained in proteinous foods.
Nodules-part of lymphatic system; also known as nodes.
Nonfunctional cells-cell that do not grant permission to life.

Nonshivering thermogenesis-heat produced w/o shivering.
Nourishment-positive food energy that fuels anabolism.
Obesity-slowdown in metabolic & vital organ function.
Occlusion, occluded-closed off/restriction of flow.
Old age-product of catabolism, dis-ease, loss of vital function.
Open pollinated seeds-seeds that can produce true to type.
Opportunistic-bacteria/viruses that manifest if the terrain is correct; all diseases are opportunistic; a condition.
Organic-a misnomer; a molecule containing carbon.
Organic poisons-poisons built on a carbon skeleton.
Osteoporosis-honey combing of the bones; loss of bone mass.
Ovaries-glands that produce female reproductive cells (egg).
Oxidation-flameless burning of glucose (sugars) in the body.
Oxygen-element of oxidation; positive energy, anabolism.
Ozone-O_3; therapeutic; bactericidal to pathogenic organisms.
P-P Factor-pellagra preventive agent; part of the B-complex; known as B-3, niacin; most commercial sources are synthetic.
Palliation-relief of signs/symptoms without cure of cause.
Pallor-poor color; abnormal color.
Pancreas-vital organ; digestion, hormonal, and metabolic functions; both duct and ductless.
Paradigm-a new model along side an older model.
Paralysis-loss of muscle function; degenerative; see soy/rape.
Parasympathetic nervous system-that part of our system over which we have no control.
Parathyroid-four tiny glands next to the thyroid; (ductless).
Parenchyma cells-functional cells of a gland or organ.
Pathogenic-pertaining to dis-ease; dis-ease causing.
Patriarchal society-blood line follows the male.
Pavlov's dog-salivated at the ringing of the bell; involuntary.
Peer review-undressing in public; submission to convention; following the protocols of "legitimate" medical science; control.
Pellagra-B-complex vitamin deficiency dis-ease; see niacin.
Pendulum-an antenna; a tuning device; a transmitter; a tool.
Peristalsis-intestinal wave-like motions that move food/waste.
Pesticide-organic poison; man-made; attached to carbon atom.
pH scale-normally from 1-14; 7 is neutral; ea. # increases 10x.
Phagocyte-a cell that eats the body's invading enemies.
Phenols-toxic whole molecules produced/absorbed in the gut.
PHG-phytohemaglutinin; a vegetable protein glue; soy beans.
Phytohemaglutinin-see PHG.
Plants-nature's antennas; mediate cosmic energy; build soil.
Pituitary-important ductless gland; linked to all other glands.
Plicae circularis-undulating folds in the walls of the gut.
Plaque-toxic waste deposits in the artery walls; dental plaque.
Poison-carcinogenic; deadly; produces negative effects.
Polar molecule-the water molecule; a bent molecule.
Polluted-toxic; loaded with poisonous waste; tap water.
Positive energy-right-spin; anabolic.
Positive thinking-mind over matter; helpful if real; no hype.
Post mortem-after death; examination after death.
Potassium-necessary element; + charge; sodium's twin; "K".
Precipitate-formation of a solid & settling out of solution.
Precursor-a substance that precedes another; beta carotene/vitamin A.
Proof-something medical science demands, but can't deliver.
Prostate-male ejaculatory organ; surrounds urinary tube.
Portal-an exit.
Protein-one of three food forms; also: fat, carbohydrates.
Proanthocyanidins (PAC)-plant derived antioxidant/free radical scavengers.
Puberty-onset of secondary sex charistics (breasts/body hair).
Pulmonary system-related to the lungs; blood to lungs.
Pulse rate-how fast your heart beats.
Pure water-water w/o any poison or mineral passengers; highly charged molecule; an energy molecule; positive energy.
Purine-a nitrogenous protein waste from the digestion of animal tissue, or self

digestion of body tissue; catabolic; composed of adenine, guanine; nucleic acid end product.

Pyridine ring-a synthetic organic molecule used to make artificial B-vitamins; left-spin; will not support life.

Pyridostigmine Bromnide-A drug given to Gulf War soldiers; blocks normal nerve function; produces Gulf War Syndrome.

R-group-a chemical group that gives an organic molecule its characteristic(s); for example DDT, dioxin, PCBs, etc.

RNA-Ribonucleic acid; nucleic acid; genetic template material.

Radiation-energy radiating from a source; nuclear is left-spin energy and catabolic; right-spin is anabolic.

Radionics-broadcasting of energy frequencies in agriculture.

Radiomemetic-substances which mimic the damaging effects of nuclear radiation; toxic chemicals are radiomemetic.

Ragweed-a weed that grows on toxic energy.

Rape oil-same as canola oil; extremely toxic; do NOT eat.

Rebounder-a mini trampoline.

Refractometer-device for determining sugar/mineral levels in the juices of plants; indicator of vitality; measures in brix.

Regeneration-see limb regeneration; growth of new parts.

Rejuvenate-to rebuild; start anew; anabolism.

Remedies-homeopathic energy fields that neutralizes negative dis-ease energy frequencies.

Replication-multiplication; reproduction.

Resiliency-return to previous condition; bounce back.

Respiration, external-O_2/CO_2 exchange in the lungs.

Respiration, internal-O_2/CO_2 exchange in the cells.

Reticular-fine network of tissues that form the glands/organs.

Retrovirus-a virus capable of using a reverse enzyme to access the host; HIV virus is said to be a retrovirus.

Reverse aging process-step-by-step process in reverse.

Right-spin energy-anabolic; positive; aerobic.

Rouleau effect-toxic waste energies in blood; clumping of blood corpuscles.

Root canal-removal of tooth's nerve; retention of dead tooth.

Rotenone-a toxic poison from the soy bean.

Roten-Japanese for derris: plant family to which soy belongs.

Rhythm-scheduled; systematic; regular; habit.

Rhymicity-routine; systematic; regular lifestyle and habits.

Saliva-secretion of the salivary glands; digestive juice.

Salt-combination of halogen and metal ions.

Satiety-fullness beyond desire; nutritionally full.

Saponification-soap making; the hydrolysis or splitting of fat by an alkali; hydrolysis of an ester; (*sapo*-soap;*facere*-to make).

Scrapie-the virus blamed for animal dementia/blindness in Europe; the real problem was rape/canola oil.

Scar tissue-a negative energy memory field; dysfunction in the skin's parenchymal cells during repair due to low energy state.

Scientific Method-medical sciences oficial system of information gathering.

Sea water-naturally balanced mineral ion water; right-spin.

Sedentary lifestyle-lack of exercise/oad bearing work.

Senility-loss of mental faculties.

Shallow breathing-insufficient exchange of lung gases.

Signature, energy-4th Dimension energy profile; combination of spin and intensity; specific to all substances and organisms.

Signs-measurable dis-ease conditions; will support diagnosis.

Silica-important element; body transmutes to calcium.

Similar(s)-energy formula that cancels offending dis-ease field.

Single factor analysis-for each effect there is a single cause; for every disease there is a single pathogen responsible; a form of scientific myopia; "head in the sand."

Silver Water (harmonic)-homeopathic type silver ion solution.

Sixth sense-intuition; Fourth Dimension; extension of mind.

Skatols-toxic whole molecules produced/absorbed via the gut.

Skin-our outer tube; halographic; an organ; exit portal.

Sky-Heart-interactive artificial intelligence device.

Sleep-detoxification period, recharge, and energy conversion.
Smoking-oxidation of dried tobacco via flame.
Snacking-small meals between main meals; create stress.
Sodium-an element; a metal; needed only in minute amounts; always involved in cancer; unbalanced lionic compound.
Soft drink-sugar + unbalanced ions; used in place of pure water; toxic to body; upsets body's mineral ratios.
Soil-live dirt; will support microbes, yeasts, fungi; right spin.
Solar energy-anionic energy; right spin; anabolic; life giving.
Solvent-dissolves substances into solution; alcohol dissolves fats; water dissolves minerals into solution.
Soy bean-toxic plant of Derris family; (Japanese for destroy).
Soy bean oil-deadly; carcinogenic; degenerative.
Space-extension of the mind; related to Time.
Sperm-solution containing male reproductive cells.
Spin-indicates left/right effect of substance; an indicator.
Spinach-an alkaloid; a Goosefoot; eat with vinegar/lemon.
Spirulina-a complete algae protein; good nutrient energy.
Sprouts-sprouted seeds; avoid alfalfa sprouts—toxic.
Spurs-mineral/body waste deposits in joints/on bones.
Standard-a defined reference point; a known yardstick.
Stannous-a tin containing compound.
Stannous fluoride-a toxic fluoride/tin containing compound.
Static-standing still; not changing; no motion; synchronized.
Steam bath-a good skin and body detoxifier.
Stomach-food receptacle; digestive organ.
Stomach, distended-out of place or shape.
Stress-effect of negative energy on the bio-electric body.
Stroma cells-nonfunctional cells of the glands; structural.
Sub-atomic-below atom level; fusion; transmutation; alchemy.
Sub-clinical-not diagnosable; symptoms; symptomatic.
Sub-cutaneous-below the dermis or dermal layer of skin; into the connective tissues (collagen, reticular, and elastic fibers).
Sugar-energy molecule; a compound; may be right/left-spin.
Sun-source of anionic energy; life giver; causes Earth to spin.
SUPER Mikrowater-BEV water + ionized Mikrowater.
Supplement-vitamin, minerals, and food additions to diet.
Sweat-a waste product; extracellular fluid; heat regulator.
Swiss chard-an alkaloid; a Goosefoot; eat with vinegar/lemon.
Symbiotic-one life form helps the other; buddy system.
Sympathetic nervous system-under our conscious control.
Symptoms-subclinical; undiagnosable; early stages of dis-ease; Fourth Dimensional; bio-electric; energy related.
Synchronization-neutralization of energy; slowing of energy transfer; aging is partial synchronization, death is total.
Synergy-the coming together of two or more energy forces.
Systemic-affecting the entire body; fever for example.
Synthesis-energy forces coming together to form a new substance; anabolic; simple substances that become comlex.
Synthetic-artifically prepared; man-made.
T-cells-defense cells of the immune/lymphatic system.
Tartar-calculus; dental plaque.
Terrain-the total state of the bio-electric body; determines opportunistic conditions for the manifestation of dis-ease.
Testes, testicles-glands that produce male reproductive cells, (sperm).
Therapeutic-having healing qualities; promotes health.
Therapeutic touch-healing through energy transfer.
Thermogenic hyperphagia-production of heat & the eating of body WAT (fat) through oxidation by mitochondria in brown fat.
Thymus-gland of the immune system and lymphatic systems.
Thyroid-Master gland of the body; central endocrine function.
Time-extension of mind; related to Space; Fourth Dimension.
Time & aging-passing of Time defines speed of aging.
Time made visible-signs of aging in the mirror.
Tin-stannous; see fluoride; toothpaste.

Tissue-cells of the body; grouped by type, function, and organ.
Tobacco-richest source of natural, complete B-vitamin complex in the world; up to 30%; alkaloid when green; acid when dry; a good food; Indian tobacco best; must grow your own.
Tone-resistance of muscles to elongation or stretch; that state in which body functions/parts are healthy and normal.
Toothpaste-next to tap water, greatest source of toxic fluoride.
Toxic-producing toxic effects on the bio-electric body.
Toxins-poisonous; negative effects of excess body waste.
Trace minerals-minerals needed in minute but balanced amounts; electrolytes; the two primary sources of bio-active trace minerals are: sea water or organic food.
Transmutation-conversion of one mineral into another in the gut/solar plexus, or liver of animals, or in soil by bacteria.
Trophy-change related to nutritional deficiencies or excesses.
TRUTH-something that can be ignored, but not denied.
Tumors-abnormal energy fields in the body; cancer.
TVP-textured vegetable protein.
Uric acid-a waste product of nitrogen tissue breakdown.
Urine-primary waste of the body.
Vaccines-live or attenuated microbes in animal protein serum; toxic.
Vascularization-blood vessel invasion into tissue or bone.
Vibrational medicine-manipulation of energy for healing.
Villi-finger-like projections of the gut wall.
Vinegar-acidic; hydrogen source; therapeutic; apple cider vinegar best; wine vinegar good; never use common store type.
Virus-a non-life form; parasitic; steals converts body's energy; proliferate when the terrain is supportive; opportunistic.
Visible -tangible; length, width, and height; Third Dimension.
Vital organs-ductless glands: ovaries/testes, pancreas, thymus, thyroid, pituitary, parathyroid:—critical to good health.
Vital force-the effect generated by the vital organs.
Vitamins-co-factors; important to health and vitality; should come from live organic food; avoid any vitamin not derived directly from a food source; see index and book.
Waste-byproducts of metabolism; toxic if not disposed of.
Water-important to ageless living; most important food; pure water is BEV; solvent to body waste removal; energy source.
Water molecule-H_2O if "pure"; otherwise contains toxic waste and mineral passengers, impure water is partially synchronized water, polluted water; one oxygen and two hydrogens.
Water substitutes-soft drinks, beer, milk, etc. ; no liquid is an acceptable substitute for water; BEV is world standard.
Weeds-negative energy antenna; detoxify the air and soil.
White blood cells-part of the immune defense system.
Whole molecules-substances that bypass decomposition; pass directly into body tissues and circulation.
Wildcats-name give to the halogens (fluorine, chlorine).
Wrinkles-confirmation of the passing of Time; aging of the vital organs; toxicity in the dermal/subcutaneous skin.

Index

IMPORTANT EXERCISES FOR KEEPING THE EXTERNAL AND THE INTERNAL MUSCLES OF THE ABDOMEN - FIRM AND HEALTHY.

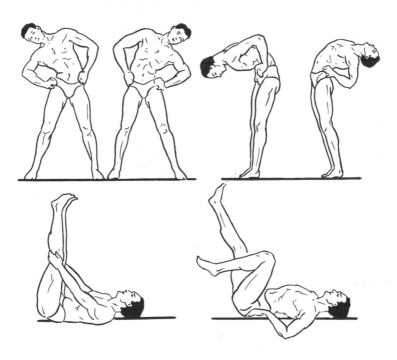

"Nothing transforms a person as much as changing from a negative to a positive attitude."
Paul C. Bragg

Source Index

Orders & Information Packets
Please Call

Plexus Press
1-800-659-1882
P.O. Box 827
Kelso WA 98626-0072
(360) 423-3168

Quantity Purchases

This book is available at special discounts for quantity purchases for gifts, business premiums, sales promotions, educational use or for resale.

Books Make Great Gifts!

Take time for 12 things

1   *Take time to* **Work** –
     it is the price of success.

2   *Take time to* **Think** –
     it is the source of power.

3   *Take time to* **Play** –
     it is the secret of youth.

4   *Take time to* **Read** –
     it is the foundation of knowledge.

5   *Take time to* **Worship** –
     *it is the highway of reverence and
     washes the dust of earth from our eyes.*

6   *Take time to* **Help and Enjoy Friends** –
     it is the source of happiness.

7   *Take time to* **Love** –
     it is the one sacrament of life.

8   *Take time to* **Dream** –
     it hitches the soul to the stars.

9   *Take time to* **Laugh** –
     it is the singing that helps life's loads.

10 *Take time for* **Beauty** –
     it is everywhere in nature.

11 *Take time for* **Health** –
     it is the true wealth and treasure of life.

12 *Take time to* **Plan** –
     *it is the secret of being able to have time
     to take time for the first eleven things.*